GAY & BISEXUAL MEN LIVING WITH PROSTATE CANCER

from diagnosis to recovery

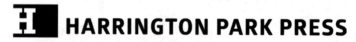

HARRINGTON PARK PRESS

NEW YORK, NY • USA

GAY & BISEXUAL MEN LIVING WITH PROSTATE CANCER

from diagnosis to recovery

EDITED BY

JANE M. USSHER

JANETTE PERZ

B. R. SIMON ROSSER

Harrington Park Press
Box #331
9 East 8th Street
New York, NY 10003

http://harringtonparkpress.com

Library of Congress Cataloging-in-Publication Data
Names: Ussher, Jane M., 1961– editor. | Perz, Janette, 1968– editor. |
    Rosser, B. R. Simon, editor.
Title: Gay and bisexual men living with prostate cancer : from diagnosis to
    recovery / edited by Jane Ussher, Janette Perz, and B. R. Simon Rosser.
Description: New York, NY : Harrington Park Press, [2018] | Includes
    bibliographical references and index.
Identifiers: LCCN 2018002814 (print) | LCCN 2018004235 (ebook) | ISBN
    9781939594266 (ebook) | ISBN 9781939594259 (pbk. : alk. paper) | ISBN
    9781939594242 (hardcover : alk. paper)
Subjects: | MESH: Prostatic Neoplasms—psychology | Homosexuality, Male |
    Bisexuality | Sexual and Gender Minorities | Attitude of Health Personnel
    | Long Term Adverse Effects | Cancer Survivors—psychology
Classification: LCC RC280.P7 (ebook) | LCC RC280.P7 (print) | NLM WJ 762 |
    DDC 616.99/463008663—dc23
LC record available at https://lccn.loc.gov/2018002814

Manufactured in the United States of America

We dedicate this book to the memories
of our fathers, Harry Ussher, Joseph Perz,
and Des Rosser.

CONTENTS

SECTION TWO:
CANCER CARE AND SUPPORT FOR GAY AND BISEXUAL MEN WITH PROSTATE CANCER

SECTION THREE:
PERSONAL EXPERIENCES

FOREWORD

Jonathan Bergman and Mark S. Litwin

In Lin-Manuel Miranda's Pulitzer, Tony, and Grammy Award–winning musical *Hamilton*, Angelica Schuyler promises to fight to overcome the second-class citizenship offered to everyone other than white males. As she tells her sisters, Eliza and Peggy: "You want a revolution? I want a revelation. So listen to my declaration: 'We hold these truths to be self-evident that all men are created equal.' And when I meet Thomas Jefferson, I'm 'a compel him to include women in the sequel!'"

The stains of sexism, racism, and homophobia remain indelible in 2017, two and a half centuries after Alexander Hamilton helped found the United States. Medical science has conspicuously—and shamefully—been complicit in valuing straight white men above all others. Women, racial minorities, and members of the lesbian, gay, bisexual, transgender, and questioning/queer (LGBTQ) communities are underrepresented in clinical trials, which limits our ability to identify their needs and to respond to them thoughtfully. Not all of us are deemed important enough to include. Congress responded to this injustice in 2012 by passing Section 907 in the Food and Drug Administration Safety and Innovation Act (FDASIA), tasking the FDA with identifying such disparities and taking action.

As Rosser and colleagues highlight in chapter 1 of this book, in no disease is this inequality better encapsulated than in prostate cancer. Of the hundreds of thousands of studies devoted to prostate cancer, 88 small-scale efforts have focused on understanding the experiences of gay, bisexual, and transgender individuals with prostate cancer. That the needs of this community are so self-evidently likely to be unique only highlights the degree to which we have abrogated our duty to care for them properly.

As practicing urologists, we recognize that understanding the experiences of GBTQ men with prostate cancer is likely to help all men with prostate cancer. Wittmann (chapter 3) astutely highlights the need to communicate about sexual needs and adapt an individual's and a couple's sexual repertoire after a prostate cancer diagnosis. Few communities are more adept at adapting their sexual arsenals than those comprising GBTQ men, whose inchoate sexual endeavors rarely hewed closely to the borders drawn by their parents or health educators. How often do we counsel a straight man about the options his sex life might offer even if he was not fully potent, and how his sex life might evolve in exciting and creative ways after prostate cancer treatment? By better understanding how sexual activity evolves in gay and bisexual men with prostate cancer, we can improve the care we provide all men.

As the authors of the later chapters note, progress is on the horizon. Innovative, comprehensive models of care that center on shared decision making, communication, and individualized care are being developed. We are starting to hear the stories like that of the man in chapter 17 who wondered whether anyone was listening to him when he was diagnosed with prostate cancer as a 46-year-old single gay man. If we are to make progress toward equality, we must listen to men like him and value his humanity as tenderly as we would his straight male counterpart. We must understand his individual needs and respond to them. In so doing, we improve the quality of care for all men with prostate cancer.

GAY & BISEXUAL MEN LIVING WITH PROSTATE CANCER

from diagnosis to recovery

INTRODUCTION

Jane M. Ussher, Janette Perz, and B. R. Simon Rosser

Gay and bisexual men, and other men who have sex with men (GBM) have always been part of the population of men who experience prostate cancer. Until relatively recently their needs and experiences have not been acknowledged in prostate cancer research, clinical practice, or policy, which has led to the description of GBM with prostate cancer as a "hidden population"[1] or an "invisible diversity."[2] This book makes visible that which has been neglected for too long—the specific needs and concerns of GBM and their partners living with prostate cancer. This book provides an overview of research and practice, interweaving the personal narratives of GBM who have experienced prostate cancer. Our intention is twofold. By providing insight into the unique experiences and concerns of GBM, we seek to inform future research, clinical practice and supportive care, and policy, ensuring that GBM are recognized and included on the prostate cancer agenda. We also seek to provide a frame of reference that normalizes the experiences of GBM and their families who are facing a prostate cancer diagnosis, undergoing treatment, or living with the aftermath of both. Knowing that you are not alone, and having information about how others in a similar situation have responded and coped, is central to coping with and surviving cancer.[3, 4]

Prostate cancer is a serious concern for all men.[5] It represents 26% of all new cancer diagnoses in men,[6] has the highest incidence of any cancer (aside from non-melanoma skin cancer), and is the second leading cause of cancer death after lung cancer.[7] Approximately 14% of men will be diagnosed with prostate cancer at some point in their lifetimes,[8] a similar incidence to breast cancer in women.[9] No precise estimate of the number of GBM and transgender women (TGW) with prostate cancer exists, as sexual orientation is rarely and inconsistently recorded in medical records,[10] the result being scarce information about cancer disparities in sexual minorities.[11] Population estimates suggest that a considerable number of GBM are affected. Take the case of the United States, where 2,795,592 men were known to be living with

Ussher, Jane M., Perz, Janette, Rosser, B. R. Simon, eds., *Gay & Bisexual Men Living with Prostate Cancer*
dx.doi.org/10.17312/harringtonparkpress/2018.06.gbmlpc.00b
© 2018 Harrington Park Press

prostate cancer in 2012.[8] The Centers for Disease Control and Prevention (CDC) estimates 3.5–4.4% of U.S. men have had sex with a man in the last five years,[12] of whom 40–60% are in sexual relationships.[13,14] By extrapolation, between 97,845 and 123,006 GBM are living with a diagnosis of prostate cancer, including 39,138 to 73,804 men in male couples.[15] One in six GBM and one in three male couples in the United States will receive a prostate cancer diagnosis in their lifetimes. In Australia, where 94,114 men were living with a prostate cancer diagnosis (2012 data),[16] using similar estimates for the size of the gay community, between 3,293 and 4,141 GBM are prostate cancer survivors, and 700 to 880 new cases are diagnosed in GBM each year.

But these are broad estimates. Because some men refuse to acknowledge their same-sex behavior to researchers, and because social research systematically usually excludes men in same-sex populations (e.g., prisons, armed forces), these are probaby underestimates. On the other hand, over half a million GBM have died of HIV/AIDS in the United States alone, which has significantly reduced the size of the older gay community. For TGW, it is impossible to estimate the prevalence of prostate cancer. Because the development of prostate cancer after orchidectomy is rare,[17] the number of TGW with prostate cancer in a country is probably a function of the availability of gender-reassignment surgery and hormone therapy.

While prostate cancer treatments have had a dramatic positive effect on five-year survival rates, which currently stand at between 84% and 92%,[18, 19] such treatments can have a long-term negative influence on men's sexual functioning, quality of life, and psychological well-being. These negative effects include erectile difficulties, non-ejaculatory orgasms, and decreases in desire and sexual satisfaction,[20] often accompanied by bowel and urinary incontinence.[21] These sexual changes have been associated with anxiety and depression,[22] as well as threats to masculine identity[23] and relationships.[24] Until recently, research examining the effects of prostate cancer has focused on heterosexual men or has not asked about sexual identity or orientation, assuming heterosexuality and heterosexual coital sex to be the norm.[25] There have been calls for health promotion and education to acknowledge that GBM with prostate cancer may experience health concerns differently from heterosexual men.[1, 26, 27] However, recent reviews of prostate cancer educational resources and lesbian, gay, bisexual, and transgender (LGBT) primary care guidelines report a dearth of such information,[28, 29] with a few notable exceptions,[30, 31] and an absence of research to inform its future development. The failure of science to conduct studies specifically on LGBT populations results in health disparities in some diseases, including prostate cancer.[32] Clearly, clinicians cannot practice evidence-informed medicine without the studies being conducted to inform their practice.

LGBT communities have been described as experiencing an "ignored epidemic"[33] and characterized as a "growing and medically underserved population"[34] in the area of cancer care. Research on cancer in sexual minorities is an emerging field of study;[34] existing evidence, though limited, suggests that LGBT cancer survivors have unique needs and greater levels of distress on most variables. These unique needs include greater stigma associated with cancer in LGBT communities, limited support from family, challenges to sexual identity, and higher cancer-related distress,[34, 35] all of which compound the higher rates of distress found generally in the LGBT population.[36] Health and access to healthcare services are adversely affected by social marginalization: up to 30% of LGBT adults do not seek healthcare services or lack a regular health service provider, compared with 10% of the non-LGBT population.[34] LGBT individuals often delay or avoid health screening, which results in later-stage cancer detection and a worse prognosis.[37]

LGBT cancer survivors also report difficulties in disclosing their sexual identity to cancer care providers, lower satisfaction with healthcare, and difficulties in accessing support services.[34, 35] When sexual identity is not disclosed to healthcare providers, there are poorer health outcomes.[38] This lack of disclosure promotes "invisibility" of LGBT cancer survivors and neglect of LGBT-specific needs and health risks.[39] Same-sex partners can also feel or be excluded from health consultations, which leaves many LGBT individuals to face difficult and stressful situations alone.[40] Fear of discrimination[40] or internalized stigma on the part of LGBT individuals[41] may prompt this lack of disclosure. Lack of knowledge or embarrassment about LGBT concerns by cancer health professionals can also make disclosure difficult.[40, 42]

There are significant gaps in knowledge about LGBT cancer survivorship and care. Previous research has been small-scale, with an emphasis on documenting disparities in diagnoses or health outcomes, and little attention has been paid to LGBT experiences of survivorship and cancer care.[34, 35] In recent years, research on GBM with prostate cancer has started to address many of these limitations, as evidenced by the many contributions to this book and the growing body of published research that is referenced and discussed throughout the chapters.[35] Leading international researchers, differing in their approaches and methods, have examined GBM's and TGW's experiences of prostate cancer from a variety of perspectives, and they provide new insights into the experience of living with prostate cancer as a sexual or gender minority.

The first section of the book provides an overview of the current research evidence base, beginning with a detailed review of published research on GBM and prostate cancer (chapter 1). We then examine in detail the consequences of prostate cancer treatment on GBM's sexual relationships and identity, drawing on a series of qualitative studies (chapters 2 and 6). We present a model of understanding psychological adjustment (chapter 5) and examine couple dynamics and coping (chapters 3 and 4).

In the second section, we examine cancer care and support, including identity disclosure and heterocentrism in clinical encounters (chapter 8), as well as treatment decision making for GBM in relation to sexual modes and functioning (chapter 9). We consider the specific effects of radiation treatment on GBM (chapter 13) and examine the range and utility of medical and sexual aids to address changes in sexual functioning (chapters 10 and 11). A model of social support and the influence of illness intrusiveness are explored in chapter 12. This section concludes with the presentation of a comprehensive model of prostate cancer care for GBM and TGW (chapter 14) and the case of a GBM support group and network, Malecare (chapter 15).

The final section of the book shares the personal experiences of GBM who are living with or have had prostate cancer. These chapters include Gary W. Dowsett's account, "Losing My Chestnut" (chapter 16), reflecting on diagnosis and treatment ten years later; Ross Henderson's question "What about Me?" (chapter 17), in which he recounts his experience as a gay man with prostate cancer; and Perry Brass describing his experience of prostate cancer as "An Invader in the Pleasure Dome" (chapter 18). In 2005 Gerald Perlman and Jack Drescher published an edited book, *A Gay Man's Guide to Prostate Cancer*,[43] the first substantive publication in this field. Today Gerald Perlman reflects on his own experience of prostate cancer and of leading a support group for GBM (chapter 19). Finally, Simon Rosser, William West, and Badrinath Konety explore a shared decision-making approach to assessing prostate cancer risk through the account of the senior author's own diagnosis (chapter 20).

We are aware that we have not included the experiences of bisexual men and transwomen with prostate cancer. There is scant research on these populations, as we note throughout the book, and unfortunately we were not able to obtain personal narratives.

We hope that this book will inform, inspire, and provide insight into the needs, concerns, and challenges facing GBM with prostate cancer and their families. It may no longer be the case that GBM with prostate cancer can be described as an "invisible diversity,"[2] as the contributions to this book demonstrate the growing body of research in this field. There is still very little knowledge of this research and its implications, however, outside the group of pioneering researchers we are privileged to include as contributors to this book. Our intention is for this book to redress this imbalance through making public and accessible our collective research findings, insights into GBM-centered clinical practice and supportive care, and reflections on the experience of GBM who live with and have survived prostate cancer. We also identify future research directions, highlighting the need for prostate cancer treatment and rehabilitation tailored to address the needs of GBM and TGW. If this book encourages future research on GBM and TGW with prostate cancer, we will have succeeded in our endeavors.

REFERENCES

1. Filiault SM, Drummond MJN, Smith JA. Gay men and prostate cancer: Voicing the concerns of a hidden population. *Journal of Men's Health.* 2008; 5 (4): 327–332.
2. Blank TO. Gay men and prostate cancer: Invisible diversity. *Journal of Clinical Oncology.* 2005; 23 (12): 2593–2596.
3. Ussher JM, Kirsten L, Butow P, Sandoval M. What do cancer support groups provide which other supportive relationships do not? The experience of peer support groups for people with cancer. *Social Science & Medicine.* 2006 (62): 2565–2576.
4. Perz J, Ussher JM, Australian Cancer and Sexuality Study Team. A randomised trial of a minimal intervention for sexual concerns after cancer: A comparison of self-help and professionally delivered modalities. *BMC Cancer.* 2015; 15 (629): 1–16, doi 10.1186/s12885-015-1638-6.
5. Griggs J, Maingi S, Blinder V, et al. American Society of Clinical Oncology Position statement: Strategies for reducing cancer health disparities among sexual and gender minority populations. *Journal of Clinical Oncology.* 2017; 35 (19): 2203–2208.
6. Siegel RL, Miller KD, Jemal A. Cancer statistics. *CA: A Cancer Journal for Clinicians.* 2015; 65 (1): 5–29.

7. National Cancer Institute. Prostate cancer. 2015; www.cancer.gov/types/prostate. Accessed June 8, 2015.

8. National Cancer Institute. Surveillance Epidemiology and End Results Program (SEER). Cancer statistics. 2015; http://seer.cancer.gov/statfacts/html/prost.html. Accessed June 8, 2015.

9. Latini DM, Hart SL, Coon DW, Knight SJ. Sexual rehabilitation after localized prostate cancer: Current interventions and future directions. *Cancer*. 2009; 15 (1): 34–40.

10. Bowen DJ, Boehmer U. The lack of cancer surveillance data on sexual minorities and strategies for change. *Cancer Causes & Control*. 2007; 18 (4): 343–349.

11. Boehmer U, Miao X, Ozonoff A. Cancer survivorship and sexual orientation. *Cancer*. 2011; 117 (16): 3796–3804.

12. Purcell DW, Johnson C, Lansky A, et al. Estimating the population size of men who have sex with men in the United States to obtain HIV and syphilis rates. *Open AIDS Journal*. 2010; 6: 98–107.

13. Kurdek LA. Are gay and lesbian cohabitating couples *really* different from heterosexual married couples? *Journal of Marrriage and Family*. 2004; 66: 880–900.

14. Kurdek LA. What do we know about gay and lesbian couples? *Current Directions in Psychological Science*. 2005; 14 (5): 251–254.

15. Rosser BRS, Capistrant BD, Iantaffi A, et al. Prostate cancer in gay, bisexual and other men who have sex with men: A review. *Journal of LGBT Health*. 2016; 3 (1): 32–41.

16. Australian Institute of Health and Welfare (AIHW). Prostate cancer in Australia. 2017; https://prostate-cancer.canceraustralia.gov.au/statistics/. Accessed October 9, 2017.

17. Miksad RA, Bubley G, Church P, et al. Prostate cancer in a transgender woman 41 years after initiation of feminization. *Journal of the American Medical Assocation (JAMA)*. 2006; 296 (19): 2312–2317.

18. Australian Institute of Health and Welfare. *Australia's health 2012*. Australia's Health series no.13. Cat. no. AUS 156. Canberra: AIHW; 2012.

19. Cancer Research UK. Cancer survival for common cancers. 2015; www.cancer researchuk.org/health-professional/cancer-statistics/survival/common-cancers-compared#heading-One. Accessed September 4, 2015.

20. Chung E, Brock G. Sexual rehabilitation and cancer survivorship: A state of art review of current literature and management strategies in male sexual dysfunction among prostate cancer survivors. *Journal of Sexual Medicine*. 2013; 10: 102–111.

21. Danile A, Haddow S. Erectile dysfunction after prostate cancer. *Clinical Advisor*. 2011; March: 64–68.

22. Perz J, Ussher JM, Gilbert E. Feeling well and talking about sex: Psycho-social predictors of sexual functioning after cancer. *BMC Cancer*. 2014; 14 (1): 228–247.

23. Zaider T, Manne S, Nelson C, et al. Loss of masculine identity, marital affection,

and sexual bother in men with localized prostate cancer. *Journal of Sexual Medicine.* 2012; 9 (10): 2724–2732.

24. Manne S, Badr H, Zaider T, et al. Cancer-related communication, relationship intimacy, and psychological distress among couples coping with localized prostate cancer. *Journal of Cancer Survivorship.* 2010; 4 (1): 74–85.

25. Asencio M, Blank T, Descartes L, Crawford A. The prospect of prostate cancer: A challenge for gay men's sexualities as they age. *Sexuality Research and Social Policy.* 2009; 6 (4): 38–51.

26. Filiault SM, Drummond MJ, Riggs DW. Speaking out on GBT men's health: A critique of the Australian government's Men's Health Policy. *Journal of Men's Health.* 2009; 6 (3): 158–161.

27. Galbraith ME, Crighton F. Alterations of sexual function in men with cancer. *Seminars in Oncology Nursing.* 2008; 24 (2): 102–114.

28. Duncan D, Watson J, Westle A, et al. *Gay men and prostate cancer: Report on an audit of existing resources and websites providing information to men living with prostate cancer in Australia.* Melbourne: Australian Research Centre in Sex, Health and Society, La Trobe University; 2011.

29. McNair RP, Hegarty K. Guidelines for the primary care of lesbian, gay, and bisexual people: A systematic review. *Annals of Family Medicine.* 2010; 8 (6): 533–541.

30. Wong WK, Lowe A, Dowsett GW, Duncan D, O'Keeffe D, Mitchell A. *Prostate cancer information needs of Australian gay and bisexual men.* Sydney, NSW: Prostate Cancer Foundation of Australia; 2013.

31. Buchting FO, Margolies L, Bare MG, et al. *LGBT best and promising practices throughout the cancer continuum.* Fort Lauderdale, Fla.: LGBT HealthLink; 2015; www.lgbthealthlink.org/. Accessed July 2017.

32. Institute of Medicine. *The health of lesbian, gay, bisexual and transgender people: Building a foundation for a better understanding.* 2011; https://www.ncbi.nlm.nih.gov/books/NBK64795/. Accessed October 9, 2017.

33. Boehmer U, Elk R. LGBT populations and cancer: Is it an ignored epidemic? *LGBT Health.* 2016; 3 (1): 1–2.

34. Quinn GP, Sanchez JA, Sutton SK, et al. Cancer and lesbian, gay, bisexual, transgender/transsexual, and queer/questioning (LGBTQ) populations. *CA: A Cancer Journal for Clinicians.* 2015; 65: 384–400.

35. Rosser S, Merengwa E, Capistrant BD, et al. Prostate cancer in gay, bisexual, and other men who have sex with men: A review. *LGBT Health.* 2016; 3 (1): 32–41.

36. Pitts M, Smith A, Mitchell A, Patel S. *Private lives: A report on the health and wellbeing of GLBTI Australians.* Melbourne: Australian Research Centre in Sex, Health and Society, La Trobe University; 2006.

37. Charlton BM, Corliss HL, Missmer SA, et al. Reproductive health screening disparities and sexual orientation in a cohort study of U.S. adolescent and young adult females. *Journal of Adolescent Health.* 2011; 49 (5): 505–510.

38. Durso L, Meyer I. Patterns and predictors of disclosure of sexual orientation to healthcare providers among lesbians, gay men, and bisexuals. *Sexuality Research and Social Policy.* 2013; 10 (1): 35–42.

39. Quinn GP, Schabath MB, Sanchez JA, et al. The importance of disclosure: Lesbian, gay, bisexual, transgender/transsexual, queer/questioning, and intersex individuals and the cancer continuum. *Cancer.* 2015; 121 (8): 1160–1163.

40. Rose D, Ussher JM, Perz J. Let's talk about gay sex: Gay and bisexual men's sexual communication with healthcare professionals after prostate cancer. *European Journal of Cancer Care.* 2017; 26 (1).

41. Wilkerson JM, Rybicki S, Barber CA, Smolenski DJ. Creating a culturally competent clinical environment for LGBT patients. *Journal of Gay & Lesbian Social Services.* 2011; 23 (3): 376–394.

42. Wassersug RJ, Lyons A, Duncan D, et al. Diagnostic and outcome differences between heterosexual and nonheterosexual men treated for prostate cancer. *Urology.* 2013; 82 (3): 565–571.

43. Perlman G, Drescher J. *A gay man's guide to prostate cancer.* Binghamton, N.Y.: Haworth Medical Press; 2005.

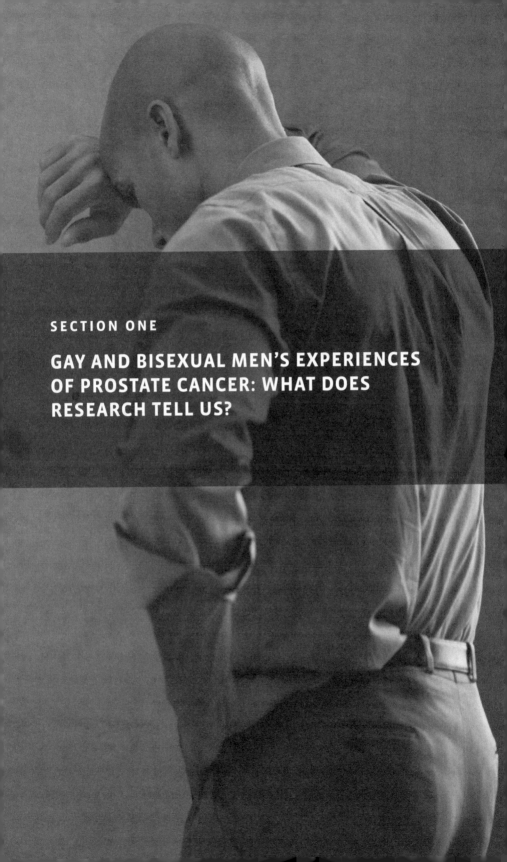

GAY AND BISEXUAL MEN'S EXPERIENCES OF PROSTATE CANCER: WHAT DOES RESEARCH TELL US?

CHAPTER 1

Understanding Prostate Cancer in Gay, Bisexual, and Other Men Who Have Sex with Men and Transgender Women

A Review of the Literature

B. R. Simon Rosser, Shanda L. Hunt, Benjamin D. Capistrant, Nidhi Kohli, Badrinath R. Konety, Darryl Mitteldorf, Michael W. Ross, Kristine M. Talley, and William West

CHAPTER SUMMARY

Prostate cancer in sexual and gender minorities is an emerging medical and public health concern. The purpose of this review is to summarize the state of the science on prostate cancer in gay, bisexual, and other men who have sex with men (GBM) and transgender women (TGW). We undertook a literature review of all publications on this topic through February 2017. With 88 unique papers (83 on prostate cancer in GBM and 5 case reports of prostate cancer in TGW), a small but robust literature has emerged. The first half of this review critiques the literature to date, identifying gaps in approaches to study. The second half summarizes the key findings in eleven areas. In light of this admittedly limited literature, GBM appear to be screened for prostate cancer less than other men, but they are diagnosed with prostate cancer at about the same rate. Compared to other men, GBM have poorer urinary, bowel, and overall quality-of-life outcomes but better sexual outcomes after treatment; all these findings need more research. Prostate cancer in TGW remains rare and underresearched, as the literature is limited to single-case clinical reports.

KEY TERMS

bisexual, cancer, gay, prostate, sexual rehabilitation

Ussher, Jane M., Perz, Janette, Rosser, B. R. Simon, eds., *Gay & Bisexual Men Living with Prostate Cancer*
dx.doi.org/10.17312/harringtonparkpress/2018.06.gbmlpc.001
© 2018 Harrington Park Press

INTRODUCTION

Research on prostate cancer in sexual and gender minorities is an emerging field of study. In the United States, improving the health of lesbian, gay, bisexual, and transgender (LGBT) individuals is a Healthy People 2020 goal.[1] The failure of science to conduct studies specifically on LGBT populations, however, results in health disparities in some diseases, including prostate cancer.[2] Clearly, clinicians cannot practice evidence-informed medicine without studies being conducted to inform their practice.

The purpose of this review is to provide an informed overview of the state of the science regarding prostate cancer in gay, bisexual, and other men who have sex with men (GBM) and transgender women (TGW). Some of the studies reviewed in this chapter are described in more detail in subsequent chapters in this book. This review contextualizes all the studies' findings in relation to one another, identifying areas for future research.

In February 2017 we performed a systematic literature search and review.[3] Database searching was conducted using MEDLINE via Ovid and PubMed, EMBASE, PsycINFO, and Social Work Abstracts. The search yielded 52 unique citations focused on prostate cancer in GBM or TGW. A supplemental search of bibliographies added 39 references. Excluding three duplicate citations, the complete search yielded a total of 88 original works. Of these, 83 focused on prostate cancer in GBM and 5 on prostate cancer in TGW. Allowing for multiple papers from the same study, there were 28 case studies (table 1.1), 8 qualitative studies (table 1.2), and 8 quantitative studies (table 1.3).

THE KEY QUESTIONS

The main results of the literature to date have addressed the following eleven key questions.

1. How many GBM are living with a prostate cancer diagnosis? No precise estimate of the number of GBM and TGW living with prostate cancer exists. Prostate cancer is the second-most common cancer among men; 2,795,592 men in the United States were living with prostate cancer in 2012.[4] The Centers for Disease Control and Prevention (CDC) estimates that 3.5–4.4% of U.S. men have had sex with a man in the last five years,[5] of whom 40–60% are in sexual relationships.[6,7] By extrapolation, between 97,845 and 123,006 GBM are living with a

TABLE 1.1

Literature on Prostate Cancer in Gay and Bisexual Men and Transgender Persons (N = 88 citations)

Number and Type of Contribution	Operational Definition	Citations
Works Containing Original Data or Original Scientific Contributions		
Case Report (N = 28)	$N \leq 5$ participants on GBM	34, 38, 48, 52–54, 61, 63, 67, 72–86
	$N \leq 5$ participants on TGW	9, 87–90
Qualitative Study Report (N = 11)	Study with > 5 participants (to inform saturation) using qualitative analyses	28, 29, 42–44, 62, 68, 91–96
Quantitative Study Report (N = 19)	a. Surveillance: study analyzing secondary data from large data set	10, 14, 20, 97, 98
	b. Observational: study with > 5 participants generating original data using quantitative methods and/or analyses	25–27, 30, 59, 99–105
	c. Treatment: study with > 5 participants where the focus is on testing a new treatment or rehabilitation	106
Works Not Reporting Original Data or Formal Studies		
Review (N = 9)	Paper reporting findings from multiple studies to review the literature	8, 11, 60, 107–112
Clinical Observation and/or Educational Articles (N = 13)	Focus is on treatment, rehabilitation, patient education, or lessons learned at a broad level without detailed description of participants, studies, or results	35–37, 52–54, 56, 63, 113–123
Commentary (N = 5)	Introduces other papers or topics or comments on other studies/works (including book reviews)	55, 124–127
Other (N = 2)	Category of last resort for citations not fitting into the above; includes books	128, 129

diagnosis of prostate cancer, including 39,138 to 73,804 men in male couples.[8] One in six GBM and one in three male couples will receive a diagnosis in their lifetimes. It is impossible to estimate the prevalence of prostate cancer among TGW. Because the development of prostate cancer after orchidectomy is rare,[9] the number of TGW with prostate cancer in a country is probably a function of the availability of gender-reassignment surgery and hormone therapy.

2. **Do GBM engage in prostate cancer screening at different rates from other men?** In the only study of PSA screening (N = 19,410 men in the California Health Interview Survey), GBM had lower odds of having an up-to-date prostate-specific antigen test than did heterosexual men (OR = 0.61; CI = 0.42, 0.89), and bivariate analyses showed African American GBM as having lower rates than either heterosexual African American men or white GBM.[10] More research is needed.

3. **Are GBM at disproportionately greater risk for prostate cancer than other men?** Santillo and Lowe[11] identify six "lifestyle co-factors" that theoretically could increase the risk of prostate cancer in GBM: use of testosterone supplements and anabolic steroids, use of finasteride (Propecia) for hair loss, HIV status and antiretroviral (ARV) treatment, a fatty diet, the effects of anal sex on prostate-specific antigen (PSA) testing, and poor doctor-patient communication.[11] Because GBM are disproportionately at greater risk for HIV and other sexually transmitted infections (STI), comparative studies of prostate cancer incidence by orientation need to control for HIV and STI history.[12]

Three epidemiologic case-control studies inform this question, and their conclusions differ. One study comparing men with prostate cancer with a control group of men matched on age and race found that members of the prostate cancer group were more likely to have a history of STIs, and more likely to report homosexual partners, than the control group.[13] A second study determined that prostate cancer risk increased with lifetime numbers of female partners and with a history of gonorrhea; however, orientation identity, anal sex, and a history of male partners were not associated with increased risk.[14] A third study found that men with 20 or more lifetime female sexual partners were at lower risk of prostate cancer than men with fewer female partners, whereas men with 20 or more lifetime male partners were at a slightly higher risk. Though sex with 20 or more men was associated with elevated risk, neither history of STIs nor sexual orientation identity as gay or bisexual was significantly associated with risk.[15]

4. **Does an HIV diagnosis or treatment change GBM's risk for prostate cancer?** Yes. Though early studies suggested an increased risk of prostate cancer among HIV-positive than among HIV-negative men,[16, 17] studies in the era of ARV treatment show an inverse association.[18–20] A cohort study of men with clinical AIDS found no difference in prostate cancer

TABLE 1.2

Qualitative Studies with $N > 5$ Participants (N = 8 Studies)

	Study Logistics	Methods (Design, Recruitment, Participants, Procedures)	Key Results
1	**PI:** Fergus **Year of study:** 2002 **Site:** Toronto, Canada **Language:** English **Funding:** Canadian Institutes of Health Research (CIHR)	**Design:** In-person, in-depth interviews **Participants:** N = 18 participants, including 14 heterosexual (including 4 Afro-Canadian) and 4 homosexual (all Euro-Canadian) **Procedures:** Sample recruited from local prostate cancer support group, through advertisements in the gay and black media, GP referral, and personal contacts **Inclusion/exclusion criteria:** Must have lived with prostate cancer diagnosis for minimum of one year	**Sexual effects:** Using grounded theory, one core category emerged (labeled "preserving manhood") with 5 themes: (1) enhancing the odds; (2) disrupting a core performance; (3) baring an invisible stigma; (4) effortful-mechanical sex; and (5) working around the loss. No formal comparison of heterosexual versus gay survivors seems to have been performed; authors concluded that the commonalities, not differences, were striking. Authors note that all the heterosexual men were partnered, whereas only 1 of the 4 gay men were, and that black heterosexual men were particularly concerned about loss of sexual ability and perhaps less willing to participate in treatment.[44]
2	**PI:** Asencio **Year of study:** Not specified (pre-2009) **Site:** Hartford, Conn. **Language:** English and Spanish **Funding:** Private foundation and internal	**Design:** 5 focus groups (3 mixed, 1 African American, and 1 bilingual in Spanish) **Participants:** 36 gay men (not prostate cancer survivors) **Procedures:** Flyers in community organizations and at Gay Pride **Inclusion/exclusion criteria:** No requirement to have prostate cancer	**Sexual effects:** Gay men have little understanding of the prostate and sexual challenges of treatment. Some hold beliefs that rough sex can cause (or prevent) prostate cancer. In Latino and black gay men, machismo and medical skepticism may prevent screening, respectively. Gay men overstressed prostate cancer being fatal. About half would seek treatment and half stated they would avoid treatment to preserve sexual functioning; older white men preferred treatment over function. Black and Latinos described more pressure to preserve sexual function.[91]
3	**PIs:** Dowsett & Wassersug **Year of study:** 2010–2011 **Site:** Online international (respondents from 17 countries) **Language:** English **Funding:** Unfunded	**Design:** Controlled online survey with open-ended questions about sexual activity before and after prostate cancer treatment **Participants:** 96 nonheterosexual and 460 heterosexual men **Recruitment:** Unvalidated sample recruited from 40 prostate cancer support organizations, including online support groups; no compensation **Criteria:** No exclusions	**Sexual effects:** Results not formally analyzed or broken out by sexual orientation. However, the authors in the discussion describe nonheterosexual men as more "adventurous" in exploring novel sexual options than heterosexual men.[30]

TABLE 1.2

Qualitative Studies with N > 5 Participants (N = 8 Studies)

	Study Logistics	Methods (Design, Recruitment, Participants, Procedures)	Key Results
4	**PI:** Doran **Year of study:** Not specified (pre-2015) **Site:** U.K. **Language:** English **Funding:** Not specified	**Design:** 12 semistructured interviews **Participants:** 12 gay men **Procedures:** Not specified (abstract) **Inclusion/exclusion criteria:** Not specified (abstract)	**General life effects:** Using Merleau-Ponty's four life world existentials, themes that emerged include: (1) *corporeality*: bodily effect of the disease, including violation of identity, assault of the physical body, and power of potency; (2) *temporality*, including threat to eternal youth; living in a state of flux; disrupted lives; and past, present, and future horizons; (3) *relationality*, including quest for mutual respect and equality, locating information, to tell or not to tell, changes and challenges, friendship and pursuit of peers; and (4) *spatiality*, including yearning for community, the power of proximity, and isolation.[92]
5	**PI:** Thomas **Year of study:** Not specified (pre-2013) **Site:** Australia **Language:** English **Funding:** Not specified	**Design:** Asynchronous online focus group transcript analysis **Participants:** 10 GBM **Recruitment:** Informally through prostate cancer support groups for GBM **Inclusion/exclusion criteria:** Had to be Australian diagnosed with prostate cancer within last 7 years	**General effects:** Some participants reported a positive perspective post-diagnosis and adopted a sense of empowerment. Participants spoke about emotional responses to a diagnosis of prostate cancer, accessing help and support, the effect of incontinence, the influence of sexual changes on identify, a reevaluation of life, changed sexual relationships, the need to find the most suitable healthcare professionals, and identification of current needs to improve quality of care. Authors conclude that the psychological effects of prostate cancer may be quite significant over an extended time frame.[42]
6	**PI:** Lee **Year of study:** Not specified (pre-2015) **Site:** Vancouver, B.C. **Language:** Not specified **Funding:** Canadian Association of Radiation Oncology Award; Canadian Institutes of Health; Eli Lilly	**Design:** 14 in-depth semistructured in-person interviews and 2 videophone interviews **Participants:** 16 MSM **Recruitment:** From clinics, gay Pride events, Facebook and Craigslist **Exclusion criterion:** Restricted to < 75 years	**Sexual effects:** Treatment resulted in (1) erectile, urinary, ejaculation, and orgasmic dysfunctions; (2) challenges to intimate relationships; and (3) lack of MSM-specific oncological and psychosocial support for survivors. Negative effects on quality of life can be severe for MSM and require targeted attention.[93]

(continued)

TABLE 1.2 *(continued)*

Qualitative Studies with *N* > 5 Participants (*N* = 8 Studies)

Study Logistics	Methods (Design, Recruitment, Participants, Procedures)	Results
7 **PIs:** Rosser & Capistrant **Name of study:** Restore **Year of study:** 2015 **Site:** U.S. and Canada **Language:** English **Funding:** National Cancer Institute (NCI, R21); American Cancer Society	**Design:** In-depth semistructured telephone interviews **Participants:** 30 GBM treated for prostate cancer: 19 with radical prostatectomy, 6 with radiation; 5 systemic **Recruitment:** Online support group **Inclusion/exclusion criteria:** Must have received surgery, radiation, or systemic treatment for prostate cancer; must be resident in the United States or Canada	**Social support:** GBM receive variable but generally low social support during diagnosis and treatment. Compared to heterosexual survivors who rely on spouse and biological family, GBM rely more on self, partner, and chosen family.[62] **Sexual effects (*N* = 19 GBM with radical prostatectomy):** Major challenges to sexual functioning included anatomical changes to the penis, loss of ejaculate, climacturia, erectile dysfunction, and possibly decreased libido. All forms of sexual behavior with other men, not just penetrative sex, appeared affected and affected across all stages of the sexual response cycle. Some GBM reported shifting their role-in-sex after surgery; others engaged in novel substitution behaviors.[29] **Mental health, identity, and relationships (*N* = 19 radical prostatectomy):** Five emotional themes emerged: (1) shock at the diagnosis, (2) a reactive depression, (3) sex-specific situational anxiety, (4) grief, and, (5) an enduring loss of sexual confidence. Identity challenges included loss of a sense of maleness and manhood, changes in strength of sexual orientation, role-in-sex identity, and immersion into sexual subcultures. Identified relationship challenges included disclosing the sexual effects of treatment to partners, loss of partners, and renegotiation of sexual exclusivity. Most to all of these effects stem from sexual changes.[68]

TABLE 1.2

Qualitative Studies with $N > 5$ Participants ($N = 8$ Studies)

	Study Logistics	Methods (Design, Recruitment, Participants, Procedures)	Results
8	**PIs:** Ussher & Perz **Year of study:** 2015-2016 **Site:** Global (mainly Australia, U.S., U.K.) **Language:** English **Funding:** Prostate Cancer Foundation of Australia (PCFA)	**Design:** Mixed methods using answers to open-ended and closed questions plus in-person or video interviews **Participants:** 124 GBM and 21 male partner survey respondents, and 46 GBM and 7 partners interviewed **Recruitment:** Cancer support groups, cancer research databases, clinicians, social media, and GB community and health organizations **Inclusion:** Diagnosis of prostate cancer	**Sexual effects:** 72% of survey respondents reported erectile dysfunction, which was associated with emotional distress, negative effect on gay identity, and feelings of sexual disqualification. Other sexual concerns included loss of libido, climacturia, loss of sensitivity or pain during anal sex, non-ejaculatory orgasms, and reduced penis size. Many of these outcomes led to feelings of exclusion from the gay community. Other men reported being reconciled to sexual changes, identified no challenge, and engaged in sexual renegotiation.[43] **GBM-physician communication:** Four themes emerged: (1) cancer-centered care negates sexual needs; (2) healthcare professionals assume heterosexuality of their patients; (3) navigating sexual orientation disclosure (avoidant vs. hesitant vs. forthright); and (4) healthcare professionals' responses to disclosure and requests for gay-specific information (rejecting vs. lack of knowledge or interest vs. acknowledgment and interest).[94]

incidence compared to the general population during the pre-PSA (and pre-ARV) time period (before 1992) but a significant twofold reduction in risk among those with AIDS during the PSA era (1992–2007).[20]

Why HIV-positive men would be at less risk for prostate cancer than HIV-negative men warrants more investigation. Unfortunately, the HIV studies to date have not reported data on sexual orientation, so it is impossible to tease out what may be HIV effects from effects due to sexual orientation. A Chicago-based study found that HIV-positive men were as likely to receive treatment for prostate cancer, less likely to undergo a radical prostatectomy, and more likely to be overtreated compared to HIV-negative men.[21] The authors concluded that while the rate of AIDS-defining cancers among HIV-positive men continues to fall, as HIV-positive men live longer, the rate of non-AIDS-defining cancers (such as prostate cancer) may rise. Though HIV and immuno-

TABLE 1.3

Key Results from Quantitative Studies of Prostate Cancer Outcomes in GBM
(*N* = 12 Papers from 8 Studies)

Study Logistics	Methods	Prostate Cancer Sexual, Urinary, Bowel, Hormonal Outcomes	Other Results
PI: Motofei **Year of study:** 2008 **Site:** Bucharest, Romania **Language:** Romanian **Funding:** Not specified	**Design:** Comparative drug treatment trial with 5-week follow-up **Participants:** 12 homosexual and 17 heterosexual **Recruitment:** From local hospital **Eligibility validation:** From hospital records **Criteria:** Diagnosed, treatment-naive prostate cancer patients presenting at local hospital	GBM had worse sexual functioning than heterosexual men following treatment with bicalutamide.[106]	—
PIs: Allensworth-Davies & Clark **Year of study:** 2010 **Site:** U.S. **Language:** English **Funding:** National Cancer Institute (NCI, R03)	**Design:** Uncontrolled, cross-sectional survey **Participants:** 111 gay-identified men **Recruitment:** Through gay print magazines **Validation:** None **Criteria:** Minimum 50 years of age; self-identify as gay only; must have been treated for at least one year for localized prostate cancer	Gay men report significantly lower urinary and bowel functioning than 341 heterosexual men.*	Younger gay prostate cancer survivors and men who reported recent severe stigma report lower masculinity self-esteem scores than men 75+ years old.[99]
PI: Lee **Year of study:** 2011–2012 **Site:** Ottawa, Canada **Language:** Not specified **Funding:** Unfunded	**Design:** Uncontrolled cross-sectional mailed pen-and-paper survey **Participants:** 15 MSM **Recruitment and validation:** From urology and oncology departments at local hospital **Criteria:** Must have received prostate cancer treatment; excluded if had androgen deprivation within 18 months or had chemotherapy/noncutaneous malignancies	GBM have worse urinary, bowel, ejaculatory function and sexual bother than published norms.[27]	—

TABLE 1.3

Key Results from Quantitative Studies of Prostate Cancer Outcomes in GBM
(N = 12 Papers from 8 Studies)

Study Logistics	Methods	Prostate Cancer Sexual, Urinary, Bowel, Hormonal Outcomes	Other Results
PI: Hart **Year of study:** Not specified (pre-2011) **Site:** Online U.S. and Canada **Language:** Not specified **Funding:** University internal funding	**Design:** Uncontrolled cross-sectional online survey **Participants:** 92 self-identified gay or bisexual men **Recruitment:** Through listservs, community centers, support groups, and advertisements in local media **Eligibility validation:** By phone screening **Criteria:** Diagnosis of prostate cancer within last 4 years; no exclusions	GBM have worse urinary, bowel, and hormonal functioning and bother than published norms, worse mental health functioning, greater fear of cancer recurrence, and better sexual functioning than published norms.[25, 59]	Outness (as GBM) mediates anxious attachment and more illness intrusiveness. Facilitating GBM to be out may benefit illness adjustment.[100] Worse bowel, hormone, and sex function predicts fear of prostate cancer recurrence, mediated by self-efficacy and satisfaction with care.[103]
PIs: Dowsett & Wassersug **Year of study:** 2010–2011 **Site:** Online international (respondents from 17 countries) **Language:** English **Funding:** Unfunded	**Design:** Controlled online survey **Participants:** 96 nonheterosexual and 460 heterosexual men **Recruitment:** Sample recruited from 40 prostate cancer support organizations, including online support groups; no compensation **Eligibility validation:** Sample not validated for eligibility **Criteria:** No exclusions	GBM have lower Gleason scores and greater ejaculatory bother than heterosexual men. No differences on incidence of urinary incontinence, bone pain, or antidepressant use.[26]	GBM versus heterosexual survivors differ by country of residence and relationship status. Many GBM cope with ED by changing their role-in-sex.[30]
PI: Mitteldorf **Year of study:** 2015 **Site:** U.S. **Language:** English **Funding:** Unfunded	**Design:** Controlled online survey **Participants:** 148 GBM and 632 heterosexual men **Recruitment:** Sample recruited from large online prostate cancer support group **Eligibility validation:** Sample not validated for eligibility **Criteria:** Inclusion criteria not specified (abstract only)	——	In unadjusted analyses, GBM report more early-stage treatments but fewer advanced-stage treatments than heterosexual men.[101]

(continued)

TABLE 1.3 *(continued)*

Key Results from Quantitative Studies of Prostate Cancer Outcomes in GBM
(*N* = 12 Papers from 8 Studies)

Study Logistics	Methods	Prostate Cancer Sexual, Urinary, Bowel, Hormonal Outcomes	Other Results
Study: Restore Aim 1 **PI:** Rosser **Year of study:** 2015 **Site:** Online U.S. and Canada **Language:** English **Funding:** National Cancer Institute (NCI, R21)	**Design:** Natural experiment: GBM offered screening and interview online, by Skype, or by phone **Participants:** *N* = 74 GBM screened and 30 interviewed **Eligibility validation:** Validated through in-depth interview** **Recruitment:** From e-mails sent to online support groups **Criteria:** Must have been treated for prostate cancer, residing in U.S. or Canada; compensated	——	**Research methods:** For qualitative interviews, GBM with prostate cancer preferred being screened online but interviewed by phone.[102]
Study: Restore Aim 3 **PI:** Rosser **Year of study:** 2015–2016 **Site:** Online U.S. and Canada **Language:** English **Funding:** National Cancer Institute (NCI, R21)	**Design:** Uncontrolled online survey **Participants:** 193 self-identified GBM **Recruitment:** Through large online prostate cancer support group **Eligibility validation:** Sample was cross-validated through de-duplication and cross-validation protocol (55% excluded) **Criteria:** Must have been treated for prostate cancer; residing in U.S. or Canada; compensated	GBM have worse urinary and hormonal function and worse hormonal bother, but better sexual function and less bother than published norms.[130]	66.6% describe their sexual function posttreatment as fair to poor. ED was common, severe, and pervasive across sexual behavior; it was also a major reason for not using condoms. 33.3% reported receptive anal sex difficulties. ED, non-condom use, anodyspareunia, and all sexual functions were problematic.[130] Needs assessment shows high interest in an online sexual recovery program tailored to GBM with prostate cancer.[131]

TABLE 1.3

Key Results from Quantitative Studies of Prostate Cancer Outcomes in GBM
(N = 12 Papers from 8 Studies)

Study Logistics	Methods	Prostate Cancer Sexual, Urinary, Bowel, Hormonal Outcomes	Other Results
PIs: Ussher & Perz **Year of study:** 2015–2016 **Site:** Australia, U.S., U.K., and global **Language:** English **Funding:** Prostate Cancer Foundation of Australia (PCFA)	**Design:** Controlled online survey **Participants:** 124 MSM and 225 heterosexual men **Recruitment:** MSM recruited through urology and general practice clinics, prostate cancer support groups, and social media. Heterosexual comparison group recruited through cancer research volunteer databases **Eligibility validation:** Sample not validated for eligibility **Criteria:** Must have been diagnosed with prostate cancer	GBM report lower quality of life; higher psychological distress; lower masculine self-esteem; lower sexual confidence and sexual intimacy; lower satisfaction with treatment; and ejaculatory concern.[105]	GBM prostate cancer survivors were significantly younger than heterosexual sample. ED was reported in 72% of GBM. Loss of libido, climacturia, anodyspareunia, orgasm, and penile size are all problematic.[105]

*This is an unpublished thesis result, noted in two other published papers.[25, 107]
** Eligibility validation denotes a best practice in online survey research to confirm that the surveys come from eligible, valid, unique participants. Methods of validation include some combination of external validity checks (e.g., hospital records, driver's license), electronic validation (e.g., Captcha), telephone validation, and cross-validation and de-duplication protocols.[132, 133]

deficiency may alter the risk of prostate cancer[11, 12, 22, 23] and cancer virulence,[11] ARV treatment appears to be protective.[24]

5. Do GBM have different treatment outcomes from other men? Yes. GBM appear to have worse urinary and possibly bowel outcomes, but better sexual outcomes, than published norms.[25–27] Why GBM report poorer urinary and bowel function than heterosexual men is not clear. Some studies conclude that the better sexual outcomes GBM report compared to heterosexual peers may be due to GBM being more open, innovative, or committed to restoring their sexual function.[28, 29] Substantial differences in role-in-sex, pre- and post-treatment, have also been reported,[25] which may also influence outcomes. GBM report more bother as a result of the inability to ejaculate than heterosexual men.[26, 105]

6. Do GBM receive different treatment from heterosexual men? Possibly. In one study, Gleason scores were significantly lower for GBM than for heterosexual men, which suggests that GBM may be diagnosed earlier than heterosexual men.[26, 30] While the authors speculate that GBM may be more likely to undergo regular health checkups, this explanation is at odds with the data reporting lower, not higher, PSA testing among MSM.[10] Because vigorous stimulation of the prostate may significantly affect the serum PSA,[31] GBM and TGW should be warned to refrain from receptive anal stimulation for at least 48 hours before a PSA test.[11] Studies of how clinicians test PSA in GBM are needed to examine whether invalid PSA testing is contributing to this disparity. A second hypothesis is that physical trauma to the prostate (e.g., from repeated receptive anal sex) could increase serum PSA levels.[15]

LGBT health disparities in accessing medical care exist.[2] GBM may experience prostate cancer treatment as heteronormative.[32-34] GBM with prostate cancer report that healthcare providers fail to ask about sexual orientation during initial consultations, may assume they are not sexually active, or assume they are heterosexual.[35] Goldstone notes that in his experience as a surgeon, gay men may be embarrassed to ask about sexual function.[36, 37] There remains a lack of prostate cancer educational resources tailored to gay men (see also chapter 6 in this book).[38]

7. What are the known psychological effects of treatment on GBM?
Like other men, GBM report reduced sense of masculinity,[39-41] identity,[42, 43] or self-esteem (or a combination of these).[44-47] The sexual effects of prostate cancer carry a stigma leading some GBM to conclude they are less sexually desirable than other GBM.[42] Prostate cancer in GBM intersects with issues of minority status,[35, 48] discrimination,[35] stigmatization,[35, 44] less familial support,[6, 7, 49-51] and less social support.[7, 49-51] Though some GBM may develop "an inner strength to meet the challenges of prostate cancer,"[42] others report profound shame at their own ignorance about prostate cancer,[52] grief at the diagnosis,[42] poor body image after treatment,[53] and premature aging.[54] For HIV-positive GBM, prostate cancer may be one more medical complication to address in an already medicalized life.[48]

8. What are the specific challenges of prostate cancer treatment for GBM? While prostate cancer affects GBM in many of the same ways as heterosexual men, GBM prostate cancer survivors face unique challenges, including the loss of the prostate as a site for sexual pleasure in receptive sex,[11, 49] loss of ejaculate (which authors emphasize is more central in gay sex),[35, 52, 54] persistent rectal irritation or pain sufficient to prevent receptive anal sex,[36, 55] and erections too weak for insertive anal sex.[52] Anal penetration is estimated to require 33 percent more rigidity than vaginal penetration.[56] In one study, most (59%) GBM reported changes in anal intercourse after treatment; almost half (46%) ceased it.[30] Weak erections may prevent GBM treated for prostate cancer from using condoms, increasing the risk of HIV transmission.[57] And changes in role-in-sex can occur. Before treatment, 58 GBM were insertive partners; of these, 14 (24%) changed to being exclusively receptive partners after treatment. None of the GBM who were exclusively receptive before treatment changed roles afterward.[30]

9. What do we know about interventions to assist mental health and quality of life for GBM? Prostate cancer and its treatment have significant effects on mental health[35, 58] as well as quality of life.[59] Race or ethnicity and sexual minority status are significant negative predictors of quality of life after treatment for prostate cancer.[60] Case studies of GBM with prostate cancer confirm significant post-treatment mental health challenges.[61] Blank concludes that though the poorer sexual outcomes for GBM need research, the negative quality-of-life effect of treatment adds urgency.[55]

10. What social supports do GBM receive? Compared to heterosexuals, GBM experience less familial[6, 7, 49–51] and social support.[7, 49–51] Social support is structured differently for GBM with prostate cancer.[38, 62] Because GBM are less likely than heterosexuals to have a partner, children, or religion-based support systems, they are more likely to go through treatment either alone or by relying on parents, chosen family, or hired help.[62] For GBM, case reports affirm the importance of talking to other GBM about their cancer.[35, 58, 63, 64] However, general support groups for men with prostate cancer may adversely affect GBM if GBM feel alienated from discussing their sexual concerns.[63] While support groups specifically for GBM with prostate cancer may be ideal, in all but the largest cities they may not be viable.[64] Instead, one-on-one peer support from a GBM prostate cancer survivor[63] and online support groups for GBM[58, 64] appear to be the two forms of prostate cancer support most commonly accessed. The effects of such support have not been evaluated.

11. How does prostate cancer change gay relationships? Some relationship researchers term prostate cancer a "couple's disease" because the illness and treatments affect the well-being of both the patients and their partners.[65] Partner involvement in prostate cancer treatment in heterosexual couples improves outcomes;[66] however, GBM may be less likely to involve their male partners in treatment.[49] We found three case reports documenting effects of prostate cancer on gay male couples.[61, 63, 67] Gay couples may engage in novel accommodation practices, including change in roles-in-sex and open relationships, that have not been noted in heterosexual couples.[67, 68] More research is needed to include the effects of prostate cancer treatment on partners, relationships, and gay couples' agreements.[63] Given gender differences, the literature on female partners of men with prostate cancer should be extrapolated to male partners only with extreme caution. Male partners may have unique concerns, such as fear of infectivity, that female partners may not experience. Caring for a partner with prostate cancer may be experienced differently by male spouses.[63] In addition, prostate cancer's effect on single GBM[49] and casual sex partners needs more research.[35, 55]

DISCUSSION

Multiple studies all describe prostate cancer in GBM as a severely under-researched area.[2, 8] As evidenced by 88 unique citations, that situation is changing. The key finding of this review is that a small but robust literature is emerging on the experience of GBM prostate cancer survivors. The same cannot be said of TGW, where the literature is limited to a single case report every two to three years. Multiple challenges have stymied research in this area. Health research on GBM for the last 30 years has focused on HIV/AIDS, which has left chronic diseases in GBM almost unstudied.[2] Now, because ARV treatments have greatly reduced AIDS mortality, large cohorts of GBM are entering age groups in which prostate cancer is commonly diagnosed. Recruitment of GBM in meaningful numbers for study is also a barrier, exacerbated by a lack of sexual history taking as standard practice, as well as clinical systems not collecting systematic data on sexual orientation or gender of sexual partners. This situation leaves GBM with prostate cancer as an invisible, geographically dispersed, hard-to-recruit population.

Language is a separate challenge. As tables 1.2 and 1.3 show, there is no consistent term used for GBM, and whether TGW are included or excluded varies across studies. Similarly, prostate cancer professionals may use the term *survivor* for patients five or more years out, whereas GBM created, and are more familiar with, the nomenclature *persons living with [HIV]*.[69] GBM may not agree with or endorse *survivor* as an identity label. Heterocentric definitions of sexual functioning and scales limited to penetrative sex are problematic. Until recently, erectile functioning in prostate cancer treatment was operationalized as "sufficient for vaginal penetration."[55, 70, 71] Population-appropriate measures and definitions will need to be developed before the effects of prostate cancer treatment in GBM can be enumerated.

Six directions for future research are identified. First, methodological research is needed to identify ways to locate, recruit, and retain GBM with prostate cancer in studies and to develop population-appropriate definitions and measures. Second, as the results detail, more formative research in specific areas is needed. Third, empirical studies to quantify the prevalence and incidence of problems, and the effects of different treatments, will be critical to informing clinical care. Fourth, comparative studies of treatment preferences for GBM and heterosexual men should confirm whether GBM are more likely than, as likely as, or less likely than heterosexuals to choose surgical intervention. Fifth, intervention studies to address the rehabilitation needs of GBM with prostate cancer are critical to develop evidence-based interventions tailored to this population. Finally, the training needs of urologists, surgeons, oncologists, and other specialists providing services to GBM with prostate cancer remain to be identified, and curricula developed, to ensure culturally competent providers capable of addressing the sexual health needs and care of this population.

ACKNOWLEDGMENTS

This chapter was developed as part of the Restore study, a National Cancer Institute–funded grant award titled "Understanding the Effects of Prostate Cancer on Gay and Bisexual Men" (grant no. CA182041; principal investigator B. R. S. Rosser). The authors warmly acknowledge Angelique Lele (executive assistant) in helping to develop this manuscript.

REFERENCES

1. U.S. Office of Disease Prevention and Health Promotion. Healthy people 2020. 2010; www.healthypeople.gov/. Accessed March 8, 2017.

2. Institute of Medicine. The health of lesbian, gay, bisexual and transgender people: Building a foundation for a better understanding. March 31, 2011; www.nationalacademies.org/hmd/Reports/2011/The-Health-of-Lesbian-Gay-Bisexual-and-Transgender-People.aspx. Accessed December 8, 2017.

3. Grant MJ, Booth A. A typology of reviews: An analysis of 14 review types and associated methodologies. *Health Information & Libraries Journal.* 2009; 26 (2): 91–108.

4. National Cancer Institute. Surveillance Epidemiology and End Results Program (SEER). Cancer statistics. 2015; http://seer.cancer.gov/statfacts/html/prost.html. Accessed June 8, 2015.

5. Purcell DW, Johnson C, Lansky A, et al. Estimating the population size of men who have sex with men in the United States to obtain HIV and syphilis rates. *Open AIDS Journal.* March 2010; 6: 98–107.

6. Kurdek LA. Are gay and lesbian cohabiting couples *really* different from heterosexual married couples? *Journal of Marrriage and Family.* 2004; 66: 880–900.

7. Kurdek LA. What do we know about gay and lesbian couples? *Current Directions in Psychological Science.* 2005; 14 (5): 251–254.

8. Rosser BRS, Capistrant BD, Iantaffi A, et al. Prostate cancer in gay, bisexual and other men who have sex with men: A review. *Journal of LGBT Health.* 2016; 3 (1): 32–41.

9. Miksad RA, Bubley G, Church P, et al. Prostate cancer in a transgender woman 41 years after initiation of feminization. *Journal of the American Medical Assocation (JAMA).* 2006; 296 (19): 2312–2317.

10. Heslin KC, Gore JL, King WD, Fox SA. Sexual orientation and testing for prostate and colorectal cancers among men in California. *Medical Care.* 2008; 46 (12): 1240.

11. Santillo VM, Lowe FC. Prostate cancer and the gay male. *Journal of Gay and Lesbian Psychotherapy.* 2005; 9 (1–2): 9–27.

12. Crum N, Hale B, Utz G, Wallace M. Increased risk of prostate cancer in HIV infection? *AIDS.* 2002; 16 (12): 1703–1704.

13. Mandel JS, Schuman LM. Sexual factors and prostatic cancer: Results from a case-control study. *Journal of Gerontology.* 1987; 42 (3): 259–264.

14. Rosenblatt KA, Wicklund KG, Stanford JL. Sexual factors and the risk of prostate cancer. *American Journal of Epidemiology.* 2001; 153 (12): 1152–1158.

15. Spence AR, Rousseau MC, Parent ME. Sexual partners, sexually transmitted infections, and prostate cancer risk. *Cancer Epidemiology.* 2014; 38 (6): 700–707.

16. Crum NF, Spencer CR, Amling CL. Prostate carcinoma among men with human immunodeficiency virus infection. *Cancer.* 2004; 101 (2): 294–299.

17. Burgi A, Brodine S, Wegner S, et al. Incidence and risk factors for the occurrence of non-AIDS-defining cancers among human immunodeficiency virus–infected individuals. *Cancer.* 2005; 104 (7): 1505–1511.

18. Marcus JL, Chao CR, Leyden WA, et al. Prostate cancer incidence and prostate-specific antigen testing among HIV-positive and HIV-negative men. *Journal of Acquired Immune Deficiency Syndromes.* 2014; 66 (5): 495–502.

19. Mani D, Aboulafia DM. Screening guidelines for non-AIDS defining cancers in HIV-infected individuals. *Current Opinion in Oncology.* 2013; 25 (5): 518–525.

20. Shiels MS, Goedert JJ, Moore RD, et al. Reduced risk of prostate cancer in U.S. Men with AIDS. *Cancer Epidemiology Biomarkers & Prevention.* 2010; 19 (11): 2910–2915.

21. Murphy AB, Bhatia R, Martin IK, et al. Are HIV-infected men vulnerable to prostate cancer treatment disparities? *Cancer Epidemiology Biomarkers and Prevention.* 2014; 23 (10): 2009–2018.

22. Cooksley C, Hwang L, Waller D, Ford CA. HIV-related malignancies: Community-based study using linkage of cancer registry and HIV registry data. *International Journal of STDs and AIDS.* 1999; 16: 1703–1704.

23. Santos J, Palacios R, Ruiz J, et al. Unusual malignant tumours in patients with HIV infection. *International Journal of STDs and AIDS.* 2002; 13: 674–676.

24. Crum-Cianflone N, Hullsiek KH, Marconi V, et al. Trends in the incidence of cancers among HIV-infected persons and the impact of antiretroviral therapy: A 20-year cohort study. *AIDS.* 2009; 23 (1): 41.

25. Hart TL, Coon DW, Kowalkowski MA, et al. Changes in sexual roles and quality of life for gay men after prostate cancer: Challenges for sexual health providers. *Journal of Sexual Medicine.* 2014; 11 (9): 2308–2317.

26. Wassersug RJ, Lyons A, Duncan D, et al. Diagnostic and outcome differences between heterosexual and nonheterosexual men treated for prostate cancer. *Urology.* 2013; 82: 565–571.

27. Lee TK, Breau RH, Eapen L. Pilot study on quality of life and sexual function in men-who-have-sex-with-men treated for prostate cancer. *Journal of Sexual Medicine.* 2013; 10 (8): 2094–2100.

28. Wassersug RJ, Westle A, Dowsett GW. Men's sexual and relational adaptations to erectile dysfunction after prostate cancer treatment. *International Journal of Sexual Health.* 2016: 1–11.

29. Rosser BRS, Capistrant BD, Torres B, et al. The effects of radical prostatectomy on gay and bisexual men's sexual functioning and behavior: Qualitative results from the *Restore* study. *Journal of Sex and Relationship Therapy.* 2016; 31 (4): 432–445.

30. Dowsett GW, Lyons A, Duncan D, Wassersug RJ. Flexibility in men's sexual practices in response to iatrogenic erectile dysfunction after prostate cancer treatment. *Sexual Medicine.* 2014; 2 (3): 115–120.

31. Klein L, Lowe F. The effects of prostatic manipulation on prostate-specific antigen levels. *Urology Clinics of North America.* 1995; 24: 293–297.

32. Burns MN, Kamen C, Lehman KA, Beach SR. Minority stress and attributions for discriminatory events predict social anxiety in gay men. *Cognitive Therapy and Research.* 2012; 36 (1): 25–35.

33. Meyer IH. Prejudice and discrimination as social stressors. *In* Meyer IH, Northridge ME, eds. *The health of sexual minorities.* Washington, D.C.: APA; 2007.

34. Perlman G. Prostate cancer, the group, and me. *Journal of Gay & Lesbian Psychotherapy.* 2005; 9 (1): 69–90.

35. Mitteldorf D. Psychotherapy with gay prostate cancer patients. *Journal of Gay and Lesbian Psychotherapy.* 2005; 9 (1–2): 56–67.

36. Goldstone SE. The ups and downs of gay sex after prostate cancer treatment. *Journal of Gay and Lesbian Psychotherapy.* 2005; 9 (1–2): 43–55.

37. Goldstone SE, Tal R. Gay sex after treatment for prostate cancer. *In* Perlman G, ed. *What every gay man needs to know about prostate cancer.* New York: Magnus Books; 2013: 76–90.

38. Dowsett GW. "Losing my chestnut": One gay man's wrangle with prostate cancer. *Reproductive Health Matters.* 2008; 16 (32): 145–150.

39. Blank TO, Bellizzi K, Murphy K, Ryan K. How do men "make sense" of their prostate cancer? Age and treatment factors. *Gerontologist.* 2003; 43 (1): 342–343.

40. Gotay CC, Holup JL, Muraoka MY. Challenges of prostate cancer: A major men's health issue. *International Journal of Men's Health.* 2002; 1: 59–66.

41. Gray RE, Fitch MI, Fergus KD, Mykhalovskiy E. Hegemonic masculinity and the experience of prostate cancer: A narrative approach. *Journal of Aging and Identity.* 2002; 7: 43–62.

42. Thomas C, Wootten A, Robinson P. The experiences of gay and bisexual men diagnosed with prostate cancer: Results from an online focus group. *European Journal of Cancer Care.* 2013; 22: 522–529.

43. Ussher JM, Perz J, Rose D, et al. Threat of sexual disqualification: The consequences of erectile dysfunction and other sexual changes for gay and bisexual men with prostate cancer. *Archives of Sexual Behavior.* 2017; 46 (7): 2043–2057.

44. Fergus KD, Gray RE, Fitch MI. Sexual dysfunction and the preservation of manhood: Experiences of men with prostate cancer. *Journal of Health Psychology.* 2002; 7 (3): 303–316.

45. Chapple A, Zieband S. Prostate cancer: Embodied experience and perceptions of masculinity. *Sociology of Health and Illness.* 2002; 24: 820–841.

46. Blank TO. The challenge of prostate cancer: "Half a man or man and a half?" *Generations.* 2008; 32 (1): 68–72.

47. Eton DT, Lepore SJ. Prostate cancer and health-related quality of life: A review of the literature. *Psycho-Oncology.* 2002; 11: 307–326.

48. Jackson L. Surviving yet another challenge. *Journal of Gay & Lesbian Psychotherapy.* 2005; 9 (1): 101–107.

49. Smith JA, Filiault SM, Drummond MJN, Knappman RJ. The psychosocial impact of prostate cancer on patients and their partners. *Medical Journal of Australia*. 2007; 186 (3): 159–160.

50. Kurdek LA. Gay men and lesbians: The family context. *In* Coleman M, Ganong LH, eds. *Handbook of contemporary families: Considering the past, contemplating the future*. Thousand Oaks, Calif.: Sage; 2004: 96–115.

51. Kurdek LA. Differences between heterosexual-nonparent couples and gay, lesbian and heterosexual-parent cohabitating couples. *Journal of Marriage and Family*. 2001; 60: 553–568.

52. Harris J. Living with prostate cancer: One gay man's experience. *Journal of Gay and Lesbian Psychotherapy*. 2005; 9 (1–2): 109–117.

53. Miller M. Identity and prostate cancer: Comments on a messy life. *Journal of Gay & Lesbian Psychotherapy*. 2005; 9 (1–2): 119–129.

54. Martinez R. Prostate cancer and sex. *Journal of Gay & Lesbian Psychotherapy*. 2005; 9 (1–2): 91–99.

55. Blank TO. Gay men and prostate cancer: Invisible diversity. *Journal of Clinical Oncology*. 2005; 23 (12): 2593–2596.

56. Gebert S. Are penile prostheses a viable option to recommend for gay men? *International Journal of Urological Nursing*. 2014; 8 (3): 111–113.

57. Varghese B, Maher JE, Peterman TA, et al. Reducing the risk of sexual HIV transmission: Quantifying the per-act risk for HIV on the basis of choice of partner, sex act, and condom use. *Sexually Transmitted Diseases*. 2002; 29 (1): 38–43.

58. Mitteldorf DM, Perlman G, Latini D. Gay, bisexual and transgender male cancer survivorship. *In* Schneider JS, Silenzio VMB, Erickson-Schroth L, eds. *Gay and Lesbian Medical Association handbook on LGBT health* (vol. 2). Santa Babara, Calif.: Praeger; 2018.

59. Hart S, Coon D, Kowalkowski M, Latini D. Gay men with prostate cancer report significantly worse HRQOL than heterosexual men. *Journal of Urology*. 2011; 185 (4S): e68–e69.

60. Kleinmann N, Zaorsky NG, Showalter TN, et al. The effect of ethnicity and sexual preference on prostate-cancer-related quality of life. *Nature Reviews Urology*. May 2012; 9 (5): 258–265.

61. Parkin RP, Girven H. Together with prostate cancer. *Journal of Gay and Lesbian Psychotherapy*. 2005; 9 (1–2): 137–146.

62. Capistrant BD, Torres B, Merengwa E, et al. Caregiving and social support for gay and bisexual men with prostate cancer. *Psycho-Oncology*. 2016; 25 (11): 1329–1336.

63. Higgins G. A gay man and his partner face his prostate cancer together. *Journal of Gay and Lesbian Psychotherapy*. 2005; 9 (1–2): 147–153.

64. Mitteldorf D. Ten lessons from gay cancer survivor support groups. *In* Perlman G, ed. *What every gay man needs to know about prostate cancer*. New York: Magus Press; 2013.

65. Wittmann D, Northouse L, Foley S, et al. The psychosocial aspects of sexual recovery after prostate cancer treatment. *International Journal of Impotence Research*. 2009; 21 (2): 99–106.

66. Navon L, Morag A. Advanced prostate cancer patients' ways of coping with the hormonal therapy's effect on body, sexuality, and spousal ties. *Qualitative Health Research*. 2003; 13 (10): 1378–1392.

67. Hartman ME, Irvine J, Currie KL, et al. Exploring gay couples' experience with sexual dysfunction after radical prostatectomy: A qualitative study. *Journal of Sex & Marital Therapy*. 2014; 40 (3): 233–253.

68. Rosser BRS, Capistrant BD, Torres B, et al. The effects of radical prostatectomy on gay and bisexual men's mental health, sexual identity, and relationships: Qualitative results form the *Restore* study. *Journal of Sex & Relationship Therapy*. 2016; 31 (4): 446–461.

69. Morolake O, Stephens D, Welbourn A. Greater involvement of people living with HIV in health care. *Journal of the International AIDS Society*. 2009; 12 (1): 4.

70. Hong EK, Lepor H, McCullough AR. Time dependent patient satisfaction with sildenafil for erectile dysfunction (ED) after nerve-sparing radical retropubic prostatectomy (RRP). *International Journal of Impotence Research*. 1999; 11 (S1): S15–S19.

71. Latini DM, Penson DF, Colwell HH, et al. Psychological impact of erectile dysfunction: Validation of a new health related quality of life measure for patients with erectile dysfunction. *Journal of Urology*. 2002; 168 (5): 2086–2091.

72. Filiault SM, Drummond MJN. Gay men and prostate cancer: Voicing the concerns of a hidden population. *Journal of Men's Health*. 2008; 5 (4): 327–332.

73. "Charles Godfry." Coping with advanced prostate cancer as a gay man. *In* Perlman G, ed. *What every gay man needs to know about prostate cancer*. New York: Magnus Books; 2013: 271–282.

74. "James Larson." Dealing with prostate cancer in my fortieth year. *In* Perlman G, ed. *What every gay man needs to know about prostate cancer*. New York: Magnus Books; 2013: 215–224.

75. "Mark Red." Active surveillance/anxious surveillance: A gay man chooses watchful waiting. *In* Perlman G, ed. *What every gay man needs to know about prostate cancer*. New York: Magnus Books; 2013: 143–153.

76. "Paul Jarod." Suggestions for those considering invasive procedures. *In* Perlman G, ed. *What every gay man needs to know about prostate cancer*. New York: Magnus Books; 2013: 185–194.

77. MacKellar DA, Valleroy LA, Secura GM, et al. Unrecognized HIV infection, risk behaviors, and perceptions of risk among young men who have sex with men:

Opportunities for advancing HIV prevention in the third decade of HIV/AIDS. *Journal of Acquired Immune Deficiency Syndromes.* 2005; 38 (5): 603–614.

78. Dalzell J. A method for identifying the best doctor and treatment for prostate cancer. *In* Perlman G, ed. *What every gay man needs to know about prostate cancer.* New York: Magnus Books; 2013: 154–165.

79. Davenport J. Treating erectile dysfunction after prostate cancer surgery: A gay man's experience of getting a penile implant. *In* Perlman G, ed. *What every gay man needs to know about prostate cancer* New York: Magnus Books; 2013: 250–262.

80. Jackson L. A sex-positive gay man compares the challenges of being HIV-positive, and having prostate cancer. *In* Perlman G, ed. *What every gay man needs to know about prostate cancer.* New York: Magnus Books; 2013: 225–236.

81. John F. A good outcome to my experience with penile implant surgery. *In* Perlman G, ed. *What every gay man needs to know about prostate cancer.* New York: Magnus Books; 2013: 263–270.

82. Martinez R. Prostate cancer treatment changes my attitudes and behaviors concerning sex. *In* Perlman G, ed. *What every gay man needs to know about prostate cancer.* New York: Magnus Books; 2013: 237–249.

83. Sonday M. Personal issues to consider before and after radical prostatectomy. *In* Perlman G, ed. *What every gay man needs to know about prostate cancer.* New York: Magnus Books; 2013: 166–184.

84. Tunnell G. Robotic radical prostatectomy. *In* Perlman G, ed. *What every gay man needs to know about prostate cancer.* New York: Magnus Books; 2013: 195–214.

85. Santillo VM. Prostate cancer diagnosis and treatment of a 33-year-old gay man. *Journal of Gay and Lesbian Psychotherapy.* 2005; 9 (1–2): 155–171.

86. Schaffner B. Prostate cancer at age 84. *Journal of Gay & Lesbian Psychotherapy.* 2005; 9 (1): 131–136.

87. Dorff TB, Shazer RL, Nepomuceno EM, Tucker SJ. Successful treatment of metastatic androgen-independent prostate carcinoma in a transsexual patient. *Clinical Genitourinary Cancer.* 2007; 5 (5): 344–346.

88. Thurston A. Carcinoma of the prostate in a transsexual. *BJU International.* 1994; 73 (2): 217.

89. Turo R, Jallad S, Cross WR, Prescott S. Metastatic prostate cancer in transsexual diagnosed after three decades of estrogen therapy. *Canadian Urological Association Journal.* 2013; 7 (7–8): 544–546.

90. Van Haarst EP, Newling DWW, Gooren HA, Prenger DM. Metastatic prostatic carcinoma in a male-to-female transsexual. *British Journal of Urology.* 1998; 81 (5): 776.

91. Asencio M, Blank T, Descartes L, Crawford A. The prospect of prostate cancer: A challenge for gay men's sexualities as they age. *Sexuality Research and Social Policy.* 2009; 6 (4): 38–51.

92. Doran D, Beaver K, Williamson S, Wright K. "It's not just about prostate cancer, it's about being a gay man": A phenomenological study of the lived experiences of gay men with prostate cancer. *European Journal of Cancer*. 2015; 51 (Suppl. 3): S248–S249.

93. Lee TK, Handy AB, Kwan W, et al. Impact of prostate cancer treatment on the sexual quality of life for men-who-have-sex-with-men. *Journal of Sexual Medicine*. 2015; 12 (12): 2378–2386.

94. Rose D, Ussher JM, Perz J. Let's talk about gay sex: Gay and bisexual men's sexual communication with healthcare professionals after prostate cancer. *European Journal of Cancer Care*. 2017; 26 (1).

95. Ussher J, Perz J, Rose D, Chambers S, Williams S. Gay and bisexual men's experiences of sexuality, identity and relationships after prostate cancer: A qualitative analysis. *Asia-Pacific Journal of Clinical Oncology*. 2015; 11: 41–42.

96. Ussher JM, Rose D, Perz J. Mastery, isolation, or acceptance: Gay and bisexual men's construction of aging in the context of sexual embodiment after prostate cancer. *Journal of Sex Research*. 2017; 56: 802–812.

97. Boehmer U, Miao X, Ozonoff A. Cancer survivorship and sexual orientation. *Cancer*. 2011; 117 (16): 3796–3804.

98. Boeri L, Capogrosso P, Ventimiglia E, et al. Lower urinary tract symptoms among Caucasian-European men who have sex with men: Findings from a real-life survey. *Prostate Cancer and Prostatic Diseases*. 2015; 18 (4): 376–381.

99. Allensworth-Davies D, Talcott JA, Heeren T, et al. The health effects of masculine self-esteem following treatment for localized prostate cancer among gay men. *LGBT Health*. 2016; 3 (1): 49–56.

100. Crangle CJ, Latini DM, Hart TL. The effects of attachment and outness on illness adjustment among gay men with prostate cancer. *Psycho-Oncology*. 2015; 26 (4): 500–507.

101. Mitteldorf D. Treatment disparities between heterosexual and gay and bisexual men diagnosed with prostate cancer. *Journal of Clinical Oncology*. 2016; 34 (15): e16548.

102. Rosser BRS, Capistrant BD. Online versus telephone methods to recruit and interview older gay and bisexual men treated for prostate cancer: Findings from the Restore study. *Journal of Medical Internet Research — Cancer*. 2016; 2 (2): e9.

103. Torbit LA, Albiani JJ, Crangle CJ, et al. Fear of recurrence: The importance of self-efficacy and satisfaction with care in gay men with prostate cancer. *Psycho-Oncology*. 2015; 24 (6): 691–698.

104. Ussher J, Perz J, Chambers S, et al. Sexual wellbeing and quality of life after prostate cancer: A comparison of gay/bisexual men and heterosexual men. *Asia-Pacific Journal of Clinical Oncology*. 2015; 11 (52): 28.

105. Ussher JM, Perz J, Kellett A, et al. Health-related quality of life, psychological distress, and sexual changes following prostate cancer: A comparison of gay

and bisexual men with heterosexual men. *Journal of Sexual Medicine.* 2016; 13 (3): 425–434.

106.   Motofei IG, Rowland DL, Popa F, et al. Preliminary study with bicalutamide in heterosexual and homosexual patients with prostate cancer. *British Journal of Urology.* 2010; 108: 110–115.

107.   Amiel GE, Goltz HH, Wenker EP, et al. Gay men and prostate cancer: Opportunities to improve HRQOL and access to care. *In* Boehmer U, Elk R, eds. *Cancer and the LGBT community: Unique perspectives from risk to survivorship.* New York: Springer; 2015: 159–168.

108.   Doran D, Beaver K, Williamson S, Wright K. An exploration of the psychosocial impact of prostate cancer on gay men: A review of the literature. *Psycho-Oncology.* 2013; 22 (S1): 1–29.

109.   Blank T, Descartes L, Ascensio M. Cancer screening in gay and bisexual men and transgender people. *In* Boehmer U, Elk R, eds. *Cancer and the LGBT community: Unique perspectives from risk to survivorship.* New York: Springer; 2015: 99–110.

110.   Bowen DJ, Boehmer U. The lack of cancer surveillance data on sexual minorities and strategies for change. *Cancer Causes & Control.* 2007; 18 (4): 343–349.

111.   Doran D, Beaver K, Williamson S, Wright K. An exploration of the psychosocial impact of prostate cancer on gay men: A review of current literature. *Psycho-Oncology.* 2013; 22: 1–29.

112.   Matheson L, Rivas C, Nayoan J, et al. Marginalised men with prostate cancer: A qualitative metasynthesis exploring the impact on younger, gay and unpartnered men with prostate cancer. *Psycho-Oncology.* 2016; 25: 4.

113.   Descartes L, Asencio M, Blank TO, Crawford A. Gay men's knowledge of prostate cancer. *In* Perlman G, ed. *What every gay man needs to know about prostate cancer.* New York: Magnus Books; 2013: 17–38.

114.   Lemer M. Incontinence and prostatic health. *In* Perlman G, ed. *What every gay man needs to know about prostate cancer.* New York: Magnus Books; 2013: 91–104.

115.   Lowe FC. A straight urologist discusses working with gay men diagnosed with prostate cancer. *In* Perlman G, ed. *What every gay man needs to know about prostate cancer.* New York: Magnus Books; 2013: 136–139.

116.   Mitteldorf D. Coming out to doctors. *In* Perlman G, ed. *What every gay man needs to know about prostate cancer.* New York: Magnus Books; 2013: 115–127.

117.   Mitteldorf D. What I have learned from working with gay men who have prostate cancer. *In* Perlman G, ed. *What every gay man needs to know about prostate cancer.* New York: Magnus Books; 2013: 128–134.

118.   Santillo VM, Lowe FC. Quality-of-life and cancer control after prostate cancer treatment. *In* Perlman G, ed. *What every gay man needs to know about prostate cancer.* New York: Magnus Books; 2013: 39–46.

119. Tal R. Prostate cancer and sexual dysfunction in gay men. *In* Perlman G, ed. *What every gay man needs to know about prostate cancer.* New York: Magnus Books; 2013: 47–75.

120. Wosnitzer MS, Lowe FC. Prostate cancer in HIV-positive patients in the era of highly-active antiretroviral therapy (HAART). *In* Perlman G, ed. *What every gay man needs to know about prostate cancer.* New York: Magnus Books; 2013: 106–114.

121. Cheron-Sauer M-C, Wong T. The establishment of PCFA affiliated gay/bi-sexual prostate cancer support groups in Australia. *Asia-Pacific Journal of Clinical Oncology.* 2014; 10: 78–79.

122. Spillare A, Metcalfe R, Thomas C, et al. "There is no information for us": The development of the first Victorian gay men's prostate cancer support group. *Asia-Pacific Journal of Clinical Oncology.* 2012; 8: 251–252.

123. Cornell D. A gay urologist's changing views of prostate cancer. *Journal of Gay and Lesbian Psychotherapy.* 2005; 9 (1–2): 29–41.

124. Hoyt MA. Book review: *What every gay man needs to know about prostate cancer: The essential guide to diagnosis, treatment, and recovery.* Edited by Gerald Perlman. Magnus Books, New York, NY, 2013. *Psycho-Oncology.* 2016; 25 (1): 119–120.

125. Latini D. Editorial comment on "The impact of prostate cancer treatment on the sexual quality of life for men-who-have-sex-with-men." *Journal of Sexual Medicine.* 2015; 12 (12): 2387.

126. Stagg K. Re: Prostate cancer in gay, bisexual, and other men who have sex with men: A review, by Simon Rosser et al. (*LGBT Health* 2016; 3 (1): 32–41) [letter to the editor]. *LGBT Health.* 2016; 3 (3): 243.

127. Perlman G. Introduction: Why a book about prostate cancer for gay men? *In* Perlman G, ed. *What every gay man needs to know about prostate cancer.* New York: Magnus Books; 2013.

128. Perlman G, Drescher J. *A gay man's guide to prostate cancer.* Binghamton N.Y.: Hawthorne Press; 2005.

129. Perlman G, ed. *What every gay man needs to know about prostate cancer.* New York: Magnus Books; 2013.

130. Rosser BRS, Kohli N, Lesher L, et al. The sexual functioning of gay and bisexual men following prostate cancer treatment: Findings from the *Restore* study. *Archives of Sexual Behavior,* under review.

131. Rosser BRS, Konety BR, Kohli N, et al. What gay and bisexual prostate cancer patients want in a sexual rehabilitation program for prostate cancer: Results of the *Restore* needs assessment. *Urology Practice.* 2017; http://dx.doi.org/10.1016/j.urpr.2017.05.001.

132. Konstan JA, Rosser BRS, Ross MW, et al. The story of Subject Naught: A cautionary but optimistic tale of Internet survey research. *Journal of Computer-Mediated Communication.* 2005; 10 (2). http://jcmc.indiana/edu/vol10/issue2/konstan.html.

133.   Grey JA, Konstan J, Iantaffi A, et al. An updated protocol to detect invalid entries in an online survey of men who have sex with men (MSM): How do valid and invalid submissions compare? *AIDS & Behavior.* 2015; 19 (10): 1928–1937.

CHAPTER 2

Threat to Gay Identity and Sexual Relationships

The Consequences of Prostate Cancer Treatment for Gay and Bisexual Men

Jane M. Ussher, Janette Perz, Duncan Rose, Gary W. Dowsett, and David M. Latini

CHAPTER SUMMARY

This chapter considers the effect of prostate cancer treatment on gay identity and sexual relationships. A total of 124 gay and bisexual men (GBM) with prostate cancer and 21 male partners completed an online survey, and a subsample of 46 men with prostate cancer and 7 partners also took part in a one-on-one interview. Erectile dysfunction, reported by 72% of survey respondents, was associated with reports of emotional distress, negative effect on gay identities, and feelings of sexual disqualification. Other sexual concerns included climacturia, pain or loss of sensitivity during receptive anal sex, non-ejaculatory orgasms, and reduced penis size. Many of these changes have particular significance in the context of gay sex and gay identities, and they can result in feelings of exclusion from a sexual community central to GBM's lives. Researchers and clinicians need to be aware of the meaning and consequences of sexual changes for GBM when designing studies to examine the influence of prostate cancer on men's sexuality, advising GBM of the sexual consequences of prostate cancer, and providing information and support to ameliorate sexual changes.

KEY TERMS

ejaculate loss, erectile dysfunction, gay and bisexual men, identity, penis size, prostate cancer, sexual functioning

Ussher, Jane M., Perz, Janette, Rosser, B. R. Simon, eds., *Gay & Bisexual Men Living with Prostate Cancer*
dx.doi.org/10.17312/harringtonparkpress/2018.06.gbmlpc.002
© 2018 Harrington Park Press

INTRODUCTION

Sexual well-being after prostate cancer treatment is an important issue: the various prostate cancer treatment options often result in erectile dysfunction, penile deformities and shrinkage, ejaculatory and orgasmic dysfunctions, reduced libido, and changes in patient and partner sexual satisfaction.[1] Erectile dysfunction is consistently reported as one of the most central concerns for prostate cancer survivors,[2,3] affecting intimate relationships[4] and psychological well-being.[5] Until recently, however, research examining the influence of prostate cancer on men's sexuality has focused on the ability to achieve and maintain an erection for penile-vaginal penetration,[6] assuming that men are in long-term heterosexual relationships and implicitly excluding the experiences of single and gay men.[7]

The primary focus of research and clinical interventions has been on the physical effects of cancer or cancer treatments on sexual functioning, which assumes that a man's experience of sexuality is limited to its embodied dimensions. This limitation serves to negate the influence of the social construction of sexuality and gender, as well as the ways in which men interpret and experience physical changes in the light of such social constructions.[8] Constructions of sexuality and masculinity are highly interwoven, meaning that loss of sexual functioning may pose a significant threat to manhood and masculinity.[9-12] But until recently there has been a dearth of research on the meaning of such sexual changes and the potential effect of prostate cancer on the identity or masculinity of gay and bisexual men (GBM). In one qualitative study examining knowledge about prostate cancer in healthy gay men,[7] participants speculated that gay men would be more able than heterosexual men to come to terms with challenges to their masculinity because gay men belong to a sexual minority. Conversely, the quantitative arm of the study found lower rates of masculine self-esteem in GBM with prostate cancer in comparison with heterosexual men with prostate cancer.[13] It has been also posited that gay men may ascribe different priorities and meanings to sexual changes after prostate cancer,[14] including the importance of the prostate as a site of pleasure during anal sex, the significance of visible ejaculate for "semen exchange" during sex, the need for a firmer erection for anal sex in comparison with vaginal sex, and the consequences of anal discomfort and incontinence for receptive partners.[15,16] These concerns, however, have been described as "speculative," and "future research [is] needed to ascertain the impact of prostate cancer on the lives of gay men."[15]

The aim of this chapter is to address these gaps and inconsistencies in the research literature by examining the meaning and consequences of sexual changes following prostate cancer for GBM, drawing on the findings of a study that used a combination of an online survey and one-on-one interviews.

THE STUDY

One-hundred and twenty-four GBM who currently have, or had, prostate cancer, and 21 male partners of men with prostate cancer participated in the survey, and 53 took part in semistructured interviews (46 GBM with prostate cancer and 7 partners). The methods are detailed elsewhere.[3, 13, 17, 18] The average age of men with prostate cancer was 64.25 years, and of their partners 55.57 years. Prostate cancer had been diagnosed five years previously on average; it resulted in a range of treatments, the majority of participants currently being monitored post-treatment. Participants were recruited primarily within Australia (71%), and a minority was recruited from the United States (21%) and the United Kingdom (8%). The survey items used in this analysis consisted of a series of closed and open-ended questions examining the nature of sexual changes experienced by GBM with prostate cancer.[13] The items reported in this chapter include erectile functioning ability and concerns; sexual desire levels and concerns; ejaculatory ability and concerns; and difficulty in urinating. The open-ended survey questions asked for additional comments on how sexuality has changed since the onset of prostate cancer; whether there have been any significant changes to relationships; and whether there were any other issues about prostate cancer and sexuality that the participant would like to comment on. One-on-one semistructured telephone interviews, lasting approximately one hour, were conducted to examine the subjective experience, meaning, and consequences of sexual changes following prostate cancer treatment. Frequency data and percentages were collected for responses to the closed survey items. The analysis of open-ended survey responses and interviews was conducted using theoretical thematic analysis.[19]

EFFECT OF PROSTATE CANCER TREATMENT ON GAY IDENTITY: "THE IMPACT ON MY LIFE AS A GAY MALE HAS BEEN REALLY PROFOUND, IN A NEGATIVE SENSE"

ERECTILE DYSFUNCTION: "IT'S A BIG THING FOR A MAN, NOT BEING ABLE TO HAVE ERECTIONS"

Loss of erectile functioning during the preceding four weeks was reported by 72% of survey respondents; 40% of this group reported that they could not achieve an erection, and 32% reported only a partial erection. Most men (81%) who reported loss or change in erectile functioning over the preceding four weeks rated it as a problem that had a "great emotional impact" and was experienced as "depressing," "very difficult," "an enormous loss," or a cause of "great sadness." For example, David (64, gay) said, "I feel devastated; the erection functioning is a really emotional thing for me," and Jonny (54, bisexual) said, "It's quite a big thing for a man, especially for a younger man, at 49, not being able to have erections."

The magnitude of loss of erectile functioning and ability to engage in penetrative sex across the sample was comparable to that reported in previous population studies of men with prostate cancer.[20, 21] The rate of distress associated with erectile dysfunction, however, was substantially higher than that reported in heterosexual men of a comparable age,[22] which confirms previous reports of significantly higher rates of psychological distress in GBM with prostate cancer who experience the associated sexual changes.[13, 23] This outcome could be explained by the finding that men who engage in more frequent sexual activity report significantly lower tolerance for living with erectile dysfunction,[24] as more frequent sexual activity is found in population studies of gay men.[25]

Many of the participants in this study emphasized the importance of sexual activity to their identities as a gay man, and that threat to identity was exacerbated by erectile dysfunction. Some of our participants described themselves as "not feeling whole" or feeling "cheated" of some core aspect of their masculinity as a result of erectile changes. For example, Graham (74, gay) said, "I am not the man I was, never will be," and Alex (62, gay) told us, "I don't see myself as a full man." The magnitude of this sense of loss is illustrated by Scott (59, gay), who said, "If I had the choice again, I would take my risks with the cancer, and not have the operation"; he described the loss of erections after robotic prostatectomy as "a defining moment in my life . . . the impact on my life as a gay male has been really profound, and in a negative sense."

While erectile dysfunction is widely recognized as having a potential effect on *masculine* identities, it is the influence on *gay* identities that is identified in Scott's account of changes to his life as a "gay male." As a result of what Mark (45, gay) described as a "crisis" in identity, some men said that they did not "feel so good about being gay anymore" (Benjamin, 63, gay), that they felt "outside the sexual community" (Jason, 49, gay), or that they felt as if they had been "forcibly retired from the gay human race" (Scott, 59, gay). The significance of an erect penis for gay identity cannot be underestimated,[7] as one man noted: "Previously I'd been a top and I was a good-looking male. I had a big cock and I could get whatever I wanted. All of a sudden it was all taken away. I'm no longer a man. You know, I've got a cock that doesn't work anymore" (Finn, 69, gay).

Absence of erection is problematic whether GBM prefer the insertive or receptive mode in anal intercourse.[16] This is not only because an erection may enhance sexual satisfaction,[26] but also because erections signal to other GBM arousal, attraction, interest, and pleasure.[27, 28] As Mark (45, gay) explained, "Partners would comment, 'Aren't you turned on, aren't you into this, don't you want to do this?'" Graham (74, gay) said, "It's a very, very flattering thing when somebody gets an erection in your company." There is also reciprocity in many sex acts between men, such as mutual oral sex or swapping insertive and receptive modes in anal intercourse.[28] Loss of erectile function is therefore a significant loss to participation in that reciprocity.

REDUCTION IN PENIS SIZE: "IT'S A BLOW TO THE EGO"

In the interviews and open-ended surveys, many participants reported significant reductions in penis size following cancer treatment. Some men estimated the reduction numerically: for example, going from "a normal 6½-, 7-inch penis . . . to 2–3 inches . . . literally, a couple of fingers and the thumb" (Gareth, 65, gay), and losing "about half the length and half the diameter" (Mark, 45, gay). Others described the loss of size qualitatively: "like in fantastically cold weather and it's like that all the time" (Stanley, 78, gay), or "slowly but surely disappearing. . . . It's not long before I'll have a string on the end of it to find it to go to the toilet" (Pete, 73, gay). These reductions in size were described as "bloody terrible," "a blow to the ego," "the most dramatic thing" to follow treatment, and a cause of suicidal ideation: "I would like to know the statistics of the suicides for guys, because, generally, the adjustment is absolutely mind blowing . . . because your dick shrinks and your diameter diminishes" (Drew, 64, gay).

Visibility and comparison of penis size with other gay men, linked to negative consequences of penis size reduction, were evident in many accounts. For example, Scott (59, gay) said, "For a gay male, you know, we notice things like that [loss of penis size], and other people do, too." Drew (64, gay) described comparing himself to his friends: "[I felt] bloody terrible, because I've always had a fairly decent dick . . . and a couple of our friends have got small dicks, so I thought, I've always thought, 'You poor bastards,' and now I'm in the same boat as them."

The effect of loss of penis size on successfully engaging in sexual encounters and new relationships was evident in men's accounts. Euan (66, gay) described the "shame" of walking around naked in the sauna. "You've got this bloody now little dick, it's awful." Mark (45, gay) described "losing the positive commentary," as his penis had previously been "a fair bit bigger than average," which "was always a bit of a talking point when I had sex." Scott (59, gay) said, "People used to be attracted to me" because of penis length, and that it was a "calling card" that was now "gone." Cameron (65, bisexual) described being embarrassed about the fact that his penis was "often drawn right back into" his body, speculating, "If I go into a relationship with someone, I will have to say, 'Well, look, honestly, it used to be bigger than this' [laughter]." These accounts demonstrate the negative meanings ascribed to real changes to the penis in terms of self, gay identity, and sexual relationships.

Reduction in penis size has been reported as a concern for many heterosexual men[29, 30] and GBM[12] treated for prostate cancer. There are specific issues with regard to penis size for GBM.[31] In gay male culture, the size of a man's penis can be part of what signifies sexual attractiveness and sexual viability, as penises are "seen, compared, [and] contrasted,"[32] and a below-average-sized penis is associated with lower psychosocial adjustment.[33] In contrast, a large penis is representative of heightened masculinity,[32] and so emasculation in the social domain following prostate cancer treatment is the potential result, as the accounts of the participants in the present study attest.

These concerns about reduced sexual desirability associated with penis size are not unfounded. Previous research has reported that many gay men have a preference for partners with large penises;[34]

smaller penis sizes sometimes are linked to sexual dissatisfaction owing to being "boring" or not being able to be "felt": "In a gay world, the bigger the dick, usually the more people want to have sex with you."[32] Penis size can also be associated with men's preferred sexual mode in anal sex, as men who have smaller penises are more likely to take the receptive mode.[33, 35] This suggests that change in penis size after prostate cancer surgery may also affect some GBM's preferred sexual modes, encouraging them to try a receptive mode in anal sex.[36]

The quantitative arm of our study found that in comparison with heterosexual men, GBM reported significantly lower masculine self-esteem and higher psychological distress, as well as higher sexual functioning and sexual confidence.[13] While previous research has recognized the influence of prostate cancer treatment on heterosexual men's idea of masculinity,[10] feelings of a relative inadequacy may be different for gay men. Gay masculinity is already marginalized or "subordinated"[37] in relation to hegemonic masculinity; gay men are often not considered to be "real men,"[38] and gay masculinity stands as "the repository of whatever is symbolically expelled from hegemonic masculinity."[39] This means that for gay men living with erectile dysfunction and other difficulties in sex following prostate cancer treatment, their already marginalized masculinity may take another blow, through the loss of ability to affirm the self through contact within a sexual community, one where they were among equals or peers as GBM, which results in a challenge to both gay masculinity and gay identity. Thus, our findings question the prediction that gay men may be more able to come to terms with challenges to their particular sense of masculinity following prostate cancer treatment,[7] suggesting that the relationship between sexual functioning and gay masculinities is complex and multifaceted.

EFFECT OF PROSTATE CANCER TREATMENT ON GBM SEXUAL RELATIONSHIPS: "DISQUALIFICATION IN THE SEXUAL EXPERIENCE"

Erectile dysfunction was described by many participants as resulting in feeling "sexually inferior," or being "a eunuch," which led to a sense of "disqualification in the sexual experience."[3] These descriptions demonstrate that erectile dysfunction can significantly influence GBM's sexual and social interactions, and the consequences of dysfunction can play out in a relational context, as discussed in chapters 3, 4, and 6 in this book.

Many men gave accounts of avoiding sexual encounters with new or casual partners because of these concerns. As Grant (72, gay) said, "I don't even like to think of trying to interest a new prospective partner in sex with me because of my limited ability to perform." Mason (68, gay) said that he was "desperate" to be in a relationship but would not feel "worthy" because he was "worried that will affect my ability to find a partner." For men who performed an insertive mode in anal intercourse, the inability to achieve or maintain an erection had the potential to influence their sexual engagement with others. For some, the consequence was cessation of sex. For example, Scott (59, gay) described himself as having been "fortunate to have a bit of a following" whereby regular partners knew what they could expect "in terms of satisfaction," but that since his prostatectomy, "I've become a basically inactive gay male without the sex part." The result was social and sexual isolation.

In ongoing relationships, participants found ways of communicating desire and pleasure through touch or talk. These methods, however, were described as more difficult in the context of casual sex: "If you're not putting out all signs that you might be interested, then people get the wrong message" (Euan, 67, gay); "If you can't get an erection, guys tend to turn away" (Cameron, 65, bisexual). The consequence of erectile dysfunction for many participants was a sense of sexual inadequacy in comparison with other gay men, particularly in the context of casual encounters. As Andy (61, gay) commented, "As a gay man and interacting with other gay men, yeah . . . I'd feel a little bit worthless." David (64, gay) said that he tended "to withdraw somewhat when there is lighthearted banter between guys about their [sexual] experiences . . . because I can't experience that anymore," and he also felt "inadequate" as a result.

These accounts demonstrate that the threat of sexual disqualification that results from erectile dysfunction is particularly acute during casual encounters, when "flexible"[40] or "renegotiated"[41] sexual practice intentions or desires are not always discussed expressly or are difficult to discern,[27] and rejection by prospective partners, accompanied by embarrassment or shame on the part of the man with prostate cancer, is anticipated. As GBM are more likely than heterosexual men to engage in casual sexual encounters[13, 42] or to have concurrent partners,[43] this concern is likely to be more common among GBM than heterosexual men.

Many GBM are versatile in terms of sexual modes during anal

intercourse.[28] For this reason, pursuing flexibility in sexual modes following prostate cancer–induced erectile dysfunction may offer further sexual options for some GBM[16] and accommodate some experiences of inadequacy and distress. Secondary self-labeling in relation to preferences in sexual modes during anal intercourse, however, is an important aspect of identity for some GBM,[44] and changing sexual mode is not always desirable.[7, 45] A number of men in this study were reluctant to become the receptive partner because of what it meant to them in terms of sexual mode, not wanting to take on what can be regarded by some men as a submissive position, or not finding it a pleasurable experience: "It doesn't appeal to me at all" (Damon, 52, gay); "It was like an unevenness in the sexual relationship. The sex became more about the other person and their enjoyment of it and it was something I was almost doing just for them" (Mark, 45, gay).

In addition, because the prostate is an erogenous zone for many gay men,[15] loss of pleasure or discomfort during anal sex following prostate cancer may deter men from engaging in receptive anal intercourse, regardless of their preferred sexual mode before prostate cancer treatment. "It's a very sensitive part of a man's body, and it is a great part of the enjoyment of anal sex . . . and so without [the prostate], a great deal of the enjoyment disappears" (Jack, 59, gay); "In terms of penetrative sex, when I'm the receiver, the pleasure that I had for that has basically gone" (Rick, 59, gay). These quotes suggest that some men may cease being receptive after treatment because of a lack of pleasure. Conversely, for a minority of men, anal sensitivity was described as having increased following prostate cancer treatment; for example, Bruce (61, gay) suggested that the "intense sexual gratification" provided by the prostate had masked other areas of sensitivity that he had "not necessarily realized or engaged," meaning "the simple act of being on the receptive end of sex is somehow more satisfying than it used to be." Thus, while men may have the "physiological capacity to both penetrate and be penetrated (through anal intercourse),"[35,] the corporeality of the body, as well as the meanings attributed to anal sexual modes, will determine whether some GBM continue to engage in anal intercourse, whether they change anal sexual modes, and whether they focus on other sexual practices after prostate cancer treatment. Consequently, the effect of erectile dysfunction on casual sexual relationships may differ significantly among GBM, depending on their ability, willingness, and physical comfort in adopting a receptive mode during anal sex.

ABSENCE OF EJACULATE: "IT'S MORE DIFFICULT TO TALK ABOUT THAN ERECTION ISSUES"

Seventy-one percent of survey participants reported complete loss of ejaculation at orgasm following prostate cancer treatment, and an additional 13% of men reported that they ejaculated "rarely" or "sometimes." Fifty-two percent of survey participants reported being "somewhat" (21%) or "very" (31%) concerned about their ability to ejaculate. Many men gave accounts of loss of sensation and pleasure as a result of ejaculatory loss. "Climax doesn't feel complete without the feeling of ejaculation," and "I don't ejaculate any more. I never will. I miss it a great deal," related two survey participants. For some men, the magnitude of this loss was unforeseen. "Lack of semen has affected me much more than I expected. . . . It's more difficult to talk about than erection issues" (Greg, 53, gay).

The absence of semen in sexual encounters and the potential effect on partners was a major concern: GBM reported significantly higher ejaculatory concern than heterosexual men in the quantitative arm of our research.[13] Ejaculation of semen stands as visible evidence of sexual completion, satisfaction, and excitement for GBM.[46] As Clive (70, gay) commented, "Ejaculation is an essential part of sexual enjoyment to both partners." Absence of ejaculate was also associated with partner disappointment, as following accounts attest: "Happy not to clean up. Not happy with partner's disappointment" (Michael, 69, gay); "I miss the sensation of ejaculating and I think it disappoints my male partner" (Boris, 68, bisexual). Other men were concerned about disappointing future partners if they could not provide the "gift" of semen: "Semen is important to some prospective partners; this has restricted the number of potential partners" (Greg, 53, gay); "I miss the sensation of pumping ejaculate. I am also concerned that some guys really enjoy swallowing a load or being ejaculated on and will be disappointed when I cannot provide that" (Arnold, 57, gay). These concerns were borne out in the accounts of a number of partners we interviewed, who described missing the visible evidence of pleasure signified by ejaculation. As Anton (54, gay, partner) said: "When you ejaculate, you watch someone's face and you hear the noises they make, you know that they are effectively engaged in that process and enjoying it to a degree, whereas when that's not present it makes it a little bit more unknown."

The consequence was that many men worried that they would lose face or could be judged a failure as a result of lack of ejaculate: "My fear is that they think less of me. Ah, in the fact that I can no longer ejaculate" (Lucian, 51, gay); "I worry in my mind that I'm judged that I haven't been enjoying the other person" (Mason, 68, gay). The result was avoidance of casual sex, during which the absence of semen, often combined with erectile difficulties, would have to be explained. As Andy (61, gay) said, "It would be too hard to kind of disclose or to pick up somebody and say, 'Well, nothing is going to happen on my part, you know . . . I can't cum.'"

It has previously been reported that most heterosexual men with prostate cancer "are not bothered by absence of ejaculate" but that it may interfere with sexual satisfaction.[47] In addition to loss of sexual pleasure during non-ejaculatory orgasms, GBM with prostate cancer also grieve the absence of the ejaculate itself.[48] Semen is of erotic significance during gay male sex,[49] and exchange of semen is a central objective of sex for some GBM.[50] Exchange or "gifting"[50] of semen signifies intimacy, mutual satisfaction, and connection with partners;[51] partner disappointment often results from absence of ejaculate, which provides an explanation for previous accounts that gay men report higher rates of ejaculatory bother after prostate cancer than heterosexual men do.[3, 52]

URINARY INCONTINENCE AND CLIMACTURIA: "YOU LOSE YOUR BODY MANAGEMENT"

Of the survey participants, 65% of survey participants reported changes in urinary patterns, primarily urinating more often following prostate cancer; 40% reported that problems with urinating limited their activities, and 25% said that they had difficulties urinating. In the open-ended survey items and interviews, men focused on the implications of urinary incontinence in the sexual and social arena. Many men reported climacturia (urinating during climax). As Pete (73, gay) commented, "It comes out, about the normal time of having an orgasm, but it just comes out in high pressure wee, instead of the normal white stuff [semen]." Others reported urinary leakage during arousal or anal sex. Clive (70, gay) said, "When you get a bit excited, you tend to leak a bit. You seem to lose your body management a bit."

Many participants reported avoidance of casual sex because explaining urination in sex was "too difficult," "unsexy," "humiliating," or "embarrassing." Negative reactions from prospective casual partners who were being informed of potential leakage of urine were common. Gordon

(56, bisexual) explained that in meeting men online, he would say, "When I climax, there's usually some spurting of urine," which he said was a turnoff, and sex would not result. Avoidance of sex with a regular or long-term partner was also reported, because of the practical difficulties of negotiating the consequences of urinary leakage during sex: "I just had to put up with being incontinent for three years and wear pads and all that kind of thing, so in terms of sexual activity, you can imagine it's extremely limited. . . . I'd finish up very wet and I'd have to have towels all over the bed, and, you know, hardly worth doing, basically" (Morris, 74, gay).

Cultural ideals of masculinity and youth are associated with bodily control,[53] and urinary incontinence can disrupt a sense of control during sexual activity for men with prostate cancer. Previous research has reported that urinary incontinence[12, 54] and climacturia[55] are associated with distress in men with prostate cancer, and that for some men urinary incontinence is worse than erectile dysfunction.[9] Our finding that difficulty in negotiating climacturia with casual or new partners was of concern for some GBM suggests that this is a difficulty that might affect a proportion of GBM with prostate cancer, given the varied nature of these relationships.

CONCLUSION

This study has demonstrated that while GBM experience the same physical sexual changes after prostate cancer treatment that have been reported by heterosexual men, there are a number of GBM-specific meanings and psychological and physical consequences attached to sexual changes that need to be considered by researchers and clinicians, in the context of the construction of gay sex, identity, and relationships. When designing studies to examine the effects of prostate cancer on any man's sexuality and quality of life, researchers need to ask about sexual orientation and include questions on anal sex, ejaculatory bother, climacturia, reduction in penis size, and types of sexual relationships—concerns that are often overlooked. Equally, when clinicians are advising men of the sexual consequences of prostate cancer treatment, they need to provide information and support relating to the broad spectrum of sexual changes, in addition to information on erectile dysfunction and incontinence. Clinicians also need to be aware of the specific meaning of sexual changes for GBM, in the context of both long-term sexual relationships and casual sexual encounters, and to avoid heteronormative assumptions about their patients. Only then will we be able to address the concerns and needs of the hitherto "hidden population"[15] of GBM with prostate cancer.

ACKNOWLEDGMENTS

This study was funded by the Prostate Cancer Foundation of Australia (PCFA), in the form of a new concept grant, no. NCG 0512, in partnership with Australian and New Zealand Urogenital and Prostate (ANZUP) Cancer Trials Group. Sections of this chapter draw on a previously published paper: Ussher, J.M., Perz, J., Rose, D., Dowsett, G.D., Chambers, S., Williams, S., Davis, S., Latini, D. (2016). Threat of Sexual Disqualification: The Consequences of Erectile Dysfunction and Other Sexual Changes for Gay and Bisexual Men with Prostate Cancer, *Archives of Sexual Behavior*, 2017; 46 (7): 2043–2057.

REFERENCES

1. Chung E, Brock G. Sexual rehabilitation and cancer survivorship: A state of art review of current literature and management strategies in male sexual dysfunction among prostate cancer survivors. *Journal of Sexual Medicine*. 2013; 10 (S1): 102–111.

2. Sivarajan G, Prabhu V, Taksler GB, et al. Ten-year outcomes of sexual function after radical prostatectomy: Results of a prospective longitudinal study. *European Urology*. 2014; 65 (1): 58–65.

3. Ussher JM, Perz J, Rose D, et al. Threat of sexual disqualification: The consequences of erectile dysfunction and other sexual changes for gay and bisexual men with prostate cancer. *Archives of Sexual Behavior*. 2017; 46 (7): 2043–2057.

4. Badr H, Taylor CL. Sexual dysfunction and spousal communication in couples coping with prostate cancer. *Psycho-Oncology*. 2009; 18 (7): 735–746.

5. Perz J, Ussher JM, Gilbert E. Feeling well and talking about sex: Psycho-social predictors of sexual functioning after cancer. *BMC Cancer*. 2014; 14 (1): 228–247.

6. Wittman D, Northouse L, Foley S, et al. The psychosocial aspects of sexual recovery after prostate cancer treatment. *International Journal of Impotence Research*. 2009; 21: 99–106.

7. Asencio M, Blank T, Descartes L, Crawford A. The prospect of prostate cancer: A challenge for gay men's sexualities as they age. *Sexuality Research and Social Policy*. 2009; 6 (4): 38–51.

8. Gilbert E, Ussher JM, Perz J, et al. Men's experiences of sexuality after cancer: A material discursive intra-psychic approach. *Culture, Health & Sexuality*. 2013; 15 (8): 881–895.

9. Fergus KD, Gray RE, Fitch MI. Sexual dysfunction and the preservation of manhood: Experiences of men with prostate cancer. *Journal of Health Psychology*. 2002; 7: 303–316.

10. Bokhour BG, Clark JA, Inui TS, et al. Sexuality after treatment for early prostate cancer: Exploring the meanings of "erectile dysfunction." *Journal of General Internal Medicine.* 2001; 16: 649–655.

11. Arrington MI. "I don't want to be an artificial man": Narrative reconstruction of sexuality among prostate cancer survivors. *Sexuality & Culture.* 2003; 7 (2): 30–58.

12. Rosser BRS, Capistrant B, Torres B, et al. The effects of radical prostatectomy on gay and bisexual men's mental health, sexual identity and relationships: Qualitative results from the Restore study. *Sexual and Relationship Therapy.* 2016; 31 (4): 446–461.

13. Ussher JM, Perz J, Kellett A, et al. Health-related quality of life, psychological distress, and sexual changes following prostate cancer: A comparison of gay and bisexual men with heterosexual men. *Journal of Sexual Medicine.* 2016; 13 (3): 425–434.

14. Thomas C. An analysis of postings on two prostate cancer discussion boards. *Gay and Lesbian Issues and Psychology Review.* 2012; 8: 15–21.

15. Filiault SM, Drummond MJN, Smith JA. Gay men and prostate cancer: Voicing the concerns of a hidden population. *Journal of Men's Health.* 2008; 5 (4): 327–332.

16. Dowsett GW, Lyons A, Duncan D, Wassersug RJ. Flexibility in men's sexual practices in response to iatrogenic erectile dysfunction after prostate cancer treatment. *Sexual Medicine.* 2014; 2 (3): 115–120.

17. Ussher JM, Rose D, Perz J. Mastery, isolation, or acceptance: Gay and bisexual men's construction of aging in the context of sexual embodiment after prostate cancer. *Journal of Sex Research.* 2017; 56 (4): 802–812.

18. Rose D, Ussher JM, Perz J. Let's talk about gay sex: Gay and bisexual men's sexual communication with healthcare professionals after prostate cancer. *European Journal of Cancer Care,* 2017; 26(1).

19. Braun V, Clarke B. Using thematic analysis in psychology. *Qualitative Research in Psychology.* 2006; 3 (2): 77–101.

20. Smith DP, King MT, Egger S, et al. Quality of life three years after diagnosis of localised prostate cancer: Population based cohort study. *BMJ.* 2009; 339: b4817.

21. Penson DF, McLerran D, Feng Z, et al. 5-year urinary and sexual outcomes after radical prostatectomy: Results from the Prostate Cancer Outcomes Study. *Journal of Urology.* 2008; 179 (5): S40–S44.

22. Roberts KJ, Lepore SI, Hanlon AL, Helgeson V. Genitourinary functioning and depressive symptoms over time in younger versus older men treated for prostate cancer. *Annals of Behavioral Medicine.* 2010; 40 (3): 275–283.

23. Hart TL, Coon DW, Kowalkowski MA, et al. Changes in sexual roles and quality of life for gay men after prostate cancer: Challenges for sexual health providers. *Journal of Sexual Medicine.* 2014; 11 (9): 2308–2317.

24. Sommers BD, Beard CJ, D'Amico AV, et al. Predictors of patient preferences and treatment choices for localized prostate cancer. *Cancer.* 2008; 113 (8): 2058–2067.

25. Pitts M, Smith A, Mitchell A, Patel S. *Private lives: A report on the health and wellbeing of GLBTI Australians*. Melbourne: Australian Research Centre in Sex, Health and Society, La Trobe University; 2006.

26. Grulich AE, de Visser RO, Smith AMA, et al. Sex in Australia: Homosexual experience and recent homosexual encounters. *Australian and New Zealand Journal of Public Health*. 2003; 27 (2): 155–163.

27. Dowsett G. *Practicing desire: Homosexual sex in the era of AIDS*. Stanford, Calif.: Stanford University Press; 1996.

28. Lyons A, Pitts M, Smith G, et al. Versatility and HIV vulnerability: Investigating the proportion of Australian gay men having both insertive and receptive anal intercourse. *Journal of Sexual Medicine*. 2011; 8 (8): 2164–2171.

29. Parekh A, Chen M-H, Hoffman KE, et al. Reduced penile size and treatment regret in men with recurrent prostate cancer after surgery, radiotherapy plus androgen deprivation, or radiotherapy alone. *Urology*. 2013; 81 (1): 130–135.

30. Powel LL, Clark JA. The value of the marginalia as an adjunct to structured questionnaires: Experiences of men after prostate cancer surgery. *Quality of Life Research*. 2005; 14 (3): 827–835.

31. Thomas C, Wootten A, Robinson P. The experiences of gay and bisexual men diagnosed with prostate cancer: Results from an online focus group. *European Journal of Cancer Care*. 2013; 22 (4): 522–529.

32. Drummond M, Filiault S. The long and the short of it: Gay men's perceptions of penis size. *Gay & Lesbian Issues and Psychology Review*. 2007; 3 (2): 121–129.

33. Grov C, Parsons JT, Bimbi DS. The association between penis size and sexual health among men who have sex with men. *Archives of Sexual Behavior*. 2010; 39 (3): 788–797.

34. Moskowitz DA, Rieger G, Seal DW. Narcissism, self-evaluations, and partner preferences among men who have sex with men. *Personality and Individual Differences*. 2009; 46 (7): 725.

35. Moskowitz DA, Hart TA. The influence of physical body traits and masculinity on anal sex roles in gay and bisexual men. *Archives of Sexual Behavior*. 2011; 40 (4): 835–841.

36. Wassersug RJ, Westle A, Dowsett GW. Men's sexual and relational adaptations to erectile dysfunction after prostate cancer treatment. *International Journal of Sexual Health*. 2017; 29 (1): 69–79.

37. Connell RW. *Masculinities*. 2nd ed. Crows Nest, N.S.W.: Allen & Unwin; 2005.

38. Nardi P. *Gay masculinities*. Thousand Oaks, Calif.: Sage; 2000.

39. Connell RW. *Masculinities*. Berkeley: University of California Press; 1995.

40. Barsky J, Friedman M, Rosen R. Sexual dysfunction and chronic illness: The role of flexibility in coping. *Journal of Sex & Marital Therapy*. 2006; 32 (3): 235–253.

41. Ussher JM, Perz J, Gilbert E, et al. Renegotiating sex after cancer: Resisting the coital imperative. *Cancer Nursing*. 2013; 36 (6): 454–462.

42. Blank TO. Gay men and prostate cancer: Invisible diversity. *Journal of Clinical Oncology.* 2005; 23 (12): 2593–2596.

43. Lyons A, Hosking W. Prevalence and correlates of sexual partner concurrency among Australian gay men aged 18–39 years. *AIDS and Behavior.* 2014; 18 (4): 801–809.

44. Wei C, Raymond H. Preference for and maintenance of anal sex roles among men who have sex with men: Sociodemographic and behavioral correlates. *Archives of Sexual Behavior.* 2011; 40 (4): 829–834.

45. Moskowitz DA, Rieger G, Roloff ME. Tops, bottoms and versatiles. *Sexual and Relationship Therapy.* 2008; 23 (3): 191–202.

46. Dowsett GW. *Practicing desire: Homosexual sex in era of AIDS.* Stanford, Calif.: Stanford University Press; 1996.

47. Benson CR, Serefoglu EC, Hellstrom WJG. Sexual dysfunction following radical prostatectomy. *Journal of Andrology.* 2012; 33 (6): 1143–1154.

48. Mitteldorf D. Psychotherapy with gay prostate cancer patients. *Journal of Gay & Lesbian Psychotherapy.* 2005; 9 (1–2): 57–67.

49. Prestage G, Hurley M, Brown G. "Cum play" among gay men. *Archives of Sexual Behavior.* 2013; 42 (7): 1347–1356.

50. Holmes D, Warner D. The anatomy of a forbidden desire: Men, penetration and semen exchange. *Nursing Inquiry.* 2005; 12 (1): 10–20.

51. Schilder AJ, Orchard TR, Buchner CS, et al. "It's like the treasure": Beliefs associated with semen among young HIV-positive and HIV-negative gay men. *Culture, Health & Sexuality.* 2008; 10 (7): 667–679.

52. Wassersug RJ, Lyons A, Duncan D, et al. Diagnostic and outcome differences between heterosexual and nonheterosexual men treated for prostate cancer. *Urology.* 2013; 82 (3): 565–571.

53. Lodge AC, Umberson D. Age and embodied masculinities: Midlife gay and heterosexual men talk about their bodies. *Journal of Aging Studies.* 2013; 27 (3): 225.

54. Punnen S, Cowan JE, Dunn LB, et al. A longitudinal study of anxiety, depression and distress as predictors of sexual and urinary quality of life in men with prostate cancer. *BJU International.* 2013; 112 (2): E67–E75.

55. Abouassaly R, Lane BR, Lakin MM, et al. Ejaculatory urine incontinence after radical prostatectomy. *Urology.* 2006; 68 (6): 1248–1252.

CHAPTER 3

Integrating Post-Prostatectomy Sexuality

The Couple's Journey

Daniela Wittmann

CHAPTER SUMMARY

This chapter addresses the sexual recovery of gay and bisexual men (GBM) with prostate cancer and their partners after surgery for prostate cancer. While the sexual function of the man with prostate cancer is primarily affected, the partner is also affected emotionally, and the couple's sexual experience is changed. Both members of the couple will probably experience grief about sexual losses. In the process of recovery, they will have to learn to communicate more explicitly about their sexual needs and may need to employ novel strategies to stay connected and maintain a satisfying level of eroticism. Currently, little support is available for GBM couples. Knowledge development is needed to ensure that GBM couples' sexual recovery proceeds toward maximizing their sexual health after prostate cancer treatment.

KEY TERMS

couples, prostate cancer, prostatectomy, sexuality, sexual recovery

INTRODUCTION

Having a partner with whom to face life's challenges has been shown to be protective, even life-saving.[1] Being in a partnership is associated with a longer life in individuals with cancer.[2] Couples support and comfort each other when a life-threatening illness intrudes and may seek sexual intimacy even in its last stages.[3] It is also a connection that can be challenging to maintain. A cancer diagnosis imposes role shifts and may cause an imbalance in the relationship's equilibrium, requiring both instrumental and emotional management.

Ussher, Jane M., Perz, Janette, Rosser, B. R. Simon, eds., *Gay & Bisexual Men Living with Prostate Cancer*
dx.doi.org/10.17312/harringtonparkpress/2018.06.gbmlpc.003
© 2018 Harrington Park Press

When prostate cancer is treated surgically, beyond the distress of the illness and role changes, the treatment side effects reach into the core of the relationship: sexuality. Problems with erections, loss of ejaculate, sometimes loss of sex drive, and urinary incontinence after prostatectomy can leave men feeling emasculated,[4] particularly if they subscribe to a traditional model of masculinity that enshrines physical strength, emotional impenetrability, and self-sufficiency.[5] Few men fully regain erectile function after surgery,[6] which means that they have to come to terms with altered sexuality. To remain sexually viable, they are pressed to create a new sexual paradigm from the functionality that remains, as outlined by chapters 2, 10, and 11 of this book.

After a man's prostatectomy, his partner is brought along on the journey, but his experiences are different. His sexual function is unchanged, but his emotional and sexual world have changed. As a caregiver, the partner will want to be supportive and loving, but as a lover, he may have needs that will now go unfulfilled.[7] He may feel resentment about the way in which his partner's cancer altered his life and worry about the future. Models of sexual recovery after cancer have suggested that couples go through a grief process together before they can develop a new way of sharing love and eroticism.[8-10]

Much of the research on couples coping with prostate cancer treatment has been conducted with heterosexual couples. Heterosexism in healthcare and in research,[11] implicit bias against sexual minorities,[12] reluctance by GBM to come out to providers for fear of discrimination,[13] lack of provider training in gay and bisexual sexuality, and providers' general discomfort with talking about sex[14] have been significant hindrances to the provision of appropriate care for gay and bisexual men and their partners. In their review of GBM sexual health, Rosser and colleagues estimate that approximately 97,845 to 123,006 GBM live in prostate cancer survivorship; of those, 39,138 to 73,804 are members of a male couple.[15] Their experiences are understudied, and they do not benefit from the limited support currently afforded to heterosexual couples. Only recently has LGBT healthcare been recognized in the United States as a health disparity.[11, 13, 16-19]

Research on GBM with prostate cancer is emerging. Recent studies have described the sexual losses that GBM face after prostate cancer treatment and the challenges that they experience in their healthcare.[7, 20-26] One study included partners;[7, 20] another was conducted with couples.[22] I have interviewed two gay couples, one in a study on the partner's role in a couple's sexual recovery after prostate cancer,[27] the other in an unpublished study of GBM with prostate cancer.[28] I work clinically with couples, including gay couples. This chapter is based on my experience and the knowledge of GBM couples' experience we have to date.

BIOPSYCHOSOCIAL SEXUALITY

A biopsychosocial perspective on sexuality reflects an understanding that after prostatectomy, sexual losses occur in three domains: (1) the loss of function, precipitated by surgery; (2) an emotional reaction on the part of both the affected man and his partner; and (3) changes in their sexual relationship.[29] The primary sexual losses are erectile dysfunction and loss of ejaculate, as described in a number of chapters in this book[7, 30, 31] (see chapters 1, 2, and 11). Additionally, urinary incontinence intrudes on sexual interactions.[31] Everything that was familiar and available sexually requires emotional adaptation, intentionality, new skill building, and reconfiguration. The transition is emotionally taxing and does not have a predictable outcome. Erectile function may require the use of sexual aids, at least temporarily, as discussed by Wibowo and Wassersug (chapter 10), and Ussher et al. (chapter 11). Psychologically, the experience of loss of control is common. Long-term studies have shown that most men, and therefore couples, do not a return to baseline sexual functioning.[6, 32] The uncertainty of the recovery can lead to chronic, ambiguous grief,[33] experienced by one or both partners; yet it can also promote creativity and solutions previously unforeseen when sex was a spontaneous activity. The following section provides examples of couples' experience of changes in their sex lives after prostatectomy.

SEXUAL LOSSES AFTER PROSTATECTOMY

In their 2016 study on the influence of sexual changes after prostate cancer treatment, Ussher and colleagues described the psychological effect of sexual losses on GBM as their feeling older, less sexually viable, and even "disqualified" in the gay community that values robust sexuality and health.[7] These responses were echoed in Wittmann and Latini's study in which a single man, yearning for a relationship but feeling undesirable, commented: "What do I write about myself [on the Match.com dating site]? 'A gay man who is a Vietnam vet against the war, against all wars, who is recovering from prostate surgery and now open-heart surgery.' [laughing] Nobody writes that shit down."[28] Rosser similarly reports the anxiety GBM experience when they face the need to disclose their sexual dysfunction to a potential new partner.[25] The possibility of a relationship for GBM with sexual dysfunction and other health problems can become elusive, at least psychologically.

In previous studies, couples acknowledged that significant changes or losses occurred in their sexual experience after radical prostatectomy.[22, 28] They reported diminished desire, erectile dysfunction, complicated feelings about the loss of ejaculate, and less frequent sexual activity.[22] They did not always feel prepared for the changes. One of the men noted: "In my case, I thought it was going to happen to everybody else, but not to me because, jeez, I'm perfectly . . . everything is just fine." His partner said, "I finally asked the question [about the loss of ejaculation] because his prostate was being removed . . . and I remember both of us looking at each other . . . for a gay couple, that is pretty dramatic news."[28]

The loss of spontaneity can be a major barrier to couples' sexual recovery because it takes away excitement and control over the sexual experience. After prostate cancer treatment, sex becomes intentional. The excitement of spontaneity can be replaced with the pleasure of anticipation, but many couples find the path from one to the other rocky and arduous: "You know what, by the time you use the pump, you use Viagra, you put a cock ring on, you know, how much interest can you have in sex?"; "Well, where you enjoyed sex and it was completely easy before and it's, excuse me, now it's not so easy and in fact, it's a lot of work."[28] When sex is experienced as work, it can be very discouraging to some couples.

For some men, coping with urinary incontinence was a barrier to initiation of sexual activity. One man, still incontinent nine years after surgery said, "Actually, the urinary is more of an issue than the erection issue." His partner was less concerned: "Um, . . . he is more embarrassed about his incontinence issues than I will ever be."[28] While the support of and acceptance by the partner is clearly a positive factor, the man's chronic sorrow about his loss of control over his physical function led to loss of confidence and diminished the experience of pleasure.

THE PARTNER'S RESPONSE TO SEXUAL LOSSES

Partners' distress about sexual issues is well documented in the heterosexual literature.[34, 35] Unlike heterosexual men with postmenopausal female partners, GBM manage a different sexual paradigm in which the partner may continue to have undiminished sexual desire and function. A male partner can have a genuine feeling of empathy. At the same time, that very empathy can lead the healthy partner to hesitate to initiate sexual activity to avoid upsetting the affected partner.[22] Or empathy may not be enough, as in the case of a partner who had already been treated for prostate cancer and was using intracavernosal injections himself. The currently affected member of the couple had been the initiator. The partner was aware that he should now maintain the couple's sexual activity by initiating: "I think that it's something that I actually need to work on more, because I do sense . . . that it's a little more difficult for him to initiate because of what he's going through."[28] From a functional point of view, the partner's comorbidities, such as a previous stroke, could also impair the partner's ability to respond actively to the sexual recovery.[22] Thus, the partner's ability to feel empathy is a great asset. At the same time, it can create distress for some partners who, for reasons either physical or psychological, feel unable to act on it in a way that furthers the couple's sexual recovery.

Ussher and colleagues found that GBM reported a variety of experiences in their partners' responses. Some were supportive and loving. While they expressed sadness about the sexual losses, they were able to move toward a more nurturing role in their relationships. Other partners found the men's inability to perform sexually after prostate cancer treatment difficult to tolerate and abandoned the relationships.[7]

It is important for couples to realize that there are generally two types of worries that they might experience. One is about the sexual "equipment." The other is about the effect of sexual changes on the relationship. Members of a couple may not always worry about the same thing at the same time. When one worries about the loss of function and the other worries about the effect of these changes on the relationship, both may feel upset about the difference in focus and fear what this means for the relationship. Communication and mutual understanding, as well as acceptance of each other's emotional response, are critical to couples' ability to cope with post-prostatectomy sexual changes with resilience and as a team.

COUPLES' COMMUNICATION

Research focused on communication in couples coping with cancer demonstrates that there is a tendency to avoid communication about upsetting, cancer-related topics. Such "protective buffering" has been associated with poorer outcomes for both the patient and the partner, and research suggests that poor communication can become a barrier to sexual recovery.[36] Protectiveness, as Hartman and colleagues suggest, may be one reason for communication problems about sexual changes. They cite a patient's dilemma about initiating sex when he knows that he will not have an erection: "What is there to talk about . . . I'm not going to, you know, rehash the whole thing and make [my partner] more upset, and it just makes me more upset."[22] Protectiveness, however, may not be the only reason couples do not talk about their sexual challenges after prostatectomy. When directly asked about sexual communication, couples in a study by Wittmann and colleagues reported that, before prostate cancer treatment, verbal communication was not a prerequisite for pleasurable and intimate sexual activity.[37] Erections communicated desire and nonverbal communication provided guidance for further activity.

Although in clinical practice I have found gay couples more open about discussing sexual practices than heterosexual men, GBM, like heterosexual men, tend to want to protect each other from feelings of grief and humiliation about sexual dysfunction and fear of abandonment. For example, in one case, the man with prostate cancer (who was much older than his partner) wanted to stop being sexually engaged and release the younger partner to sexual activity with new partners. For some couples this is a viable solution, as described below, but if it is not discussed and accepted by both members of the couple as an approach that works for both of them, the younger partner can feel rejected and the older partner may chronically grieve the loss of sexuality. In this case, the older man came to understand that he was assuming that the younger man would privilege his intact sexuality over the relationship. In fact, this was not true, and a conversation helped reassure both that they valued the relationship and would work on sexual recovery together. It is easy to see that, for some couples, not communicating about each other's preferences may lead to a loss of the relationship.

Couples' ability to communicate about prostatectomy-related sexual changes and associated feelings gives them an opportunity to examine what sexual changes mean to them. Sexuality is an integral part of masculine identity, and the ability to have erections and express pleasure through ejaculation reinforces it. For most men, hardness of erection is an important symbol of virility,[38] but for GBM, it is also necessary for anal penetration, as was discussed in chapter 2. The loss of firm erections and the loss of ejaculate have important implications for sharing pleasure. Through explicit discussion of the meaning of these experiences, couples can acknowledge sexual losses, recognize their emotional reactions, and reimagine what can become erotic and satisfying in the new context.

After prostate cancer treatment, verbal communication about sex becomes a necessity and a challenging new skill to develop. Self-disclosure and positive communication can enhance a couple's emotional intimacy and make sexual activity more connected and pleasurable in a new way. Some couples have indicated that having been able to talk it through and work toward a new sexual paradigm has made them feel closer than they were before prostate cancer treatment.[10]

MAINTAINING SEXUAL INTIMACY AND EROTIC PLEASURE

EXPANDING SEXUAL REPERTOIRE

When erectile function requires the use of sexual aids and sex becomes unspontaneous, many couples experience frustration, feeling put off by the fact that sex becomes "work." Yet some couples have found that working on sexual recovery has brought them closer together. Studies report that couples learn to focus on emotional intimacy, sensuality, and exploration of new sexual experiences.[7, 22, 39] Longer foreplay, discovery of new erotically sensitive body zones, stimulation with oral sex as a substitute for anal intercourse, expansion of the use of sex toys, and new or stronger visual stimulation can be further enhanced with sexy talk and humor. Couples can feel close when they share vulnerability, the success of new sexual stimulation, and the recognition that they are working it out despite the functional challenges brought on by prostate cancer treatment.[10] We can see that many of these issues are probably true of both heterosexual and GBM. However, GBM may need more encouragement to develop this aspect of their sexuality because GBM put a heavy emphasis on a strong penis as a source of pleasure. As a man in the Wittmann and Latini study ruefully commented: "I've been thinking about it . . . not just penetrative sex, but what alternatives there are for sexual fulfillment besides penetration, whatever, it would be interesting to have someone talk about that in an open way. Because then it widens the opportunity to be able to explore the sexual or be interested in sex in a different way rather than have it be limited to penetration." A couple observed: "Nobody really from the surgeons and from the hospital came in and talked to us about the emotional part . . . about how this is going to affect your sex life."[28] Learning to derive pleasure from non-penetrative practices and from the emotional aspects of sex and incorporate these into sexual interactions can be challenging but can, paradoxically, strengthen the relationship.

THE ROLE CHANGE IN ANAL INTERCOURSE

Losing erectile function by the man who is the top in a couple who engage in anal intercourse can lead to a dilemma when that couple has enjoyed relying on particular roles during sexual activity. It cannot be assumed that the situation can be remedied by the couple's switching roles. Hartman and colleagues found that for couples whose sexual activity was not focused on anal intercourse, the inability to have a firm erection did not present a significant barrier to resuming sexual activity.[22] Dowsett and colleagues, in their study of both nonheterosexual and heterosexual men, found that anal intercourse decreased after prostate cancer treatment. Some men were able to change from insertive to receptive intercourse, and some continued flexible approaches to being either a top or a bottom. None of the men adopted insertive intercourse for the first time. However, 12 men (in a sample of 406) in relationships adopted receptive anal sex for the first time after prostate cancer treatment.[26] This study demonstrates that, while the numbers are small, it is possible for couples to work toward an alternative sexual paradigm if they are motivated to do so. The couples that flexibly changed roles or those in which a partner adopted insertive intercourse were probably able to negotiate the change through their own process without advice or support. Ussher and colleagues found that some couples were able to successfully negotiate receptive and insertive role changes. In their study, for some GBM, anal sensitivity remained after prostatectomy. Others no longer felt anal sexual sensitivity; thus, being a bottom no longer led to sexual satisfaction.[7] Being able to change roles is a solution that also depends on how much the role is a part of one's core identity as a man and as a lover. It cannot be assumed that couples who like anal intercourse can easily switch roles and achieve comparable satisfaction. Dowsett and colleagues suggest, however, that men's willingness and ability to be flexible should not be underestimated. We can imagine that if counseling were available to help normalize flexibility and encourage couples to experiment, more couples would be able to expand their sexual repertoire and achieve satisfaction after prostate cancer treatment.

COPING WITH INCONTINENCE

It is generally the GBM with prostate cancer who is more mortified by leaking urine than the partner, as the partner quoted earlier in this chapter demonstrates. For most men, incontinence during foreplay and climacturia resolve some months after they become continent of urine, particularly if they engage in pelvic floor rehabilitation.[31] Just knowing that this is probably a temporary problem can be helpful for the couple. In clinical practice, one can discuss urine as just another body fluid that is sterile and harmless when it leaves the body. Men and partners respond well when they understand that their early training leads them to view urine as a distasteful emission. As a body fluid, it is no different from the viscous product of the Cowper's gland or semen. Couples can be encouraged to work psychologically to accept urine as a temporary nuisance that need not detract from their sexual pleasure. If needed, it can be disguised with a lubricant. I have found, in discussions with couples, that injecting humor into the conversation about urine's intrusion on sexual activity can ease tension and lighten the burden of a potentially mortifying concern. Urination then becomes just a typical, normal body function.

OPENING THE RELATIONSHIP

Opening the relationship to a new lover is a solution more easily embraced by GBM couples than heterosexual couples. When both members of the couple can feel secure and find meaning in choosing this solution, it can reduce anxiety and enhance pleasure. It can also alleviate any residual guilt that the man with prostate cancer might feel because of his sexual dysfunction. Hartman and colleagues reported that at least for one of the couples in their study, this was a solution that was acceptable to both partners.[22] Ussher and colleagues cite a man who came to regard an open relationship as a creative solution: "I recognize that he's got physical needs and I don't have a problem with that. And he comes home to me all the time, and in fact, shares part of his fantasy life with me anyway."[7] The result is not always as positive, but it can become an accepted recognition of the partner's need that does not detract from the couple's primary intimacy, as a patient in Wittmann and Latini's study reported: "And actually he brought someone home and I tried to join in but soon lost interest . . . that is what he does and you know what, I am fine with it."[28] In open relationships in which emotional intimacy remains intact, the inclusion of an additional partner may succeed as a way of optimizing sexual satisfaction without endangering the integrity of the relationship.

THE PROTECTIVE NATURE OF BEING IN A RELATIONSHIP

The support of a partner is a critical element in couples' sexual recovery, as has been demonstrated in the literature on both heterosexual and GBM couples. Ussher and colleagues give examples of partners' loving support that adds security for sexual recovery. Hartman and colleagues echo the importance of a partner. The strength of long-term relationships was expressed by a partner in Wittmann and Latini's study: "We got together as a couple later in life, if you will, and one of the things we talked about is that we, it was not, we are not in our 20's . . . we are growing older together . . . and so you expect a lot of physical changes in your life as you grow older . . . you expect to have to cope with it together."[28] The ability to cope with sexual losses as a couple, taking a long view and expressing commitment to each other, propels couples toward seeking solutions in order to maintain a sexual relationship despite sexual dysfunction.

Rosser and colleagues reported on the paucity of social support for GBM with prostate cancer and suggest that this is an area that needs more research.[15] In Wittmann and Latini's study, all three men with prostate cancer and one partner reported having been in psychotherapy before prostate cancer, but they also sought support for this experience. Though the sample is very small, it indicates that GBM may be more open to support than heterosexual men who are much more hampered by the notion of traditional masculinity.[28] At the same time, these men also indicated a concern about how they might be perceived in the gay community should their sexual dysfunction be known. Ussher and colleagues write eloquently about men feeling "sexually disqualified" after prostate cancer treatment.[7] Addressing the stigma of sexual dysfunction in the gay community could be an important contribution to supporting the sexual health of GBM recovering sexual intimacy with their partners after prostate cancer treatment. Group interventions for heterosexual couples have shown promise.[40, 41] There is no reason why GBM couples could not similarly benefit from mutual support as they navigate the prostate cancer experience. In the meantime, in the United States, sex therapists certified by the American Association of Sexuality Educators, Counselors, and Therapists, easily found on the association's website (aasect.org), can probably provide the best support for gay couples because their training includes specific focus on LGBT sexuality.

CONCLUSION

Gay and bisexual men with prostate cancer and their partners represent an important minority population of prostate cancer survivors. As sexual recovery after prostate cancer treatment gains legitimacy in prostate cancer survivorship in general, it is important to develop specific support for GBM and their partners that is based on their experience and their needs. As our understanding of the sexual health needs of GBM with prostate cancer and their partners grows through research, clinical care, and personal testimonials, it is critical that relevant and appropriate programs be developed to maximize their sexual health and reduce a health disparity that has, for too long, prevented them from achieving satisfactory sexual health adjustment in survivorship.

REFERENCES

1. Kaplan RM, Kronick RG. Marital status and longevity in the United States population. *Journal of Epidemiology and Community Health.* 2006; 60 (9): 760–765.
2. Aizer AA, Chen MH, McCarthy EP, et al. Marital status and survival in patients with cancer. *Journal of Clinical Oncology.* 2013; 31 (31): 3869–3876.
3. Blagbrough J. Importance of sexual needs assessment in palliative care. *Nursing Standard.* 2010; 24 (52): 35–39.
4. Hedestig O, Sandman PO, Tomic R, Widmark A. Living after radical prostatectomy for localized prostate cancer: A qualitative analysis of patient narratives. *Acta Oncologica.* 2005; 44 (7): 679–686.
5. Wall D, Kristjanson L. Men, culture and hegemonic masculinity: Understanding the experience of prostate cancer. *Nursing Inquiry.* 2005; 12 (2): 87–97.
6. Resnick MJ, Koyama T, Fan KH, et al. Long-term functional outcomes after treatment for localized prostate cancer. *New England Journal of Medicine.* 2013; 368 (5): 436–445.

7.   Ussher JM, Perz J, Rose D, et al. The threat of sexual disqualification: The consequences of erectile dysfunction and other sexual changes for gay and bisexual men with prostate cancer. *Archives of Sexual Behavior*. 2017; 46 (7): 2043–2057.

8.   Pillai-Friedman S, Ashline JL. Women, breast cancer survivorship, sexual losses, and disenfranchised grief—a treatment model for clinicians. *Sexual and Relationship Therapy*. 2014; 29 (4): 436–453.

9.   Wittmann D, Foley S, Balon R. A biopsychosocial approach to sexual recovery after prostate cancer surgery: The role of grief and mourning. *Journal of Sex & Marital Therapy*. 2011; 37 (2): 130–144.

10. Wittmann D, Carolan M, Given B, et al. What couples say about their recovery of sexual intimacy after prostatectomy: Toward the development of a conceptual model of couples' sexual recovery after surgery for prostate cancer. *Journal of Sexual Medicine*. 2015; 12 (2): 494–504.

11. Herek G. Avoiding heterosexist bias in psychological research. *American Psychologist*. 1991; 44 (9): 957–963.

12. Fallin-Bennett K. Implicit bias against sexual minorities in medicine: Cycles of professional influence and the role of the hidden curriculum. *Academic Medicine*. 2015; 90 (5): 549–552.

13. Crangle CJ, Latini DM, Hart TL. The effects of attachment and outness on illness adjustment among gay men with prostate cancer. *Psycho-Oncology*. 2017; 26 (4): 500–507.

14. Marwick C. Survey says patients expect little physician help on sex. *JAMA: Journal of the American Medical Association*. 1999; 281 (23): 2173–2174.

15. Rosser BRS, Merengwa E, Capistrant B, et al. Prostate cancer in gay, bisexual, and other men who have sex with men: A review. *LGBT Health*. 2016; 3 (1): 32–41.

16. Leyva VL, Breshears EM, Ringstad R. Assessing the efficacy of LGBT cultural competency training for aging services providers in California's Central Valley. *Journal of Gerontological Social Work*. 2014; 57 (2–4): 335–348.

17. Alexander R, Parker K, Schwetz T. Sexual and gender minority health research at the National Institutes of Health. *LGBT Health*. 2016; 3 (1): 7–10.

18. Makadon HJ. Ending LGBT invisibility in health care: The first step in ensuring equitable care. *Cleveland Clinic Journal of Medicine*. 2011; 78 (4): 220–224.

19. Marwick C. Survey says patients expect little physician help on sex. *JAMA: Journal of the American Medical Association*. 1999; 281 (23): 2173–2174.

20. Rose D, Ussher JM, Perz J. Let's talk about gay sex: Gay and bisexual men's sexual communication with healthcare professionals after prostate cancer. *European Journal of Cancer Care*. 2017; 26 (1).

21. Ussher JM, Perz J, Kellett A, et al. Health-related quality of life, psychological distress, and sexual changes following prostate cancer: A comparison of gay and bisexual men with heterosexual men. *Journal of Sexual Medicine*. 2016; 13 (3): 425–434.

22. Hartman ME, Irvine J, Currie KL, et al. Exploring gay couples' experience with sexual dysfunction after radical prostatectomy: A qualitative study. *Journal of Sex and Marital Therapy*. 2014; 40 (3): 233–253.

23. Hart TL, Coon DW, Kowalkowski MA, et al. Changes in sexual roles and quality of life for gay men after prostate cancer: Challenges for sexual health providers. *Journal of Sexual Medicine*. 2014; 11 (9): 2308–2317.

24. Torbit LA, Albiani JJ, Crangle CJ, et al. Fear of recurrence: The importance of self-efficacy and satisfaction with care in gay men with prostate cancer. *Psycho-Oncology*. 2015; 24 (6): 691–698.

25. Rosser BRS, Capistrant B, Torres B, et al. The effects of radical prostatectomy on gay and bisexual men's mental health, sexual identity and relationships: Qualitative results from the Restore study. *Sexual and Relationship Therapy*. 2016; 31 (4): 446–461.

26. Dowsett GW, Lyons A, Duncan D, Wassersug RJ. Flexibility in men's sexual practices in response to iatrogenic erectile dysfunction after prostate cancer treatment. *Sexual Medicine*. 2014; 2 (3): 115–120.

27. Wittmann D, Carolan M, Given B, et al. Exploring the role of the partner in couples' sexual recovery after surgery for prostate cancer. *Supportive Care in Cancer*. 2014; 22 (9): 2509–2515.

28. Wittmann D., Latini D. Gay men's sexual recovery after prostate cancer treatment: An exploratory study. Unpublished, 2010.

29. Bober SL, Varela VS. Sexuality in adult cancer survivors: Challenges and intervention. *Journal of Clinical Oncology*. 2012; 30 (30): 3712–3719.

30. Perlman G, Drescher J. *A gay man's guide to prostate cancer*. Binghamton, N.Y.: Haworth Medical Press; 2005.

31. Fode M, Serefoglu EC, Albersen M, Sonksen J. Sexuality following radical prostatectomy: Is restoration of erectile function enough? *Sexual Medicine Reviews*. 2017; 5 (1): 110–119.

32. Bernat JK, Wittman DA, Hawley ST, et al. Symptom burden and information needs in prostate cancer survivors: A case for tailored long-term survivorship care. *BJU International*. 2015; 118 (3): 372–378.

33. Boss P. *Ambiguous loss: Learning to live with unresolved grief*. Cambridge: Harvard University Press; 1999.

34. Couper JW, Bloch S, Love A, et al. Psychosocial adjustment of female partners of men with prostate cancer: A review of the literature. *Psycho-Oncology*. 2006; 15 (11): 937–953.

35. Tanner T, Galbraith M, Hays L. From a woman's perspective: Life as a partner of a prostate cancer survivor. *Journal of Midwifery and Women's Health*. 2011; 56 (2): 154–160.

36. Manne S, Ostroff J, Rini C, et al. The interpersonal process model of intimacy: The role of self-disclosure, partner disclosure, and partner responsiveness in

interactions between breast cancer patients and their partners. *Journal of Family Psychology*. 2004; 18 (4): 589–599.

37. Wittmann D, Northouse L, Crossley H, et al. A pilot study of potential pre-operative barriers to couples' sexual recovery after radical prostatectomy for prostate cancer. *Journal of Sex & Marital Therapy*. 2015; 41 (2): 155–168.

38. San Martin C, Simonelli C, Sonksen J, et al. Perceptions and opinions of men and women on a man's sexual confidence and its relationship to ED: Results of the European Sexual Confidence Survey. *International Journal of Impotence Research*. 2012; 24 (6): 234–241.

39. Perz J, Ussher JM, Gilbert E. Constructions of sex and intimacy after cancer: Q methodology study of people with cancer, their partners, and health professionals. *BMC Cancer*. 2013; 13: 270.

40. Paich K, Dunn R, Skolarus TA, et al. Preparing patients and partners for the recovery from the side effects of prostate cancer surgery: A group approach. *Urology*. 2016; 88: 36–42.

41. Wittmann D, He C, Mitchell S, et al. A one-day couple group intervention to enhance sexual recovery for surgically treated men with prostate cancer and their partners: A pilot study. *Urologic Nursing*. 2013; 33 (3): 140–147.

CHAPTER 4

"My partner is my family"

An Interdependence and Communal Coping Approach to Understanding Prostate Cancer in Same-Sex Male Couples

Charles Kamen and Lynae Darbes

CHAPTER SUMMARY

In this chapter, we describe a model for understanding the process by which same-sex male couples cope with prostate cancer. The model incorporates individual factors (e.g., sociodemographics, perceptions of cancer treatment), couple- and relationship-level factors (e.g., relationship quality, communication), and prejudice and stigma, with the goal of explaining health behavior change and treatment outcomes among sexual minority men with prostate cancer. The interplay of the various factors in the model is explored in the context of communal coping—a dyadic process thought to increase a couple's ability to respond positively to a health threat. We also discuss the importance of cancer care providers, who are a crucial factor in the patient's experience of cancer treatment. Challenges for providers include integration of same-sex partners into cancer treatment, even though partner involvement is a well-established predictor of improved patient outcomes for heterosexual patients. Throughout the chapter, we provide empirical support from the current literature, as well as quotes from a qualitative study of LGBT cancer patients, which serve to illuminate the issues discussed. Our aim is to provide a conceptual framework for future investigations into the role of partners, facilitate interventions for same-sex couples who are coping with prostate cancer, and ultimately to improve the physical and psychological health of this underrepresented and understudied population.

Ussher, Jane M., Perz, Janette, Rosser, B. R. Simon, eds., *Gay & Bisexual Men Living with Prostate Cancer*
dx.doi.org/10.17312/harringtonparkpress/2018.06.gbmlpc.004
© 2018 Harrington Park Press

KEY TERMS
bisexual, coping, couples, gay, prostate cancer, providers

INTRODUCTION

Well-publicized studies have highlighted the powerful positive effect that partner support and marriage have on cancer survivorship;[1] however, the majority of these studies have focused on heterosexual couples and have lacked data on the relationships of sexual-minority (lesbian, gay, and bisexual) persons diagnosed with cancer.[2] Given this lack of data, research on and integration of same-sex male couples into care for prostate cancer remains inconsistent, despite potential cancer-related disparities affecting this population.[3–5] Models of the processes by which same-sex male couples are affected by prostate cancer are similarly lacking. This chapter draws on a theoretical framework that has been used to explore coping with medical illness and predictors of health behavior among heterosexual and same-sex male couples, applying that framework to the experience of same-sex male couples coping with prostate cancer.[6]

Throughout this chapter, we use the term *sexual-minority men* as defined in the glossary of this book. We refer to *dyadic couplehood* when describing a romantic relationship between two sexual-minority men, but we acknowledge that other relationship configurations (e.g., polyamorous, triadic) may have beneficial effects on prostate cancer – related health. We are interested in men in same-sex relationships broadly, not only those in same-sex marriages, as not all gay and bisexual men opt to enter into legal marriage, and in some jurisdictions same-sex marriage is not possible.

The majority of sexual-minority men enter into committed romantic relationships at some point in their lives, and male partners of sexual-minority men with prostate cancer are likely to play a significant role in caregiving and providing support throughout the cancer trajectory.[7, 8] However, the importance and the unique aspects of these contributions have been overlooked in cancer care and research. In one study, Aizer discussed the protective effect of heterosexual marriage on cancer survival, outlining both pragmatic advantages (e.g., improved adherence) and emotional advantages (e.g., improved coping) conferred by couplehood.[1] This study did not overtly sample or describe the experiences of sexual-minority men or same-sex male couples. Similarly, established models of heterosexual coping with medical illness have remained mute on the experiences of same-sex couples.

Broadly speaking, couples-focused cancer research has focused on dyadic coping (see Regan et al.,[9] for a review), but it has had less of a focus on relationship dynamics (e.g., commitment, intimacy) and their influence on treatment and outcomes. The mutual influence between dyadic coping and relationship dynamics has been examined in studies of relationship-based outcomes such as divorce, but it has not been examined as much in the context of chronic illness. However, a model proposed by Lewis and colleagues[6] aimed to directly integrate dyadic coping with a relationship-focused theory (interdependence theory[10]), thereby directly addressing how the relationship context can affect the quality or presence of coping. In addition, the model includes health behavior outcomes, which are typically lacking from relationship-focused models. Therefore, the model offers a comprehensive approach to understanding ways in which relationship functioning contributes to dyadic coping, as well as how coping serves to influence subsequent health outcomes in couples. Empirical support has been found for this model from studies with both heterosexual and same-sex male couples in a variety of settings, primarily within the realm of HIV.[11-15] Here we will adapt it and extend its application to the experience of gay male couples coping with prostate cancer (the Adapted Interdependence Model, figure 4.1).[16]

Lewis's interdependence model of couples' communal coping and behavior change[6] incorporates individual- and couple-level factors that can influence the experience of medical illness. By *communal coping*, Lewis's model refers to the process by which each partner in a couple supports the other in making health-related behavior change and ensuring optimal health outcomes in the face of medical illness. At present, there have been only a few investigations into the communal coping process for sexual-minority men and their male partners,[17, 18] but initial findings have demonstrated that internalized homophobia can adversely affect communal coping. However, the model has not been applied to the experience of coping with prostate cancer. The following sections will outline components of this model, apply them to the experience of coping with prostate cancer, and then describe how these experiences may differ for sexual-minority men and same-sex male couples.

FIGURE 4.1 The Adapted Interdependence Model for sexual-minority men with prostate cancer

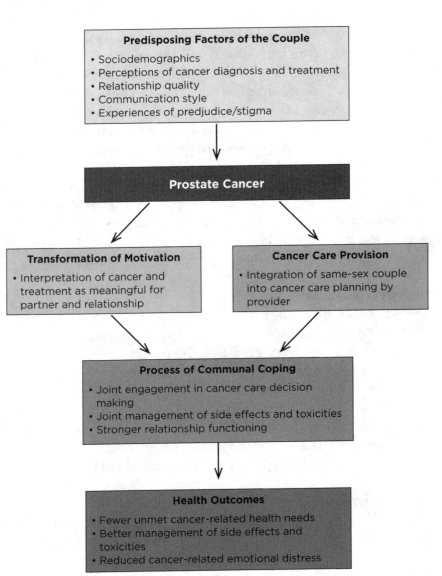

Source: Adapted from Lewis MA, McBride CM, Pollak KI, et al. Understanding health behavior change among couples: An interdependence and communal coping approach. *Social Science & Medicine.* 2006; 62 (6): 1369–1380.

OUR STUDY

We will punctuate our discussion of the model with quotes from gay and bisexual men (GBM) diagnosed with prostate cancer. These quotes are drawn from a study conducted by Marilyn Smith-Stoner (California State University, San Bernardino), Liz Margolies, LCSW (National LGBT Cancer Network), and Charles Kamen (University of Rochester).[19, 20] In this study, 311 self-identified lesbian, gay, bisexual, and transgender cancer survivors (with a range of cancer types) from around the United States completed an online survey. Data included are drawn from qualitative responses to an open-ended survey question, which asked, "If you were to give a class to healthcare workers, focused on cancer care, what would you tell them about being LGBT and being diagnosed with cancer?" A total of 84 men in this sample had been diagnosed with prostate cancer, and their responses are highlighted below. Of these 84, 47 were in romantic relationships with another man at the time of the survey; we include responses from both partnered and unpartnered men.

INDIVIDUAL- AND COUPLE-LEVEL FACTORS

The Adapted Interdependence Model for sexual-minority men posits that each partner in a couple has his own predisposing factors that may influence his experience of prostate cancer. Specifically, interpersonal factors between the couple may affect how well or how poorly the couple copes communally with external stressors, such as diagnosis of and treatment for prostate cancer. These factors include sociodemographics (gender, age, cultural background, education, etc.), perceptions of cancer diagnosis and treatment, relationship functioning (commitment, intimacy, communication, etc.), and experiences of discrimination and prejudice.

Sociodemographics. Illness perceptions and coping resources vary among individuals on the basis of a host of historical and intrapersonal factors. Socialization, upbringing, health literacy, and life stage can all influence how a man understands his own or his partner's susceptibility to prostate cancer and how well he understands and deals with the demands and consequences of cancer treatment. A man's understanding and acceptance of his prostate cancer diagnosis can influence both his own prostate cancer – related outcomes, as well as his partner's distress and outcomes.[16, 21] All these processes can be affected by the quality of coping by each partner. According to the model, to achieve optimal results both partners will enact a mutual engagement regarding the health threat (i.e., prostate cancer) and respond as a cohesive unit. This process of mutual reinforcement of coping resources is referred to as interdependence.

The influence of sociodemographics and the process of interdependence and communal coping may look different for sexual-minority men from the way it does for heterosexual men. Sexual-minority men are sociodemographically diverse. Thus, it is important to consider intersectional identities when assessing the coping resources of a sexual-minority man with prostate cancer.[22, 23] A couple composed of a man in his twenties or thirties who identifies as a bisexual, African American student and an older male partner who identifies as a gay, Caucasian businessman may have different experiences of coping, different degrees of interdependence, and a different set of couple-level resources than two men in their fifties with graduate-level educations who both identify as gay and Caucasian. Considering these overlapping or intersecting identities is critical when assessing or intervening to enhance communal coping, particularly given the potential influence of homonegativity (formally understood as homophobia) on coping, which may be expressed or experienced differently for sexual-minority men of color.[24, 25]

Gender has been shown to have a robust effect on coping at the individual and the couple level. Compared to heterosexual women, heterosexual men tend to rely more often on their spouses as a primary source of social support, and support from women spouses is strongly linked to health outcomes among men.[6, 26] By contrast, heterosexual women are more likely than heterosexual men to use interpersonal strategies to change their spouse's health-related behaviors, and they are also more likely to use intrapersonal, as opposed to interpersonal, coping strategies to deal with their own health-related issues.[27] Though some research literature details gender-based tendencies among same-sex couples,[28, 29] little is known about how these gender roles manifest themselves among sexual-minority men and their male partners coping with prostate cancer. In studies of same-sex male couples coping with HIV, disease-specific social support (i.e., support about HIV) was a more consistent and robust predictor of coping and health-related behavior than general emotional support.[11, 30] On the basis of existing literature, it could be hypothesized that sexual-minority men diagnosed with prostate cancer would be highly likely to rely on their partners for social support and would use interpersonal coping strategies to manage cancer-related distress. As one man stated: "I think there is much to be studied in how orthodox gender codes affect how patients discuss (or not) their cancer journey. I noticed men who adopted traditional masculine roles of stoicism and emotional guardedness missed out significantly on some of the vital tips and lessons that you pick up along [the way] about managing treatments and challenges. Most of all, communication styles (gendered in whatever way) govern how one socially navigates new identity issues around cancer, disease, and dying/surviving."

Perceptions of cancer diagnosis and treatment. To muster resources to cope with prostate cancer, partners must both perceive cancer as relevant and important to their relationship. According to our adapted model, if either partner views prostate cancer as being unimportant or nonthreatening, he may minimize the need to enact health-related behavior changes or impede his partner's efforts to cope.[31, 32] Some sexual-minority men view prostate cancer as extremely threatening, given its effect on sexual functioning. As one man stated: "You really need to take seriously the fact that many men are castrated to treat prostate cancer. Thus, the treatments can change their gender and sexual orientation." This man viewed prostate cancer as threatening not only to his health but also to his perception of his gender and sexuality. By contrast, another man noted: "I feel that my case was different from others. I am not sure why, but it might stem from the fact that I don't worry about dying, or maybe I was under the impression that the cancer was not going to be my demise." This man's perception may have influenced the coping resources he brought to bear on the cancer, and it may have influenced his responses to his partner (with whom he was living at the time of cancer treatment).

Relationship quality and communication. Each partner's emotional experience within the relationship can also influence the process of communal coping. Relationship quality is composed of a host of factors, including commitment, trust, satisfaction, and intimacy. Couples with better relationship quality, and those who have more finely honed communication skills, tend to use communal coping strategies more often and more successfully.[33]

Given that sexual-minority men may not be supported by biological family members, or may have support structures that are different from heterosexual men's, support from male partners may be even more critical to those who are in romantic relationships.[34] This phenomenon is exemplified by one participant's experience. He stated: "Since my biological family refuses to have any contact with me, it is essential to my health and survival that they [the medical team] understand that my partner IS MY FAMILY, and when they treat him as such my outcomes are much better. He is my advocate and can remember everything I can't (gotta love anesthesia). Good outcomes depend on his involvement, as does my emotional well-being."

Many sexual-minority men with prostate cancer may not be in committed romantic relationships, and so many are not be able to fully utilize communal coping. In the online study, for example, nearly 50% of the sample of men were not in a romantic relationship at the time they completed the survey. Future research could explore the influence of peers, friends, and other family members on the health outcomes of sexual-minority male cancer patients in order to identify the extent and effectiveness of their involvement. It may be that other types of relationships can provide benefits similar to the ones romantic relationships offer. Few studies have examined the quality of these non-intimate relationships, which could have important influences on the experience of sexual-minority men with prostate cancer.

Experiences of prejudice and stigma. Sexual-minority men may have experienced discrimination, prejudice, and stigma in previous experiences seeking healthcare, and these encounters may influence their willingness to seek care for prostate cancer. As one man in the online study said, when describing his relationship with his provider: "My experience with this doctor made me feel small, as if I was not worth his time or effort. This is not something that you ever want to make someone who is sick and going through surgery and radiation treatments to remove and prevent the return of cancer feel like." For a same-sex male couple, the historically stigmatized nature of sexual-minority identities and previous experiences of prejudice and discrimination in healthcare settings may also limit their ability to cope together, as prostate cancer patients may not feel comfortable bringing a partner to clinic visits or male partners may not feel comfortable participating in medical care,[35, 36] as Rose, Ussher, and Perz outline in chapter 8.[37] Attending a clinic visit as a same-sex couple can be a tacit form of disclosure and may raise fears of discrimination and prejudice once the patient's sexuality and relationship status are known.[38]

TRANSFORMATION OF MOTIVATION

Once a couple has perceived prostate cancer as affecting their conception of themselves as a couple, they must integrate thoughts about the disease into their dyadic coping strategies. In other words, following prostate cancer diagnosis, a "transformation of motivation" may occur, as partners shift their perspectives to perceive health threats (e.g., cancer diagnosis and treatment) as salient to themselves and the relationship. This transformation relies on robust communication and high levels of relationship quality factors (e.g., intimacy, commitment).[6] If such a transformation does occur, then cancer is no longer perceived to affect only the individual cancer patient, but rather the couple as a whole. The couple can then bring joint efforts to bear in tackling the threat represented by cancer.[10]

For same-sex male couples, this experience may involve new thoughts about same-sex sexuality (e.g., negotiating sexual positioning after prostatectomy).[39, 40] As one man stated: "I think we might be able to discuss more openly how sex and sensuality can be an important part of coping/healing/recovery processes. I thought this aspect was underplayed and even stigmatized in most environments, but to me it was one of the reasons I fought to survive. Sex can be a great motivator, and it can also be a great medicine."

CANCER CARE PROVISION

While early work drawing on Lewis's model focused solely on the role of each partner and the couple in coping with medical illness, our adaptation of this model recognizes the importance of the cancer provider in integrating both partners into the medical decision-making process. Studies of "triadic communication" have highlighted the ways in which cancer care providers respond to patients and caregivers, and the ways in which these responses affect care. Thus far, no studies of provider response have focused on providers working with sexual-minority men with prostate cancer and their partners. Cancer care providers must treat sexual-minority patients in a culturally competent fashion, integrate same-sex partners into treatment decision making, and facilitate same-sex couples' engagement with care.[41] In the field of HIV research, gay couples perceive that dyadic-focused care can facilitate "emotional, instrumental, and informational support" and that it can "provide a sense of togetherness" and "alleviate stress."[42]

Sexual-minority men with prostate cancer in the online study similarly highlighted the benefits of responsive providers who incorporated their partners into care. As one man stated: "My experience was a good one, but I feel that is because I have a very supportive primary care physician who referred me to the urologist he trusted. If I had not felt that both me and my partner were fully supported by the medical team, I would have immediately gone elsewhere." Several respondents referred to the importance of the prostate cancer team's recognizing and validating same-sex relationships. Given that same-sex marriage was legalized in the United States only in 2015, and in many countries is not legal at present, there is a long history of same-sex couples being invisible or made to feel less than equal in medical encounters. One man observed: "They [providers] need to be prepared that patients are going to be LGBT and that their reaction is crucial in how comfortable the patient is. In my case, a young resident seemed much more confused by my male partner than the much older doctor, who was always solicitous of my partner."

By contrast, men recognized when their partners were not being fully integrated into care: "It would have been appropriate and even comforting for more of the staff to have overtly recognized my partner as such and in general to have acknowledged my being gay." Another man stated: "It's relevant because the partner and familial relationship is important to the success of treatment. . . . When you are sick you may need your partner to hold your hand or kiss your cheek, and you don't want anyone to get upset at that to make you feel even worse." And some participants had specific recommendations for how care providers could ask about relationship partners: "Don't be afraid to ask all the same questions regarding a person's relationship status, and if the person has a partner, from that point ask all the same questions you would (what kind of work does your spouse/partner do, how long have you been together—taking an interest shows that healthcare workers don't look upon you in a different manner)."

COMMUNAL COPING

At its most basic level, according to the Adapted Interdependence Model proposed here, communal coping refers to the condition in which both members of a couple hold a mutual assessment of a health threat, as well as a common vision for combating it.[6] In addition, to enact communal coping, both partners must believe that responding jointly is beneficial, communicate with each other regarding the threat, and work together to achieve their health-related goals. Specifically for our purposes, the goal of these processes is to facilitate active use of coping resources by both partners to deal with the prostate cancer diagnosis and treatment. To the extent that same-sex male couples are able to shift perspective and providers are able to treat competently, the couple will experience "communal coping" as both support each other through the cancer experience, manage side effects of treatment, and develop a stronger and more intimate relationship, all of which ultimately lead to better health outcomes.[43] Communal coping implies that the couple believes that responding in a unified fashion is more advantageous than responding individually to cancer, that they are communicating openly about how cancer is affecting them, and that they are jointly involved in problem-solving efforts such as shared decision making regarding cancer treatment and care (detailed in chapter 20). Communal coping in same-sex male couples could influence health outcomes in several ways: through earlier and better access to care, better adherence to treatment, less psychological distress, and better immune function.[1]

In terms of earlier and better access to care, prostate cancer patients in same-sex male relationships may hesitate to seek treatment or may withhold information about their sexuality because of fear of discrimination.[38, 44] Lack of disclosure in this population has been shown to increase distress and negatively affect referrals to appropriate ancillary care and health outcomes.[45, 46] Engaging in communal coping could help reduce distress and could facilitate disclosure of sexual-minority identities to cancer care providers, particularly if a same-sex male partner accompanies a prostate cancer patient to clinic visits.

The same fear of exposure to prejudice that could limit male partners' attendance at clinic visits, however, also limits their inclusion in medical decision making and involvement in treatment adherence. Heterosexual couples often involve their partners in medical care decisions,[47] but it is unknown how frequently sexual-minority men involve their same-sex male partners in these decisions. If same-sex male partners are excluded from participation in prostate cancer care visits, they may be less aware of the treatment plan and thereby limited in their ability to support the patient's treatment adherence. Underscoring the importance of engaging both members of the couple is the fact that support from same-sex male partners has been shown to improve medication adherence in other disease contexts (e.g., antiretroviral treatment for HIV) when this support is overtly solicited.[48]

Engagement in a long-term relationship or marriage could influence better cancer-related outcomes by reducing cancer survivors' psychological distress and improving their well-being. Previous studies have shown that psychological distress is associated with a nearly twofold increase in cancer-related mortality.[49] This increased risk of mortality is particularly salient for sexual-minority individuals, who experience psychological distress at one and a half to three times higher rates than heterosexual individuals.[50, 51] Emerging evidence indicates that elevated distress is also seen among sexual-minority cancer patients,[52] as Hoyt and Millar describe in chapter 5. The literature on heterosexual and same-sex relationships consistently shows the benefits of couplehood, and marriage in particular, in reducing psychological distress.[53, 54] Same-sex male couples who are able to cope communally may experience reduced distress, which may reduce the risk of prostate cancer–related mortality.

In terms of improved immune function, data from heterosexual married couples indicate that marital relationship quality is associated with immune response.[55] For same-sex male couples, the additional factor of chronic stress owing to prejudice and discrimination may impinge on immune function.[56] Data from other minority groups have shown that exposure to prejudice and discrimination results in increased immune and physiological reactivity and increased inflammation.[57] Few studies have examined immune function among sexual-minority individuals. One study showed that exposure to prejudice increases inflammatory biomarkers,[56] whereas another showed that disclosure of sexual-minority identity improved inflammation.[58] Neither of these studies examined immune function in partnered sexual-minority men affected by prostate cancer.

CONCLUSION

The Adapted Interdependence Model provides a preliminary framework for considering the experience of same-sex male couples coping with prostate cancer. However, the tenets of this model have not been tested among men with prostate cancer, and sexual-minority men with prostate cancer specifically. Further empirical explorations, drawing on both qualitative and quantitative data, are needed to validate the adaptation of the Lewis model for this specific population. Thus, this chapter should be treated as exploratory rather than confirmatory and used as a basis for hypothesis generation.

On the basis of this preliminary outline, however, along with qualitative data from sexual-minority men with cancer, several recommendations can be made. First, there is a need for more research on the experience of same-sex male couples coping with prostate cancer.[5, 59, 60] This research should take the form of descriptive studies as well as randomized controlled trials of interventions to improve relationship quality and communal coping in this population.[61] Cancer care providers could also strive to ensure a nondiscriminatory clinical environment with culturally competent staff and providers, educated about the unique needs of sexual-minority patients, so that sexual-minority men feel comfortable in disclosing their identities and bringing their male partners into care. Integrating these male partners into cancer care decision making could improve treatment outcomes, and bolstering support between same-sex partners could reduce psychological distress and improve immune function.

Communal coping may play a role in the experience of many cancer survivors and their relationship partners. Unfortunately, little is known about how same-sex male relationships function in the context of cancer in general, and prostate cancer specifically, and so it is yet unknown how communal coping may affect sexual-minority men with prostate cancer. We hope that this chapter will spark interest in examining the process of communal coping with prostate cancer among same-sex male couples and lead to enhanced services for this underserved and underrepresented group.

ACKNOWLEDGMENTS

This research was supported by NIH grant nos. K07 CA190529, UG1 CA189961. All authors report that they have no conflicts of interest to disclose.

REFERENCES

1. Aizer AA, Chen MH, McCarthy EP, et al. Marital status and survival in patients with cancer. *Journal of Clinical Oncology.* 2013; 31 (31): 3869–3876.

2. Bare MG, Margolies L, Boehmer U. Omission of sexual and gender minority patients. *Journal of Clinical Oncology.* 2014; 32: 182–183.

3. LIVESTRONG Foundation. *Coming out with cancer.* Austin, Tex.: LIVESTRONG Foundation; 2010.

4. Gates G. *How many people are lesbian, gay, bisexual, and transgender?* Los Angeles: Williams Institute, UCLA School of Law; 2011.

5. Boehmer U, Miao X, Ozonoff A. Cancer survivorship and sexual orientation. *Cancer.* 2011; 117 (16): 3796–3804.

6. Lewis MA, McBride CM, Pollak KI, et al. Understanding health behavior change among couples: An interdependence and communal coping approach. *Social Science & Medicine.* 2006; 62 (6): 1369–1380.

7. Peplau LA, Fingerhut AW. The close relationships of lesbians and gay men. *Annual Review of Psychology.* 2007; 58: 405–424.

8. Ussher JM, Perz J, Kellett A, et al. Health-related quality of life, psychological distress, and sexual changes following prostate cancer: A comparison of gay and bisexual men with heterosexual men. *Journal of Sexual Medicine.* 2016; 13 (3): 425–434.

9. Regan TW, Lambert SD, Kelly B, et al. Couples coping with cancer: Exploration of theoretical frameworks from dyadic studies. *Psycho-Oncology.* 2015; 24 (12): 1605–1617.

10. Rusbult C, Van Lange P. Interdependence, interaction, and relationships. *Annual Review of Psychology.* 2003; 54: 351–375.

11. Darbes LA, Chakravarty D, Neilands TB, et al. Sexual risk for HIV among gay male couples: A longitudinal study of the impact of relationship dynamics. *Archives of Sexual Behavior.* 2014; 43 (1): 47–60.

12. Conroy AA, Gamarel KE, Neilands TB, et al. Relationship dynamics and partner beliefs about viral suppression: A longitudinal study of male couples living with HIV/AIDS (the Duo Project). *AIDS and Behavior.* 2016; 20 (7): 1572–1583.

13. Gamarel KE, Neilands TB, Dilworth SE, et al. Smoking, internalized heterosexism, and HIV disease management among male couples. *AIDS Care.* 2015; 27 (5): 649–654.

14. Montgomery CM, Watts C, Pool R. HIV and dyadic intervention: An interdependence and communal coping analysis. *PLoS One.* 2012; 7 (7): e40661.

15. Reczek C. The promotion of unhealthy habits in gay, lesbian, and straight intimate partnerships. *Social Science & Medicine.* 2012; 75 (6): 1114–1121.

16. Ellis KR, Janevic MR, Kershaw T, et al. The influence of dyadic symptom distress on threat appraisals and self-efficacy in advanced cancer and caregiving. *Supportive Care in Cancer.* 2017; 25 (1): 185–194.

17. Stachowski C, Stephenson R. Homophobia and communal coping for HIV risk management among gay men in relationships. *Archives of Sexual Behavior.* 2015; 44 (2): 467–474.

18. Capistrant BD, Torres B, Merengwa E, et al. Caregiving and social support for gay and bisexual men with prostate cancer. *Psycho-Oncology.* 2016; 25 (11): 1329–1336.

19. Margolies L, Scout NFN. LGBT patient-centered outcomes: Cancer survivors teach us how to improve care for all. National LGBT Cancer Network. April 2013;

https://cancer-network.org/wp-content/uploads/2017/02/lgbt-patient-centered-outcomes.pdf.

20. Kamen C, Margolies L, Smith-Stoner M, et al. *Correlates and outcomes of lesbian, gay, bisexual, and transgender (LGBT) identity disclosure to cancer care providers.* Miami: Multinational Association of Supportive Care in Cancer; 2014.

21. Kershaw T, Ellis KR, Yoon H, et al. The interdependence of advanced cancer patients' and their family caregivers' mental health, physical health, and self-efficacy over time. *Annals of Behavioral Medicine.* 2015; 49 (6): 901–911.

22. Bowleg L, Burkholder G, Teti M, Craig ML. The complexities of outness: Psychosocial predictors of coming out to others among black lesbian and bisexual women. *Journal of LGBT Health Research.* 2008; 4 (4): 153–166.

23. Bowleg L. "Once you've blended the cake, you can't take the parts back to the main ingredients": Black gay and bisexual men's descriptions and experiences of intersectionality. *Sex Roles.* 2013; 68 (11–12): 754–767.

24. Quinn K, Dickson-Gomez J, DiFranceisco W, et al. Correlates of internalized homonegativity among black men who have sex with men. *AIDS Education and Prevention* 2015; 27 (3): 212–226.

25. Quinn K, Dickson-Gomez J. Homonegativity, religiosity, and the intersecting identities of young black men who have sex with men. *AIDS and Behavior.* 2016; 20 (1): 51–64.

26. Cutrona CE. *Social support in couples: Marriage as a resource in times of stress.* Thousand Oaks, Calif.: Sage; 1996.

27. Baider L, Bengel J. Cancer and the spouse: Gender-related differences in dealing with health care and illness. *Critical Reviews in Oncology/Hematology.* 2001; 40 (2): 115–123.

28. Kornblith E, Green RJ, Casey S, Tiet Q. Marital status, social support, and depressive symptoms among lesbian and heterosexual women. *Journal of Lesbian Studies.* 2016; 20 (1): 157–173.

29. Gotta G, Green RJ, Rothblum E, et al. Heterosexual, lesbian, and gay male relationships: A comparison of couples in 1975 and 2000. *Family Process.* 2011; 50 (3): 353–376.

30. Darbes LA, Lewis MA. HIV-specific social support predicts less sexual risk behavior in gay male couples. *Health Psychology.* 2005; 24 (6): 617–622.

31. Mullens AB, McCaul KD, Erickson SC, Sandgren AK. Coping after cancer: Risk perceptions, worry, and health behaviors among colorectal cancer survivors. *Psycho-Oncology.* 2004; 13 (6): 367–376.

32. Jackson SE, Steptoe A, Wardle J. The influence of partner's behavior on health behavior change: The English Longitudinal Study of Ageing. *JAMA Internal Medicine.* 2015; 175 (3): 385–392.

33. Traa MJ, De Vries J, Bodenmann G, Den Oudsten BL. Dyadic coping and relationship functioning in couples coping with cancer: A systematic review. *Br Journal of Health Psychology.* 2015; 20 (1): 85–114.

34. Ryan C, Huebner D, Diaz RM, Sanchez J. Family rejection as a predictor of negative health outcomes in white and Latino lesbian, gay, and bisexual young adults. *Pediatrics*. 2009; 123 (1): 346–352.

35. Macapagal K, Bhatia R, Greene GJ. Differences in healthcare access, use, and experiences within a community sample of racially diverse lesbian, gay, bisexual, transgender, and questioning emerging adults. *LGBT Health*. 2016; 3 (6): 434–442.

36. Jackson CL, Agenor M, Johnson DA, et al. Sexual orientation identity disparities in health behaviors, outcomes, and services use among men and women in the United States: A cross-sectional study. *BMC Public Health*. 2016; 16 (1): 807.

37. Rose D, Ussher JM, Perz J. Let's talk about gay sex: Gay and bisexual men's sexual communication with healthcare professionals after prostate cancer. *European Journal of Cancer Care*. 2017; 26 (1).

38. Institute of Medicine. *The health of lesbian, gay, bisexual, and transgender people: Building a foundation for better understanding*. Washington, D.C.: National Academies Press; 2011.

39. Ussher JM, Perz J, Rose D, et al. Threat of sexual disqualification: The consequences of erectile dysfunction and other sexual changes for gay and bisexual men with prostate cancer. *Archives of Sexual Behavior*. 2017; 46 (7): 2043–2057.

40. Dowsett GW, Lyons A, Duncan D, Wassersug RJ. Flexibility in men's sexual practices in response to iatrogenic erectile dysfunction after prostate cancer treatment. *Sexual Medicine*. 2014; 2 (3): 115–120.

41. Brown C, Mayer DK. Are we doing enough to address the cancer care needs of the LGBT community? *Clinical Journal of Oncology Nursing*. 2015; 19 (3): 242–243.

42. Goldenberg T, Stephenson R. "The more support you have the better": Partner support and dyadic HIV care across the continuum for gay and bisexual men. *Journal of Acquired Immune Deficiency Syndromes*. 2015; 69 (Suppl. 1): S73–79.

43. Saita E, Acquati C, Molgora S. Promoting patient and caregiver engagement to care in cancer. *Frontiers in Psychology*. 2016; 7: 1660.

44. Boehmer U, Case P. Physicians don't ask, sometimes patients tell: Disclosure of sexual orientation among women with breast carcinoma. *Cancer*. 2004; 101 (8): 1882–1889.

45. Boehmer U, Freund KM, Linde R. Support providers of sexual minority women with breast cancer: Who they are and how they impact the breast cancer experience. *Journal of Psychosomatic Research*. 2005; 59 (5): 307–314.

46. Durso LE, Meyer IH. Patterns and predictors of disclosure of sexual orientation to healthcare providers among lesbians, gay men, and bisexuals. *Sexuality Research and Social Policy*. 2013; 10 (1): 35–42.

47. Volk RJ, Cantor SB, Cass AR, et al. Preferences of husbands and wives for outcomes of prostate cancer screening and treatment. *Journal of General Internal Medicine*. 2004; 19 (4): 339–348.

48. Johnson MO, Dilworth SE, Taylor JM, et al. Primary relationships, HIV treatment adherence, and virologic control. *AIDS and Behavior.* 2012; 16 (6): 1511–1521.

49. Hamer M, Chida Y, Molloy GJ. Psychological distress and cancer mortality. *Journal of Psychosomatic Research.* 2009; 66 (3): 255–258.

50. Meyer IH. Prejudice, social stress, and mental health in lesbian, gay, and bisexual populations: Conceptual issues and research evidence. *Psychological Bulletin.* 2003; 129 (5): 674–697.

51. Cochran SD, Mays VM, Sullivan JG. Prevalence of mental disorders, psychological distress, and mental health services use among lesbian, gay, and bisexual adults in the United States. *Journal of Consulting and Clinical Psychology.* 2003; 71 (1): 53–61.

52. Kamen C, Mustian KM, Dozier A, et al. Disparities in psychological distress impacting lesbian, gay, bisexual and transgender cancer survivors. *Psycho-Oncology.* 2015; 24 (11): 1384–1391.

53. Lick DJ, Durso LE, Johnson KL. Minority stress and physical health among sexual minorities. *Perspectives in Psychological Science.* 2013; 8 (5): 521–548.

54. Hatzenbuehler ML, McLaughlin KA, Keyes KM, Hasin DS. The impact of institutional discrimination on psychiatric disorders in lesbian, gay, and bisexual populations: A prospective study. *American Journal of Public Health.* 2010; 100 (3): 452–459.

55. Jaremka LM, Glaser R, Malarkey WB, Kiecolt-Glaser JK. Marital distress prospectively predicts poorer cellular immune function. *Psychoneuroendocrinology.* 2013; 38 (11): 2713–2719.

56. Hatzenbuehler ML, McLaughlin KA. Structural stigma and hypothalamic-pituitary-adrenocortical axis reactivity in lesbian, gay, and bisexual young adults. *Annals of Behavioral Medicine.* 2014; 47 (1): 39–47.

57. Cunningham TJ, Seeman TE, Kawachi I, et al. Racial/ethnic and gender differences in the association between self-reported experiences of racial/ethnic discrimination and inflammation in the CARDIA cohort of 4 US communities. *Social Science & Medicine.* 2012; 75 (5): 922–931.

58. Juster RP, Smith NG, Ouellet E, et al. Sexual orientation and disclosure in relation to psychiatric symptoms, diurnal cortisol, and allostatic load. *Psychosomatic Medicine.* 2013; 75 (2): 103–116.

59. Boehmer U, Miao X, Ozonoff A. Health behaviors of cancer survivors of different sexual orientations. *Cancer Causes & Control.* 2012; 23 (9): 1489–1496.

60. Kamen C, Palesh O, Andrykowski M, et al. Disparities in physical health concerns among lesbian, gay, bisexual and transgender (LGBT) cancer survivors. *Psychosomatic Medicine.* 2014; 76 (3): A101.

61. White JL, Boehmer U. Long-term breast cancer survivors' perceptions of support from female partners: An exploratory study. *Oncology Nursing Forum.* 2012; 39 (2): 210–217.

CHAPTER 5

Psychological Adjustment in Gay and Bisexual Men after Prostate Cancer

Michael A. Hoyt and Brett M. Millar

CHAPTER SUMMARY

The experience of prostate cancer can exact a psychological and physical toll. Gay and bisexual men (GBM) have been underrepresented in prostate cancer care and research and represent a subpopulation at high risk for poorer health-related quality of life and psychological adjustment following diagnosis. The physical and psychological demands of prostate cancer present new circumstances to which patients and loved ones must adjust, and GBM disproportionately experience risk factors for impaired physical and emotional functioning, including general and minority-related stressors, unmet healthcare needs, and social isolation. Psychological adjustment to chronic disease is a complex and multidimensional process that constitutes more than merely the absence of psychopathology and includes both positive and negative domains. Theories of stress and coping, self-regulation, and personal growth have informed the understanding of the dynamics of psychological adjustment and its determinants. These, coupled with considerations of the unique risk and resilience factors experienced by GBM, will inform a more inclusive model of psychological adjustment to prostate cancer. This chapter integrates existing theories of psychological adjustment to chronic illness with theories of minority stress and observations from focus groups comprising GBM with prostate cancer to identify influences on adjustment across the cancer trajectory.

KEY TERMS

gay and bisexual men, minority stress, prostate cancer, psychological adjustment, sexuality

Ussher, Jane M., Perz, Janette, Rosser, B. R. Simon, eds., *Gay & Bisexual Men Living with Prostate Cancer*
dx.doi.org/10.17312/harringtonparkpress/2018.06.gbmlpc.005
© 2018 Harrington Park Press

INTRODUCTION

Most treatments for prostate cancer carry the risk of side effects, including urinary and bowel incontinence, erectile dysfunction, and fatigue.[1] Profound health threat and such physical changes can confer substantial psychosocial effects, particularly when severe or persistent.[2] Survivorship often involves navigating numerous and overlapping challenges across life domains over a course of time that could range from several years to several decades. Because the preponderance of existing research has focused on heterosexual men, this chapter aims to explore the unique aspects of these challenges for gay and bisexual men (GBM). Although disparities have been documented for sexual minorities regarding cancer risk factors (e.g., smoking, lower likelihood of cancer screening),[3-5] research about disparities in psychological adjustment to prostate cancer has been scant.[6, 7] We offer a brief synthesis of models of psychological adjustment, unique experiences of minority stress, and unique concerns for GBM who have experienced prostate cancer, in order to establish a research agenda to better understand adjustment and its determinants.

UNDERSTANDING GAY AND BISEXUAL MEN'S PSYCHOLOGICAL ADJUSTMENT TO PROSTATE CANCER

Psychological adjustment to cancer has been conceptualized in several ways, including the successful negotiation of cancer-related adaptive tasks, the presence or absence of psychological disorder, experiences of psychological distress, and performance in functional roles.[8, 9] For various reasons, gay and bisexual cancer survivors are at heightened risk for poor adjustment; however, little research has documented cancer-related adjustment in GBM.

Epidemiological surveys have established that GBM are more likely to suffer from stress-sensitive mental health disorders—namely, depression and anxiety—than the general population.[10, 11] Sexual-minority survivors across cancer types tend to report more depression, distress, and relationship difficulties after cancer than do heterosexual survivors.[4, 12] A preliminary report of a small ($N = 92$) sample of sexual-minority men with prostate cancer showed lower health-related quality of life (HRQOL) than published norms in general samples, particularly with regard to mental health and sexual function.[13] An Australian study of gay, bisexual, and heterosexual men with prostate cancer reported similar disparities with regard to sexual functioning, higher distress, and lower treatment satisfaction.[14] Both studies point to ejaculatory bother as a particular concern, a finding that highlights the likelihood that GBM have unique priorities and concerns regarding loss of sexual function. For instance, one widely used benchmark in medical care for sufficient erectile functioning is the ability to perform vaginal intercourse. GBM who prefer insertive anal intercourse, however, may need stronger erectile functioning, whereas anal sensitivity and bowel functioning might be a greater concern for the receptive partner.[15]

Some preliminary reports suggest that sexual side effects affect GBM differently after prostate cancer surgery, as outlined by chapters 2, 3, and 6 in this book. In summary, compared to heterosexual patients, GBM report worse sexual bother, ejaculatory dysfunction, and ejaculatory bother.[13, 14, 16] Medical school curricula rarely include training in sexuality and sexual health,[17] particularly among sexual minorities.[18] Thus, limited knowledge and cultural competency among healthcare providers about sexual activity within this population during treatment decision making and symptom management may be particularly damaging to the adjustment of GBM to prostate cancer.

Interrelated contexts (e.g., disease, individual differences, macro-level and interpersonal factors) on coping processes and long-term trajectories of adjustment and quality of life are potent influences on adjustment (see figure 5.1). These include economic, gender-related, cancer-specific, and individual factors.[9, 19] Sexual minorities disproportionately experience contexts of risk, and therefore the integration of traditional models of cancer adjustment with conceptualizations of the unique experience of sexual-minority stress might yield a more comprehensive model of psychological adjustment to prostate cancer for GBM.

Minority stress theory posits that, compared to heterosexuals, gender and sexual minorities experience unique forms of social stress stemming from their devalued and stigmatized social status.[11] Early life experiences, chronic life stressors, and disproportionate experiences with discrimination and rejection increase vulnerability to diminished adjustment and are associated with health disparities across the life span.[20] The cumulative stress response manifests as sensitivity to future threats, internalization of negative societal attitudes,[21] concealment of sexual identity and behavior,[22] and self-consciousness about one's self-presentation or conformity to gender norms.[23] Research with noncancer samples of sexual-minority men has demonstrated that minority stress, in its many forms, is associated with indicators of poor HRQOL, mental and physical health problems,[24, 25] and elevated rates of substance

FIGURE 5.1 Contributors to adjustment to prostate cancer for GBM

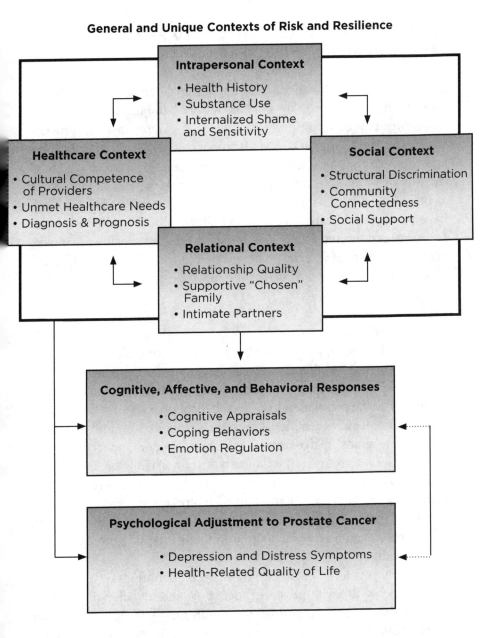

General and Unique Contexts of Risk and Resilience

Intrapersonal Context
- Health History
- Substance Use
- Internalized Shame and Sensitivity

Healthcare Context
- Cultural Competence of Providers
- Unmet Healthcare Needs
- Diagnosis & Prognosis

Social Context
- Structural Discrimination
- Community Connectedness
- Social Support

Relational Context
- Relationship Quality
- Supportive "Chosen" Family
- Intimate Partners

Cognitive, Affective, and Behavioral Responses
- Cognitive Appraisals
- Coping Behaviors
- Emotion Regulation

Psychological Adjustment to Prostate Cancer
- Depression and Distress Symptoms
- Health-Related Quality of Life

use.[26] Such minority stress factors might contribute to specific vulnerability to poor adjustment in GBM with prostate cancer.

CONTRIBUTORS TO ADJUSTMENT TO PROSTATE CANCER FOR GAY AND BISEXUAL MEN

The contributions of demographic, clinical, personality, social, and cognitive-behavioral factors (including coping) in determining adjustment are well established.[8, 9] However, there may be additional considerations that account for compromised adjustment in gay and bisexual prostate cancer survivors. Notably, GBM disproportionately experience risk factors for declining adjustment (which we discuss below). They are at increased risk for experiencing health-damaging social conditions such as prejudice, stigma, violence, and discrimination,[11 - 27] and they tend to have poorer healthcare access, lower likelihood of health insurance coverage, and limited access to culturally competent healthcare providers.[28] Thus, a set of interrelated contexts (i.e., social, relational, health are) exerts influence on adjustment to prostate cancer.

THE SOCIAL CONTEXT

Social systems and interpersonal support networks are powerful contributors to adjustment. Institutionalized (or structural) discrimination in the practices and policies that restrict employment, education, and other healthcare opportunities produces negative health outcomes and ultimately, at the population level, health disparities.[29, 30] Discrimination can produce negative emotional and stress responses[31, 32] and negatively influence relationship dynamics.[33, 34] A lack of support and receptiveness in the social environment (i.e., social constraints) contributes to diminished coping efficacy in cancer patients.[35] Such social stressors may infringe on optimal coping and diminish physical and emotional functioning of gay and bisexual patients. Therefore, understanding the role of support systems and how to appropriately integrate them into care is paramount.

Community-level resources have been identified as particularly important to GBM with prostate cancer.[36] A sense of belonging and the ability to depend on a supportive community may be critical to the health and adjustment of sexual minorities.[11, 37] Connectedness to a sexual-minority community can mitigate the negative effects of minority stress on health.[38] As a result of discrimination and rejection by families of origin, community connectedness may be a group-level coping resource in counteracting the negative effects of social stressors for many GBM.[11, 39, 40] Yet research illustrates that GBM are more likely to be single, report insufficient social support, and experience higher levels of social isolation than their heterosexual counterparts.[28, 41]

THE RELATIONAL CONTEXT

Research and practice have suggested the important role of spouses in heterosexual men's adjustment to prostate cancer.[42, 43] However, little work has characterized the dynamics of community and dyadic support transactions among GBM with chronic illness.[44] Discriminatory policies and negative prejudices surrounding same-sex relationships affect GBM's mental health,[45] as well as their experiences *within* relationships.[46]

At the same time, many studies have demonstrated the beneficial effects of supportive environments, including support from family members and intimate romantic partners, when facing a chronic illness.[47] However, traditional romantic partnering should not be assumed in gay and bisexual prostate cancer patients. Friends are equally likely to be primary caregivers following chronic illness for LGBT persons.[48] Whereas heterosexual men are more likely to rely on a spouse and biological family in the provision of caregiving and support after cancer, GBM are more likely to be single and rely on friends and "chosen" family.[41, 49]

THE HEALTHCARE CONTEXT

GBM disproportionately experience healthcare barriers and unmet needs that influence their adjustment to chronic conditions.[28, 50] Sexual minorities report experiencing refusal of treatment by healthcare providers, verbal abuse, and disrespectful behaviors, as well as other forms of failure to provide adequate and culturally competent care,[18, 51] as Rose and colleagues outline in chapter 8 in this book. As a result of internalized, interpersonal, and structural stigma and discrimination, GBM tend to report lower satisfaction with care and greater discomfort with disclosing their sexual orientation to providers,[52] including cancer care providers.[53, 54] In fact, only 68% of GBM prostate cancer survivors in a recent study were out to their cancer specialists.[55] Notably, disclosure of sexual orientation to cancer care providers is associated with better overall perceptions of one's own health.[54]

GBM face particular challenges to accessing adequate provision of prostate-related healthcare. Focus group data suggest that GBM have limited understanding of their prostate and the range of sexual challenges associated with differing prostate cancer treatments.[56] Also, GBM may have different priorities and concerns regarding loss of sexual function. In our own focus group work, one participant reported, "Being a top [i.e., the insertive partner] was part of my identity, and not being able to satisfy in that way really messed up my sense of who I was."[36] Additionally, optimal cancer care for GBM may need to be cognizant of other health challenges that are elevated in this population, such as HIV,[57] mental health problems, and substance use.[26] Such medical and physical comorbidities probably intersect with prostate cancer – specific difficulties, further affecting adjustment.

DIRECTIONS FOR RESEARCH

Cancer care professionals have identified the critical need for more research to understand and address the needs and concerns of LGBT survivors across the survivorship continuum.[58] There is much to learn about psychological adjustment to prostate cancer among sexual minorities. Longitudinal epidemiological data across multiple indicators of adjustment among gay and bisexual survivors are necessary to plotting adjustment trajectories. Further, studies that elucidate the unique contributions of connectedness to the LGBT community, dyadic coping processes within same-sex romantic and platonic relationships, experiences of systemic discrimination, and receipt of culturally competent prostate cancer care on coping and adjustment will provide opportunities to improve adjustment over time.

Given that many GBM experience prolonged minority stress in addition to general life stress, researchers should explore the synergistic consequences on cancer adjustment. For instance, cancer-related stressors (e.g., low satisfaction with care) may interact synergistically with minority stress processes (e.g., chronic experiences of discrimination) to affect adjustment negatively. Research that moves beyond betweengroup differences and examines how culturally relevant within-group processes affect adjustment will probably make the strongest contribution. For instance, understanding the pathways by which minority stress factors lead to declines in adjustment would serve to identify useful targets for intervention programs for GBM with prostate cancer. Further, managing multiple devalued identities (e.g., sexual *and* racial minority identities) exerts a compounded burden on well-being.[30, 31] However, no one has yet examined this possibility in the context of prostate cancer or related disease models.

A promising research direction includes exploring the potential of minority stress and poor prostate cancer adjustment to confer biological risk and influence progression of the disease. Prolonged exposure to social stressors, such as minority stress, fosters patterned dysregulation of pro-inflammatory activity through epigenetic markings.[59] Early work examining the biological effect of gay-related stressors revealed disclosure of sexual orientation to be associated with lower incidence of cancer and infectious disease.[60] In fact, chronic elevations in the inflammatory response associated with gay-related social stress has been identified as a likely mechanism of physical health disparities between gay and heterosexual groups.[3, 61] Elevations in pro-inflammatory biomarkers among heterosexual men have been documented.[62] Doyle and Molix identified a positive association of minority stress and biological markers of inflammation among GBM who had disclosed their sexual orientation, which suggests that minority stress might "get under the skin" and affect physical and mental well-being.[63] It will be important for exploratory work to comprehensively assess biobehavioral processes to more precisely target relevant, malleable, individual-level factors to influence behavioral responses.

Evidence supports the efficacy of psychosocial interventions for prostate cancer patients. These cover a broad spectrum of approaches and include the testing of decision aids for treatment selection,[64] cognitive-behavioral stress management interventions for HRQOL and distress,[65] couples-based supportive counseling,[66] individual psychotherapy for depression,[67] and targeted approaches to enhance coping with sexual changes.[68] Yet no intervention trial has specifically considered the needs, priorities, or concerns of GBM with prostate cancer.

Interventions are needed that account for the differing priorities of GBM in selecting medical treatment, understanding their distinct information and support needs (within and apart from the healthcare delivery system), understanding their unique internalization of sexual and other bodily changes, and identifying particular factors of resilience (such as harnessing support from one's chosen family and wider community). Identification of these factors across the disease trajectory provides opportunities for the development of new interventions and, more important, the tailoring of currently available intervention approaches. Interventions that are equipped to promote culturally competent care, identify GBM at risk for poor outcomes, foster informed medical decision making, mitigate the effect of minority stress factors, address relationship and intimacy needs, and provide individual- and community-level support will make the greatest contribution to improving adjustment in GBM living with, and living beyond, prostate cancer.

REFERENCES

1. Latini DM, Hart SL, Coon DW, Knight SJ. Sexual rehabilitation after localized prostate cancer: Current interventions and future directions. *Cancer.* 2009; 15 (1): 34–40.

2. Gore JL, Kwan L, Lee SP, et al. Survivorship beyond convalescence: 48-month quality-of-life outcomes after treatment for localized prostate cancer. *Journal of the National Cancer Institute.* 2009; 101 (12): 888–892.

3. Conron KJ, Mimiaga MJ, Landers SJ. A population-based study of sexual orientation identity and gender differences in adult health. *American Journal of Public Health.* 2010; 100 (10): 1953–1960.

4. Kamen C, Palesh O, Gerry AA, et al. Disparities in health risk behavior and psychological distress among gay versus heterosexual male cancer survivors. *LGBT Health.* 2014; 1 (2): 86–92.

5. Tang H, Greenwood GL, Cowling DW, et al. Cigarette smoking among lesbians, gays, and bisexuals: How serious a problem? (United States). *Cancer Causes and Control.* 2004; 15 (8): 797–803.

6. Blank TO. Gay men and prostate cancer: Invisible diversity. *Journal of Clinical Oncology.* 2005; 23 (12): 2593–2596.

7. Kleinmann N, Zaorsky NG, Showalter TN, et al. The effect of ethnicity and sexual preference on prostate-cancer-related quality of life. *Nature Reviews Urology.* 2012; 9 (5): 258–265.

8. Helgeson VS, Zajdel M. Adjusting to chronic health conditions. *Annual Review of Psychology.* 2017; 68: 545–571.

9. Hoyt MA, Stanton AL. Adjustment to chronic illness. In Baum AS, Revenson TA, Singer, JE, eds. *Handbook of health psychology,* 2nd ed. New York: Taylor & Francis; 2012: 219–246.

10. Cochran SD, Mays VM. Burden of psychiatric morbidity among lesbian, gay, and bisexual individuals in the California Quality of Life Survey. *Journal of Abnormal Psychology.* 2009; 118 (3): 647–658.

11. Meyer IH. Prejudice, social stress, and mental health in lesbian, gay, and bisexual populations: Conceptual issues and research evidence. *Psychological Bulletin.* 2003; 129 (5): 674–697.

12. Kamen C, Mustian KM, Dozier A, et al. Disparities in psychological distress impacting lesbian, gay, bisexual and transgender cancer survivors. *Psycho-Oncology.* 2015; 24 (11): 1384–1391.

13. Hart TL, Coon DW, Kowalkowski MA, et al. Changes in sexual roles and quality

of life for gay men after prostate cancer: Challenges for sexual health providers. *Journal of Sexual Medicine.* 2014; 11 (9): 2308–2317.

14. Ussher JM, Perz J, Kellett A, et al. Health-related quality of life, psychological distress, and sexual changes following prostate cancer: A comparison of gay and bisexual men with heterosexual men. *Journal of Sexual Medicine.* 2016; 13 (3): 425–434.

15. Gebert S. Are penile prostheses a viable option to recommend for gay men? *International Journal of Urological Nursing.* 2014; 8: 111–113.

16. Wassersug RJ, Lyons A, Duncan D, et al. Diagnostic and outcome differences between heterosexual and nonheterosexual men treated for prostate cancer. *Urology.* 2013; 82: 565–571.

17. Malhotra S, Khurshid A, Hendricks KA, Mann JR. Medical school sexual health curriculum and training in the United States. *Journal of the National Medical Association.* 2008; 100 (9): 1097–1106.

18. Graham R, Berkowitz B, Blum R, et al. *The health of lesbian, gay, bisexual, and transgender people: Building a foundation for better understanding.* Washington, D.C.: Institute of Medicine; 2011.

19. Stanton AL, Rowland JH, Ganz PA. Life after diagnosis and treatment of cancer in adulthood: Contributions from psychosocial oncology research. *American Psychologist.* 2015; 70 (2): 159–174.

20. McLaughlin KA, Hatzenbuehler ML, Keyes KM. Responses to discrimination and psychiatric disorders among black, Hispanic, female, and lesbian, gay, and bisexual individuals. *American Journal of Public Health.* 2010; 100 (8): 1477–1484.

21. Meyer IH. Minority stress and mental health in gay men. *Journal of Health and Social Behavior.* 1995; 38–56.

22. Pachankis JE. The psychological implications of concealing a stigma: A cognitive-affective-behavioral model. *Psychological Bulletin.* 2007; 133 (2): 328–345.

23. Pachankis JE, Westmaas JL, Dougherty LR. The influence of sexual orientation and masculinity on young men's tobacco smoking. *Journal of Consulting and Clinical Psychology.* 2011; 79 (2): 142–152.

24. Frost DM, Lehavot K, Meyer IH. Minority stress and physical health among sexual minority individuals. *Journal of Behavioral Medicine.* 2015; 38 (1): 1–8.

25. Hatzenbuehler ML, Nolen-Hoeksema S, Erickson SJ. Minority stress predictors of HIV risk behavior, substance use, and depressive symptoms: Results from a prospective study of bereaved gay men. *Health Psychology.* 2008; 27 (4): 455–462.

26. Corliss HL, Rosario M, Wypij D, et al. Sexual orientation disparities in longitudinal alcohol use patterns among adolescents: Findings from the Growing Up Today Study. *Archives of Pediatrics & Adolescent Medicine.* 2008; 162 (11): 1071–1078.

27. Herek G. Sexual prejudice. In Nelson T, ed. *Handbook of prejudice: stereotyping and discrimination.* New York: Psychology Press; 2009.

28. Frazer S. *LGBT health and human services needs in New York State.* Albany: Empire State Pride Agenda Foundation; 2009.

29. Cutrona CE, Russell DW, Abraham WT, et al. Neighborhood context and financial strain as predictors of marital interaction and marital quality in African American couples. *Personal Relationships.* 2003; 10 (3): 389–409.

30. Diaz RM, Ayala G, Bein E, et al. The impact of homophobia, poverty, and racism on the mental health of gay and bisexual Latino men: Findings from 3 US cities. *American Journal of Public Health.* 2001; 91 (6): 927–932.

31. Gamarel KE, Reisner SL, Parsons JT, Golub SA. Association between socioeconomic position discrimination and psychological distress: Findings from a community-based sample of gay and bisexual men in New York City. *American Journal of Public Health.* 2012; 102 (11): 2094–2101.

32. Williams DR, Neighbors HW, Jackson JS. Racial/ethnic discrimination and health: Findings from community studies. *American Journal of Public Health.* 2003; 93 (2): 200–208.

33. Meyer IH, Dean L. Internalized homophobia, intimacy, and sexual behavior among gay and bisexual men. In Greene B, Herek GM, eds. *Stigma and sexual orientation: Understanding prejudice against lesbians, gay men, and bisexuals.* Thousand Oaks, Calif.: Sage; 1998: 160–186.

34. Mohr JJ, Fassinger RE. Sexual orientation identity and romantic relationship quality in same-sex couples. *Personality and Social Psychology Bulletin.* 2006; 32 (8): 1085–1099.

35. Lepore SJ, Revenson TA. Social constraints on disclosure and adjustment to cancer. *Social and Personality Psychology Compass.* 2007; 1 (1): 313–333.

36. Hoyt MA, Frost DM, Cohn E, et al. Gay men's experiences with prostate cancer: Implications for future research. *Journal of Health Psychology.* 2017; doi: 10.1177/1359105317711491.

37. Kertzner RM, Meyer IH, Frost DM, Stirratt MJ. Social and psychological well-being in lesbians, gay men, and bisexuals: The effects of race, gender, age, and sexual identity. *American Journal of Orthopsychiatry.* 2009; 79 (4): 500–510.

38. Frost DM, Meyer IH. Measuring community connectedness among diverse sexual minority populations. *Journal of Sex Research.* 2012; 49 (1): 36–49.

39. Crocker J, Major B. Social stigma and self-esteem: The self-protective properties of stigma. *Psychological Review.* 1989; 96 (4): 608–630.

40. Major B, O'Brien LT. The social psychology of stigma. *Annual Review of Psychology.* 2005; 56: 393–421.

41. Capistrant BD, Torres B, Merengwa E, et al. Caregiving and social support for gay and bisexual men with prostate cancer. *Psycho-Oncology.* 2016; 25 (11): 1329–1336.

42. Kershaw TS, Mood DW, Newth G, et al. Longitudinal analysis of a model to predict quality of life in prostate cancer patients and their spouses. *Annals of Behavioral Medicine.* 2008; 36 (2): 117–128.

43. Song L, Northouse LL, Zhang L, et al. Study of dyadic communication in couples managing prostate cancer: A longitudinal perspective. *Psycho-Oncology.* 2012; 21 (1): 72–81.

44. Gamarel KE, Revenson TA. Dyadic adaptation to chronic illness: The importance of considering context in understanding couples' resilience. *In* Skerrett K, Fergus K, eds. *Couple Resilience*. Dordrecht: Springer; 2015: 83–105.

45. Hatzenbuehler ML, McLaughlin KA, Keyes KM, Hasin DS. The impact of institutional discrimination on psychiatric disorders in lesbian, gay, and bisexual populations: A prospective study. *American Journal of Public Health*. 2010; 100 (3): 452–459.

46. Frost DM, Meyer IH. Internalized homophobia and relationship quality among lesbians, gay men, and bisexuals. *Journal of Counseling Psychology*. 2009; 26: 97–109.

47. Revenson TA, DeLongis A. Couples coping with chronic illness. *In* S. Folkman, ed. *The Oxford handbook of stress, health, and coping*. New York: Oxford University Press; 2011: 101–123.

48. Fredriksen-Goldsen KI, Kim H-J, Muraco A, Mincer S. Chronically ill midlife and older lesbians, gay men, and bisexuals and their informal caregivers: The impact of the social context. *Sexuality Research and Social Policy*. 2009; 6 (4): 52–64.

49. Arena PL, Carver CS, Antoni MH, et al. Psychosocial responses to treatment for breast cancer among lesbian and heterosexual women. *Women & Health*. 2007; 44 (2): 81–102.

50. Jowett A, Peel E. Chronic illness in non-heterosexual contexts: An online survey of experiences. *Feminism & Psychology*. 2009; 19 (4): 454–474.

51. Quinn GP, Sanchez JA, Sutton SK, et al. Cancer and lesbian, gay, bisexual, transgender/transsexual, and queer/questioning (LGBTQ) populations. *CA: A Cancer Journal for Clinicians*. 2015; 65 (5): 384–400.

52. Bernstein KT, Liu KL, Begier EM, et al. Same-sex attraction disclosure to health care providers among New York City men who have sex with men: Implications for HIV testing approaches. *Archives of Internal Medicine*. 2008; 168: 1458–1464.

53. Katz A. Gay and lesbian patients with cancer. *Oncology Nursing Forum*. 2009; 36 (2): 203–207.

54. Kamen CS, Smith-Stoner M, Heckler CE, et al. Social support, self-rated health, and lesbian, gay, bisexual, and transgender identity disclosure to cancer care providers. *Oncology Nursing Forum*. 2015; 42 (1): 44–51.

55. Rosser BRS, Konety BR, Mitteldorf D, et al. What gay and bisexual men treated for prostate cancer are offered and attempt as sexual rehabilitation for prostate cancer: Quantitative results from the Restore study with implications for clinicians. *Urology Practice*. 2017; http://doi.org/a0.a016/j.urpr.2017.04.002.

56. Asencio M, Blank T, Descartes L, Crawford A. The prospect of prostate cancer: A challenge for gay men's sexualities as they age. *Sexuality Research and Social Policy*. 2009; 6 (4): 38–51.

57. Centers for Disease Control and Prevention. HIV among gay and bisexual men: CDC factsheet. 2015; https://www.cdc.gov/nchhstp/newsroom/docs/factsheets/cdc-msm-508.pdf.

58. Burkhalter JE, Margolies L, Sigurdsson HO, et al. The National LGBT Cancer

Action Plan: A white paper of the 2014 National Summit on Cancer in the LGBT Communities. *LGBT Health.* 2016; 3 (1): 19–31.

59. Miller GE, Chen E, Parker KJ. Psychological stress in childhood and susceptibility to the chronic diseases of aging: Moving toward a model of behavioral and biological mechanisms. *Psychological Bulletin.* 2011; 137 (6): 959–997.

60. Cole SW, Kemeny ME, Taylor SE, Visscher BR. Elevated physical health risk among gay men who conceal their homosexual identity. *Health Psychology.* 1996; 15 (4): 243–251.

61. Sandfort TG, Bakker F, Schellevis FG, Vanwesenbeeck I. Sexual orientation and mental and physical health status: Findings from a Dutch population survey. *American Journal of Public Health.* 2006; 96 (6): 1119–1125.

62. Everett BG, Rosario M, McLaughlin KA, Austin SB. Sexual orientation and gender differences in markers of inflammation and immune functioning. *Annals of Behavioral Medicine.* 2014; 47 (1): 57–70.

63. Doyle DM, Molix L. Minority stress and inflammatory mediators: Covering moderate associations between perceived discrimination and salivary interleukin-6 in gay men. *Journal of Behavioral Medicine.* 2016; 39 (5): 782–792.

64. Diefenbach MA, Mohamed NE, Butz BP, et al. Acceptability and preliminary feasibility of an Internet/CD-ROM-based education and decision program for early-stage prostate cancer patients: Randomized pilot study. *Journal of Medical Internet Research.* 2012; 14 (1): e6.

65. Penedo FJ, Molton I, Dahn JR, et al. A randomized clinical trial of group-based cognitive-behavioral stress management in localized prostate cancer: Development of stress management skills improves quality of life and benefit finding. *Annals of Behavioral Medicine.* 2006; 31 (3): 261–270.

66. Manne SL, Kissane DW, Nelson CJ, et al. Intimacy-enhancing psychological intervention for men diagnosed with prostate cancer and their partners: A pilot study. *Journal of Sexual Medicine.* 2011; 8 (4): 1197–1209.

67. Hart SL, Hoyt MA, Diefenbach M, et al. Meta-analysis of efficacy of interventions for elevated depressive symptoms in adults diagnosed with cancer. *Journal of the National Cancer Institute.* 2012; 104 (13): 990–1004.

68. Chisholm KE, McCabe MP, Wootten AC, Abbott JAM. Review: Psychosocial interventions addressing sexual or relationship functioning in men with prostate cancer. *Journal of Sexual Medicine.* 2012; 9 (5): 1246–1260.

CHAPTER 6

The Social Dimensions of Prostate Cancer in Gay Men's Sexuality

Gary W. Dowsett, Duane Duncan, Andrea Waling, Daniel R. du Plooy, and Garrett P. Prestage

CHAPTER SUMMARY

Much of the research on men and prostate cancer has neglected gay and bisexual men. Assumptions are made that gay men are men too, so they must have the same experiences as heterosexual men. Recent research, however, has shown marked differences between gay and bisexual men and heterosexual men in diagnosis, treatment, care, and support. This chapter considers the recent research that is beginning to understand gay men's different experiences of prostate cancer diagnosis and treatment, arguing that a focus on the social dimensions of gay men's sexuality is needed. Three issues are explored: gay sex and sexuality, gay relationships and gay community, and HIV infection.

KEY TERMS

gay community, gay men, gay relationships, HIV infection, sex, sex-based sociality, sexuality

INTRODUCTION

It has been suggested that living with any life-threatening illness is akin to living in a liminal space—always being on the threshold of whatever might happen next.[1] *Being* is the key word here: liminality is an existential space, an interiority. In this chapter we explore this liminal space for gay men as they cope with prostate cancer, not just as an individual experience but also as one with profound *social* dimensions. Perlman and Drescher, in a seminal volume of essays published in 2005, were the first to flag gay men's different experiences of prostate cancer.[2] At the same moment, Blank termed gay men an "invisible diversity" in prostate cancer as a medical and health field.[3] Jump to the present, and

Ussher, Jane M., Perz, Janette, Rosser, B. R. Simon, eds., *Gay & Bisexual Men Living with Prostate Cancer*
dx.doi.org/10.17312/harringtonparkpress/2018.06.gbmlpc.006
© 2018 Harrington Park Press

a recent qualitative study reported a number of current and specific concerns for gay men with prostate cancer that echo Perlman and Drescher and Blank.[4] These concerns are confirmed in recent reviews of the literature in the field (see chapter 1).

There is a hint of this liminality in the terms *survivor* and *survivorship* (basically, the person and the process), often widely used in referring to cancer. Prostate cancer is no different. The terms, however, are not liked by everyone and are resisted (see chapter 16).[5] These are not just terms; they are discursive framings of experience.[6] They can sometimes affect outcomes.[7] Many men with prostate cancer may be asymptomatic, remain undiagnosed, and die of other causes. These men are not the focus of this chapter. For other men, prostate cancer involves regular monitoring for disease progression. This monitoring is termed *active surveillance* or *watchful waiting*. The first is a technical, clinical term—it sounds professional, efficient, managed; the second implies, at the least, concern, apprehension, caution—the liminality noted earlier. If treatment intervention is undertaken and is effective, many men may be deemed, at some point, cured: cancer never returns, or it has no or little effect if it does return later in life. *Cured* is also a discursive framing of experience; it is a loaded emotive term, not just a fact, even if it is assessed objectively on various measures (e.g., five- or ten-year time frames) through regular disease recurrence monitoring (e.g., prostate-specific antigen [PSA] tests) or subjectively by getting on with life. Yet, as one participant in a study we outline later in this chapter noted: "According to my specialist, they got everything so there's nothing there to worry about, but it still sits in the back of my mind, you know. Is there another, is there another little piece that's gonna flare up?" This *fear of recurrence* is a constituent of liminality, driving anxiety, a daily looking over the shoulder. For many other men, diagnosis and treatment of prostate cancer lead to lifelong side effects of mild to major magnitude, particularly with respect to sexuality, but not disease progression. There are others for whom progression occurs and is likely to contribute to a death rate in men that is slightly greater than for women with breast cancer in Australia.

It is these diagnosed men we prefer to say are "living with prostate cancer." For these men, prostate cancer is an ongoing reality: something they monitor (active surveillance), something with early side effects (difficulty urinating), something awaiting treatment, something whose treatment side effects they fear. It is something they learn to manage during treatment and recovery, something they fear recurring even when "cured." It is something that others start to experience and ask about, something that may become part of their work—for example, in research (as is the case with a number of authors in this book), as support group leaders, as health activists. It is something they manage with and for partners, whether female or male, something they navigate with new partners. It is something that structures "getting on" with life. This is living with prostate cancer. It is endless and ever-present. It is liminal. The terms *survivor* and *survivorship* barely approximate this experience. It is the experiences of gay men living with prostate cancer every day, not just surviving it, that we address in this chapter.

With that framing in mind, we focus primarily on sexuality issues for these gay men, not just as personal experience but also in relation to their participation in the sex-based sociality of the gay community.[8] We argue that, for gay men living with prostate cancer, it is important to regard sexuality—not merely sexual function and its treatment—as a *social practice*. We suspect, and hope, that some of what we report here will be relevant to thinking about all men living with prostate cancer.

This chapter is, in part, a commentary, illustrated at times by findings from recent studies of prostate cancer in gay men (or gay and bisexual men in some studies—hereafter referred to as GBM), a number of which are reported in detail elsewhere in this book. We also draw on findings from our qualitative study of gay men and prostate cancer conducted in Australia in 2013–2015, the Moving On study, described in more detail elsewhere.[9] This study recruited 35 gay men living with prostate cancer (not bisexual men or other men who have sex with men—MSM) and 6 gay male partners of such men. Quotations from this study will be used at times to illustrate the subjective experience of gay men on a number of issues.

SEXUALITY AFTER PROSTATE CANCER

The consequences of prostate cancer treatment are well known. In relation to sexuality, depending on age, earlier sexual activity, and treatment success, 30–90% of all men diagnosed with, and treated for, prostate cancer will experience mild to severe sexual problems, such as erectile dysfunction, loss of ejaculatory capacity, decreases in sexual desire and satisfaction, loss of sexual confidence, intimacy issues, and incontinence (see chapters 1–3, 7). Mental health issues are another major concern (chapter 5). One study in the United States, for example, found that the average annual incidence of suicide for men with prostate cancer was over four times that of a comparable age- and gender-specific cohort.[10] It is known that predictors of depression after diagnosis and treatment include preexisting depression or anxiety.[11] As twelve-month and lifetime rates for depression and anxiety are higher for GBM, whether or how these two facts converge for gay men living with prostate cancer is not clear.[12] However, a recent U.S. study found a number of issues that affect GBM's mental health in relation to prostate cancer, including sexuality-related anxiety.[13]

Recent studies in the United States, Canada, and Australia found significant differences after prostate diagnosis and treatment for gay men (at times GBM/MSM) in relation to orgasm, ejaculation, sexual quality of life (QoL), functioning, and confidence.[14–16] These findings are discussed elsewhere in this volume (see chapter 1). However, gay men (or GBM/MSM) did not always receive worse scores on the measures used. For example, sexual confidence was higher, and it is possible that gay men and heterosexual men may differ on some of these issues regardless of prostate cancer. These findings on sexuality do speak to gay men's different experience, but not to broader social factors that might be affecting gay men living with prostate cancer. For example, it has been argued that the particular stigma attached to homosexuality affects QoL outcomes for gay men in general.[17] One review noted that depression and anxiety among GBM can be related to sexual orientation and identity concerns, as well as to experiences of stigma, discrimination, and other forms of social disapprobation and exclusion.[12] Research on social factors of this kind affecting gay men living with prostate cancer is relatively underdeveloped, except for contextual issues of social support and problems in healthcare and service provision (chapter 8).[18] These findings on higher sexual confidence and functioning are indicators that something else may be going on for gay men as a population, beyond individual responses to prostate cancer diagnosis and treatment. There are a number of issues to be considered that we take up in the rest of this chapter: gay sex and sexuality, gay relationships and gay community, and HIV infection.

GAY SEX AND SEXUALITY

Our qualitative data revealed experiences of sexual difficulty for gay men after diagnosis and treatment, but it was not quite as expected.

One participant said, "I don't consider it [sexual problems] anything like the problem the depression's been." In contrast, another said, "The problem wasn't between my ears, it was between my legs." In much of the literature on prostate cancer, sexuality is often regarded as an individual patient's concern and reduced to physical symptoms (e.g., erectile dysfunction, inability to ejaculate, compromised capacity for penetration). There is consideration of psychological and QoL issues, but less focus on those aspects of men's lives that link sexuality to relationality and to gay men's social worlds. In our study, one participant noted: "I just sort of think that I'd rather throw myself into work and try and forget about my gayness and my sexual problems, and try and look at other things."

Sexual problems following prostate cancer are well documented; "forgetting" gayness is an unknown phenomenon—just how does a gay man do that? Gayness and sexual problems are not two different things; they are interconnected. Trying to forget did not work for others: "Well, basically, my desire for sex has only diminished since the surgery. . . . So therein lie the mental issues. . . . 'Cause, when you're very fit and sexually active and enjoying that part of your life, when it's taken from you it's like, you know, having an amputation, really."

The category *gay* is primarily a sexual category, not just in society's eyes but for gay men themselves, who are identified by, and must identify primarily with, their sexual orientation. This is particularly so for the generation of gay men most affected by prostate cancer, the generation that fought for gay liberation, built the first openly proud gay communities, and who have been living with, and affected by, the HIV epidemic for over 35 years. For such gay men, the damaging effects of prostate cancer treatment on sexuality are not simply about erections, ejaculation, and penetration; they affect the central or core part of these men's identity—that sense of themselves as gay men: "Well, sex was a really important and enjoyable part of my life and I rarely have sex anymore. It's so, I've lost something that was really significant and important to me, and . . . not just recreationally but really as a, as part of my identity, I guess." For these men, gayness here is not just an individual's sexual orientation; gayness is a social identity, a defined—if marginal—place in the world, and it is embodied in daily practices and connections with others like them. This gayness has its own specific physical and social pleasures; losing or being wrenched from that source and experience of pleasure is a significant personal *and* social loss.

When discussing post-treatment sexual difficulties, particularly erectile dysfunction, the prostate cancer literature commonly assumes that sex usually is, and is desired to be, penile-vaginal intercourse. The great majority of men living with prostate cancer are heterosexual, so this focus on erections for coitus is understandable, but it might be a little misguided. Sexual functioning for gay men should be considered in relation to the men's sexual practices and preferences, including—but not limited to—anal intercourse. One study has reported post-treatment changes in anal intercourse among nonheterosexual *and* heterosexual men living with prostate cancer.[19] These included men in both groups changing modes (or positions)—for example, moving from insertive to receptive and vice versa—and a few even took up the practice and explored other, noncoital ways to regain sexual pleasure and connection.[20] Clearly, a focus on erectile dysfunction primarily for vaginal penetration is unhelpful for gay and bisexual men. It might be less than helpful for other men, too.

Most gay men who engage in anal intercourse are "versatile"; that is, they enjoy both modes, so swapping modes could help (see chapter 10).[21] Mode swapping, however, may be an unwelcome change for men and partners with specific modal preferences, and the fact of anal discomfort might mean that changes in mode are not possible for some men.[3, 15] Even for men with reasonable sexual function, anal intercourse does require a firmer erection than vaginal penetration. Though pharmacological and technological assistance may help (e.g., PDE5 inhibitor drugs such as Viagra, vacuum pumps, Caverject injections, or penile implants), not all men respond to or like these (see chapter 11), and their use has been found to be reduced significantly after about a year, even when reasonably effective.[22] In addition, condom use to prevent HIV transmission can compound difficulties with erectile function, even with the use of PDE5 inhibiter drugs.[23] Further, the loss of the prostate itself reduces sensation and pleasure during anal intercourse, while rectal incontinence related to radiation treatment may have serious side effects, adversely affecting the pleasures of anal intercourse for both partners. Urinary incontinence, a frequent prostate cancer treatment side effect, can also be a problem.

Finally, it has been known since the earliest days of HIV/AIDS research that the most frequent sexual practice for gay men is masturbation (alone or mutual), followed by oral sex.[24] Focusing more on these practices, which do not necessarily require erections for orgasm, might better support gay men (indeed, all men) in sexual recovery after prostate cancer treatment by creating non-erection-dependent measures of sexual success. Aside from individual masturbation, these sex practices are undertaken mostly not in solitude, but with one or more other persons. They are interpersonal, hence social, acts within often-complex relational dynamics. Though these sexual issues may be negotiated fairly successfully in a regular or primary relationship, they can be an added problem in, or even a blockage to, casual sexual encounters. It is to this issue of sexual relations we now turn.

GAY RELATIONSHIPS AND GAY COMMUNITY

The conceptualization of relationships in the prostate cancer field is, commonly, mostly of married, or at least cohabiting, heterosexual couples. Though same-sex marriage or civil union recognition has become possible in an increasing number of countries, many countries still do not have these institutional supports for gay relationships. However, gay men with primary partners in our study did report those partners as very supportive, but even solid relationships can be tested by prostate cancer: "The relationship is still fine. I, I feel that, that I'm letting him down a bit 'cause he was also very sexually active prior to me being inactive. . . . It's a monogamous relationship, to the degree that, if he feels like having sex with somebody else, I, I don't object . . . at times he's quite disappointed but he's very understanding." This participant was no longer able to achieve a satisfactory erection and was experiencing serious emotional strain as a result. He was deeply aware of what was happening for his partner. Gay men's intimate relationships are very likely to be open or nonmonogamous—if not at first, then later.[25] In this context, it was the participant who insisted that his partner have sex with others. That said, negotiating the end of an active sex life with a life partner is not a simple process, nor is negotiating nonmonogamy always as easy as this participant makes it sound.[26]

The prostate cancer research field rarely acknowledges other relational forms such as nonmonogamy, regular noncohabiting sex partners, "friends with benefits," group sex, casual sex, and encounters at sex parties and in other commercial sex-on-premises venues that constitute the social and sexual circumstances of gay men, more so than for heterosexual men.[27] Recent excellent health education websites and resources for gay men living with prostate cancer do address gay male relationships, but mostly as couples; they rarely address the variety and complexity of gay men's relational forms.[28-31]

Pursuing a sex life beyond that of a monogamous couple can be complex to negotiate. There is also little literature on prostate cancer in single men, of whatever sexual orientation.[32] Body image is a significant contributor to prostate cancer recovery, and prostate cancer can have a profound, long-term affect on men's sense of body image, self-worth, and social interactions.[33, 34] Self-worth and body image are not simply self-assessments; they also find expression and meaning in social interactions and relations. This reality may have particular consequences for gay men living with prostate cancer and their senses of self, given the literature on the importance of the body and physical appearance to gay men, and to their participation in varied sexual and relational aspects of gay community life.[35]

For some gay men living with prostate cancer, being sexually active, whether single or beyond a couple, can be daunting (see chapter 2). There are the side effects to deal with: "I'm not ashamed of it or worried about it—but it just, you know, I like to be honest and up-front. . . . I say, 'Look, I had prostate cancer. I'm all fine but I just don't ejaculate.'" It can be like coming out all over again: "But how much do you reveal on a first date I suppose? It's kind of that question. I guess I've just kind of gone with the flow a bit, to an extent, and just thought, 'Well, you know, there's no point hiding this.'" It is not only about mentioning cancer and its consequences: "It's feeling inhibited and the fact, that lack of confidence. . . . If I try to venture into a new partner, that's where I start to feel a bit inhibited, a bit, oh . . . what's the word? I can't just quite think of it but I feel a bit inferior sort of thing."

These interpersonal issues confront many men who have experienced prostate cancer, but for many gay men these issues are embedded in more varied relationalities that form gay men's broader social worlds. When some of the predictable flaws in the sexual cultures of gay communities are encountered, further complexities arise: "If I tell them it's prostate cancer, then they think you're too old." For some gay men, prostate cancer engenders a sense of resignation to the fact that a sexually active life has been brought to a close: "I was 64 when it was done so, you know, I was getting to the stage where it was, 'Thank you. Thanks for the memories.'" Those "memories" too are embedded in belonging to, and participating in, gay sexual cultures. A premature end to that participation is hard to deal with: "Yeah. I, I see myself now as an old gay man because it really makes you think of your—think about your age. . . . And it's not pleasant, especially in the gay scene, to think of yourself as a senior citizen. So, yeah, you just battle on, you know."

Prostate cancer has effects on gay men's sexual identities, relationships, and sexual senses of self,[13] all of which are compounded by a sense of premature aging.[36] The loss of access to sexual activity is a circumstance that can amount to "sexual disqualification" or "being out of sync" with gay sexual communities.[27, 32] A gay man's sense of membership of a gay community and participation in gay sexual cultures can be damaged. Gay communities—and we are not referring to LGBTIQ communities here—are unusual social formations in which sexual attraction, sexual activity, and sexual relationships (past, present, and future) often provide the social "glue" to produce a sex-based sociality.[8] This idea situates sex itself, and being seen to be a sexually active and attractive being, at the center of a gay man's social life. That life consists in a web of social activity and sexual encounters, shared with other gay men in close friendship circles, broader social and sexual networks, and the wider gay community itself. Many gay men, such as our research participants, see their sex lives as constituted in sexual cultures, rather than in sexual partnerships or couples. Most heterosexual men negotiate their experience of prostate cancer in the context of coupledom; at least, this is what can be discerned from the research literature on them, and the health-education resources directed to them. For gay men, whether in committed relationships or not, the sexual "adventure" can continue throughout their adult lives, even into their seventies.

Gay men deal with prostate cancer in the context of sexual cultures where possibilities—and the foreclosure of those possibilities—can be multifaceted. The quotations above are not just about individual experiences; they point to a *disembedding* from that sex-based sociality. None of these sexuality issues is easy for any gay man to negotiate. Each gay man's sense and experience of that sociality, of belonging to, and membership of, gay community, is deeply affected by any hint of sexual disqualification. When sexuality lies at the heart of identity and a sense of self; when sex is a social and cultural, not just interpersonal, practice; when varied relationalities have been experienced in a sex-based sociality: for gay men living with prostate cancer, any disqualification and disembeddedness result in different and difficult social consequences. Health professionals and services are barely able to conceive these social consequences.

HIV INFECTION

It is difficult to think about health issues for gay men without taking HIV infection into account. Those receiving effective treatment are living longer and, consequently, becoming prone to diseases of aging and other chronic health problems often related to their HIV infection and its treatment. A second issue is how HIV infection might intersect with prostate cancer (see chapter 1). One U.S. Navy study found higher rates of prostate cancer among HIV-positive men, and many cancer rates are higher in HIV-positive people.[37, 38] One review of the literature suggested that there is no reason treatment options for HIV-positive men with prostate cancer should be different from those available to other men, although certain effects of HIV infection on the body could influence prostate cancer treatment outcomes.[39] However, HIV-positive gay men were not specifically mentioned in that review. A PSA screening study of 200,000 men in California found that HIV-positive men, two-thirds of whom were gay, compared with HIV-negative men, had a lower incidence of prostate cancer, were more likely to be diagnosed with less advanced cancers, and had a reduced risk of prostate cancer, even though they had higher levels of PSA screening.[40] Why these differences occur is unclear. There is also research pointing to the prostate as a reservoir for HIV,[41] which may potentially complicate the treatment of both illnesses in research seeking an HIV cure. In sum, there is uncertainty ahead in dealing with gay men living with both prostate cancer and HIV infection.

Negotiating sex can become more complex if HIV has to be factored into the equation. Gay men have developed many ways in their sexual lives to work around potential or existing HIV infection for themselves and others. Using condoms has been and is the primary HIV-prevention technique of gay men; however, using condoms effectively requires a firm erection. Other strategies involve agreements on what kind of sexual practices are permitted within and beyond existing primary relationships, such as when or not to use condoms and with whom, or engaging in sex practices considered less risky. Recent dramatic improvements in antiretroviral treatments to lower HIV infection rates at individual and community levels further complicate the negotiation of sexual relations and practices. None of this is easy; nothing is foolproof; and no strategy guarantees 100% protection from transmitting or being infected with HIV. All involve levels of risk assessment and risk taking that put a strain on gay relationships and can make sex between men more complex.

Employing these strategies and technologies is not an individual or even simply an interpersonal decision, negotiation, and act. The HIV epidemic has been going on for over 35 years. Many gay men living with prostate cancer and their contemporaries have created and are living and being sexually active in communities and global gay social worlds that are suffused with HIV/AIDS as a powerful discursive, political, and cultural phenomenon. AIDS has been called an "epidemic of signification."[42] Gay sex became the central symbol of risk and danger and remains inextricably entwined with HIV/AIDS in the collective experience and culture of gay men. Add prostate cancer to the mix, particularly for the age group of gay men who have experienced both diseases, and rebuilding the sexual lives of gay men living with prostate cancer becomes more complicated than coping with individual experiences of sexual difficulty.

The additional strain of prostate cancer on all men living with HIV is likely to add to the mental health burden and sexuality issues that accompany HIV infection. There is already additional strain on gay men and other homosexually active men who report high levels of stigma and discrimination resulting from homophobia.[43] There is added stigma related to HIV infection and the long history of representing the HIV pandemic as a gay disease, a "gay plague," and the persecution attached and shame attributed to that labeling continue to this day.[44] This constituent of the social structuring of gay men's lives is best captured in the concept of "minority stress," and that framing is important and instructive for understanding the social dimensions of prostate cancer for gay men.[4, 45]

CONCLUSION

The HIV epidemic has been and is an important context for this generation of gay men living with prostate cancer. HIV/AIDS has been here for over three decades, and during that time much has been learned about gay men's sexuality and health. Assessing just how far prostate cancer as a field of research and professional practice has come in the thirteen years since we were told that gay men were that "invisible diversity" is less clear. This book would seem to confirm some progress on a number of issues. Those health education websites and resources noted above reflect a considerable advance in the state of play;[28 – 31] the research on health professionals and services suggests there is more to do.

We must first work specifically to include gay men in the category *men,* as long noted in the masculinity studies field.[46] One reason is that prostate cancer as a field of research and professional practice often invokes "masculinity" as a framing of men's sexual concerns, mostly in relation to erectile dysfunction and its consequences. This framing usually uses a singular notion of masculinity—as if it is one and the same thing, a quantity a man has more of or less of and exists only in the penis. Masculinity studies long ago reconfigured the frame as "masculini*ties,*" recognizing the significant social and cultural differences, experiences, values, and circumstances of men, including their different sexual interests.[47] Working with "masculinities" might produce better understandings of the varied sexual and social situations for all men living with prostate cancer. Using this term might be more useful than relying on simplistic binary oppositions: gay/straight or heterosexual/homosexual, bisexual being thrown in at times but usually combined with homosexual, as in "GBM." It is important in prostate cancer research, programs, and interventions that gay men be included, if only to add their clearly different experiences of prostate cancer to our understanding of the disease as a whole and how all men live with it.

Second, we can no longer work solely with simplistic notions of sexual identity, preference, or orientation in trying to investigate prostate cancer. It is not enough to change "wife" to "partner" in a pamphlet or survey and assume that covers it. Gay men's sexual lives are not singular, even if they are structured differently from heterosexual men's sexual lives. Straight men can have anal sex too, and more men might find it and other practices beyond coitus as ways to improve their sexual lives after prostate cancer treatment. There might also be some other things to learn from gay men living with prostate cancer—for example, exploring further those findings on their higher sexual confidence noted earlier.

Third, a gay man living with prostate cancer does not just live an individual life; nor is his sexuality just an individual concern. The lives of this generation of gay men are embedded in gay sexual cultures where consequences of prostate cancer are experienced and can potentially be remediated. Programs to support or intervene to achieve better outcomes for gay men living with prostate cancer need to focus not just on the specificities of gay men's sexuality, but also on their connection to the varied social and sexual relations that gay men can explore. As one research participant declared: "I think it's inexcusable that no one can really tell you anything. I think that's not acceptable and you, sort of, like—go to your GP as a woman and your GP not having any comprehension of what issues might be for women! I think that there needs to be a baseline to at least be able to explore with the person in front of you what kind of extra support, assistance, advice, information they might need, and then be able to match them to what's available."

Surely, this is not too much to ask?

ACKNOWLEDGMENTS

Research funding: beyondblue, through its National Priority Driven Research Program—Men's Stream, with support from the Movember Foundation.

In preparing this chapter, we note earlier presentations at the First Prostate Cancer Specialist Nursing Program Induction Event, Prostate Cancer Foundation of Australia, Melbourne, 2012; the Tenth Oncology Social Work Australia National Conference, Sydney, 2014; the 14th Psychosocial Oncology New Zealand Conference, Wellington, New Zealand, 2016; University of Pretoria Medical School, Pretoria, South Africa, 2017; University of Witwatersrand, Johannesburg, South Africa, 2017.

Our thanks to colleagues in this and various related projects: Richard Wassersug, Anthony Lyons, Andrew Westle, Alissar El-Murr, Marian Pitts, Tsz Kin (Bernard) Lee, Jane Ussher, Janette Perz, and Simon Rosser.

Our thanks to the research participants in the Moving On study.

REFERENCES

1. Bruce A, Sheilds L, Molzahn A, et al. Stories of liminality: Living with life-threatening illness. *Journal of Holistic Nursing.* 2014; 32 (1): 35–43.

2. Perlman G, Drescher J. *A gay man's guide to prostate cancer.* Binghamton, N.Y.: Haworth Medical Press; 2005.

3. Blank TO. Gay men and prostate cancer: Invisible diversity. *Journal of Clinical Oncology.* 2005; 23 (12): 2593–2596.

4. Hoyt MA, Carpenter KM. Sexual self-schema and depressive symptoms after prostate cancer. *Psycho-Oncology.* 2015; 24 (4): 395–401.

5. Bell K, Ristovski-Slijepcevic S. Cancer survivorship: Why labels matter. *Journal of Clinical Oncology.* 2013; 31 (4): 409–411.

6. Plummer K. *Telling sexual stories: Power, change, and social worlds.* London: Routledge; 1995.

7. Park CL, Zlateva I, Blank TO. Self-identity after cancer: "Survivor," "victim," "patient," and "person with cancer." *Journal of General Internal Medicine.* 2009; 24 (Suppl. 2): S430–435.

8. Dowsett GW, Wain D, Keys D. Good gay men don't get "messy": Injecting drug use and gay community. *Sexuality Research & Social Policy.* 2005; 2 (1): 22–36.

9. Dowsett GW, Prestage G, Duncan D, et al. *Moving on: Mental health, resilience and sexual recovery among gay men living with prostate cancer.* Melbourne: Austra-

lian Research Centre in Sex, Health and Society, La Trobe University; 2015.

10. Llorente MD, Burke M, Gregory GR, et al. Prostate cancer: A significant risk factor for late-life suicide. *American Journal of Geriatric Psychiatry.* 2005; 13 (3): 195–201.

11. Sharpley CF, Bitsika V, Wootten AC, Christie DRH. Predictors of depression in prostate cancer patients: A comparison of psychological resilience versus pre-existing anxiety and depression. *Journal of Men's Health.* 2014; 11 (3): 115–120.

12. Carman M, Corboz J, Dowsett GW. Falling through the cracks: The gap between evidence and policy in responding to depression in gay, lesbian and other homosexually active people in Australia. *Australian and New Zealand Journal of Public Health.* 2012; 36 (1): 76–83.

13. Rosser BRS, Capistrant B, Torres B, et al. The effects of radical prostatectomy on gay and bisexual men's mental health, sexual identity and relationships: Qualitative results from the Restore study. *Sexual and Relationship Therapy.* 2016; 31 (4): 446–461.

14. Wassersug RJ, Lyons A, Duncan D, et al. Diagnostic and outcome differences between heterosexual and nonheterosexual men treated for prostate cancer. *Urology.* 2013; 82 (3): 565–571.

15. Hart TL, Coon DW, Kowalkowski MA, et al. Changes in sexual roles and quality of life for gay men after prostate cancer: Challenges for sexual health providers. *Journal of Sexual Medicine.* 2014; 11 (9): 2308–2317.

16. Lee TK, Handy AB, Kwan W, et al. Impact of prostate cancer treatment on the sexual quality of life for men-who-have-sex-with-men. *Journal of Sexual Medicine.* 2015; 12 (12): 2378–2386.

17. Allensworth-Davies D, Talcott JA, Heeren T, et al. The health effects of masculine self-esteem following treatment for localized prostate cancer among gay men. *LGBT Health.* 2015; 3 (1): 49–56.

18. Capistrant BD, Torres B, Merengwa E, et al. Caregiving and social support for gay and bisexual men with prostate cancer. *Psycho-Oncology.* 2016; 25 (11): 1329–1336.

19. Dowsett GW, Lyons A, Duncan D, Wassersug RJ. Flexibility in men's sexual practices in response to iatrogenic erectile dysfunction after prostate cancer treatment. *Sexual Medicine.* 2014; 2 (3): 115–120.

20. Wassersug RJ, Westle A, Dowsett GW. Men's sexual and relational adaptations to erectile dysfunction after prostate cancer treatment. *International Journal of Sexual Health.* 2017; 29 (1): 69–79.

21. Lyons A, Pitts M, Grierson J. Versatility and HIV vulnerability: Patterns of insertive and receptive anal sex in a national sample of older Australian gay men. *AIDS and Behavior.* 2013; 17 (4): 1370–1377.

22. Walker LM, Wassersug RJ, Robinson JW. Psychosocial perspectives on sexual recovery after prostate cancer treatment. *Nature Reviews Urology.* 2015; 12 (3): 167–176.

23. Sanders SA, Milhausen RR, Crosby RA, et al. Do phosphodiesterase type 5 inhib-

itors protect against condom-associated erection loss and condom slippage? *Journal of Sexual Medicine.* 2009; 6 (5): 1451–1456.

24. Kippax S, Crawford J, Davis M, et al. Sustaining safe sex: A longitudinal study of a sample of homosexual men. *AIDS.* 1993; 7 (2): 257–263.

25. Philpot SP, Ellard J, Duncan D, et al. Gay and bisexual men's interest in marriage: An Australian perspective. *Culture, Health and Sexuality.* 2016; 18 (12): 1347–1362.

26. Bavinton BR, Duncan D, Grierson J, et al. The meaning of "regular partner" in HIV research among gay and bisexual men: Implications of an Australian cross-sectional survey. *AIDS and Behavior.* 2016; 20 (8): 1777–1784.

27. Ussher JM, Perz J, Rose D, et al. Threat of sexual disqualification: The consequences of erectile dysfunction and other sexual changes for gay and bisexual men with prostate cancer. *Archives of Sexual Behavior.* 2017; 46 (7): 2043–2057.

28. Prostate Cancer UK. Prostate facts for gay and bisexual men. https://prostatecanceruk.org/prostate-information/living-with-prostate-cancer/gay-and-bisexual-men.

29. Prostate Cancer Foundation of Australia. Gay and bisexual men. www.prostate.org.au/awareness/for-recently-diagnosed-men-and-their-families/gay-and-bisexual-men.

30. Malecare. Gay man's guide to prostate cancer and doctors. http://malecare.org/gay-prostate-cancer-and-doctors/.

31. Prostate Cancer Canada. Gay and bisexual men & prostate cancer. www.prostatecancer.ca/Prostate-Cancer/Facing-Prostate-Cancer/Gay-and-Bisexual-Men-Prostate-Cancer.

32. Matheson L, Watson EK, Nayoan J, et al. A qualitative metasynthesis exploring the impact of prostate cancer and its management on younger, unpartnered and gay men. *European Journal of Cancer Care.* 2017; doi: 10.1111/ecc.12676.

33. O'Shaughnessy P, Laws TA. Australian men's long term experiences following prostatectomy: A qualitative descriptive study. *Contemporary Nurse.* 2009; 34 (1): 98–109.

34. Taylor-Ford M, Meyerowitz BE, D'Orazio LM, et al. Body image predicts quality of life in men with prostate cancer. *Psycho-Oncology.* 2013; 22 (4): 756–761.

35. Duncan D. Embodying the gay self: Body image, reflexivity and embodied identity. *Health Sociology Review.* 2010; 19 (4): 437–450.

36. Ussher JM, Rose D, Perz J. Mastery, isolation, or acceptance: Gay and bisexual men's construction of aging in the context of sexual embodiment after prostate cancer. *Journal of Sex Research.* 2017; 54 (6): 802–812.

37. Crum NF, Hale B, Utz G, Wallace M. Increased risk of prostate cancer in HIV infection? *AIDS.* 2002; 16 (12): 1703–1704.

38. Crum-Cianflone NF, Hullsiek KH, Marconi V, et al. Trends in the incidence of cancers among HIV-infected persons and the impact of antiretroviral therapy: Authors' reply. *AIDS.* 2009; 23 (13): 1791–1792.

39. Wosnitzer MS, Lowe FC. Management of prostate cancer in HIV-positive patients. *Nature Reviews Urology.* 2010; 7 (6): 348–357.

40. Marcus JL, Chao CR, Leyden WA, et al. Prostate cancer incidence and prostate-specific antigen testing among HIV-positive and HIV-negative men. *Journal of Acquired Immune Deficiency Syndromes.* 2014; 66 (5): 495–502.

41. Smith DM, Kingery JD, Wong JK, et al. The prostate as a reservoir for HIV-1. *AIDS.* 2004; 18 (11): 1600–1602.

42. Treichler PA. AIDS, homophobia, and biomedical discourse: An epidemic of signification. *In* Crimp D, ed. *AIDS: Cultural analysis, cultural activism.* Cambridge: MIT Press; 1987: 31–70.

43. Herek GM. A nuanced view of stigma for understanding and addressing sexual and gender minority health disparities. *LGBT Health.* 2016; 3 (6): 397–399.

44. Dowsett GW. The "gay plague" revisited: AIDS and its enduring moral panic. *In* Herdt G, ed. *Moral panics, sex panics: Fear and the fight over sexual rights.* New York: New York University Press; 2009: 130–156.

45. Meyer IH. Prejudice, social stress, and mental health in lesbian, gay, and bisexual populations: Conceptual issues and research evidence. *Psychological Bulletin.* 2003; 129 (5): 674–697.

46. Dowsett GW. I'll show you mine, if you'll show me yours: Gay men, masculinity research, men's studies, and sex. *Theory and Society.* 1993; 22 (5): 697–709.

47. Connell RW. *Masculinities.* 2nd ed. Crows Nest, N.S.W.: Allen & Unwin; 2005.

CHAPTER 7

Gay Men and Prostate Cancer

Learning from the Voices of a Hidden Population

Murray Drummond, James Smith, and Shaun Filiault

CHAPTER SUMMARY

Ten years ago, we published a study on gay men and prostate cancer. The paper gave a voice to gay men with prostate cancer whose voices had been largely unheard or, in some respects, silenced. Fortunately, there has been a groundswell of work in this area since the publication of our study. This chapter begins with a personal vignette of the first author, Murray Drummond, to provide important contextual information for how gay men and prostate cancer are perceived at a primary healthcare level. We then draw on contemporary health promotion scholarship to discuss what is known about men's health promotion and describe how this promotion intersects with gay men and prostate cancer. We then use some of the concerns voiced by the original group of gay men with prostate cancer in our study to illuminate the key issues they faced—and in many cases continue to face. We then reflect on some of the legal aspects associated with these concerns in the face of the rapidly changing landscape of LGBTQI rights (and lack thereof) in contemporary Western cultures. We conclude by describing a way forward in light of the sociocultural, legal, and physical health concerns these men face with respect to their illness.

KEY WORDS

gay and bisexual men, health promotion, LGBTQI rights, prostate cancer

A PERSONAL REFLECTION

Standing behind the podium looking out toward the faces of 80 to 90 people in the audience, at an unfamiliar conference, I feel a little daunted.

Ussher, Jane M., Perz, Janette, Rosser, B. R. Simon, eds., *Gay & Bisexual Men Living with Prostate Cancer*
dx.doi.org/10.17312/harringtonparkpress/2018.06.gbmlpc.007
© 2018 Harrington Park Press

I am about to deliver a keynote presentation on gay men and prostate cancer. I was invited to present at a National Nursing Oncology Conference at which the majority of delegates are primary healthcare specialists, including oncologists, nurses, and palliative care and health promoters. It has been a while since I have felt like this. I often know at least a few faces in the crowd. However, this audience is somewhat foreign to me. I am a health sociologist with a background in sport, health, and physical activity and a specific interest in men's health and masculinities. This research has evolved from my work with men. I am hoping they "get it."

I pride myself on being a good presenter. I feel I have the audience's attention. I see a few heads nodding, which is a good sign. I am now at the "exciting" part of the presentation, where I feel I can relax, as we are now hearing the voices of the men who have been interviewed. I can see that the conference delegates are listening with intent. This information is new to them. Many of them have not previously heard this type of narrative.

As the presentation draws to a close, as a keynote speaker, I am concerned about whether I have engaged the audience enough and made them think beyond their daily professional lives. It is our role as academics to challenge, and I hope that I have achieved this. The obligatory clapping rings out around the large room, for which I am at least grateful. The first comment comes from a leading oncologist (though I do not to know this until after the presentation), who in an authoritative voice exclaims: "I would like to thank you for the wonderful presentation. You know, in all my years of working with men with prostate cancer, I have never asked them about their sexuality. Nor have I asked how their sexual attitudes and behaviors will have implications for them moving forward. I will from now on, and I thank you for that."

I have been an academic for more than 20 years, and this is certainly the most rewarding comment that I have received. It vindicates the work I have been doing and continue to do, and it highlights the significance of understanding gay men and prostate cancer. On this day I feel that the work I am doing is making a difference.

GAY MEN, PROSTATE CANCER, AND HEALTH PROMOTION

There has been a noticeable growth in global men's health promotion efforts over the past 20 years.[1-4] These efforts have included investments in health education, community and workplace health promotion programs, health screening, online health resources, and a variety of mass media and social marketing campaigns on sex-specific health issues, such as prostate cancer.[5-10] Many of these efforts have relied heavily on hegemonic constructions of masculinity to engage, or target health messages toward, men.[4, 8]

Yet there is a significant evidence base demonstrating that masculine stereotypes are detrimental to men's (and women's) health.[11-13] Indeed, it can be argued that perpetuating hegemonic masculine stereotypes through men's health promotion efforts can potentially be health-damaging.[3, 4, 14] Some commentators have been critical of health promotion approaches that categorize men in this way.[3, 4, 14] So what is the alternative?

There has been rapidly growing scholarship relating to multiple masculinities and their relationship to men's health.[15-17] Understanding this discourse is critically important for reconceptualizing the way we approach men's health promotion in Australia and elsewhere in the world. It provides scope to tailor and target men's health promotion approaches more effectively. We already know that there are notable differences in health status between men and women, as well as differences among subpopulations of men.[13, 18, 19] These differences are usually a result of social, economic, and health inequities. The concept of promoting health equity is gradually surfacing in national men's health policies across the globe, such as those in Australia, Ireland, Brazil, and Iran.[19-21] For example, in Australia the National Male Health Policy (NMHP) has an explicit focus on addressing health inequities by acknowledging the unique health needs of Australia's most marginalized and vulnerable groups of men.[19] Priority groups include indigenous men, men from socioeconomically disadvantaged backgrounds, men living in rural and remote areas of Australia, men with disabilities, and men from migrant and refugee backgrounds.[19] Gay, bisexual, and transgender men are also identified as a marginalized group.[19] While there is still tremendous diversity among these subgroups of men, these categories provide a different way of conceptualizing future men's health promotion investments. That is, a health promotion approach that pays greater attention to the social, political, and cultural contexts faced by these subpopulations of men is more likely to provide a supportive environment in which better health outcomes can be achieved. This means paying attention not only to the social construction of gender, but also to other intersecting social determinants of health.[22, 23]

In this chapter we argue that there needs to be a sharper focus on who the target audience is and the specific factors that influence the health and decision making of that audience. In other words, men's health promotion strategies need to be tailored more effectively. Understanding these strategies in the context of the health of gay and bisexual men' (GBM), and particularly in relation to prostate cancer, is important. So, what do we currently know about GBM, and how can this knowledge be used to strengthen health promotion efforts in relation to prostate cancer?

Historically, GBM are one particular subpopulation in which targeted health promotion efforts have been noted. Issues associated with sexual and reproductive health have been a prominent focus,[24] particularly in relation to the early work focused on reducing the spread of AIDS and HIV.[25] Such work has inadvertently (albeit blatantly) positioned GBM as being sexually promiscuous and risk takers.[26] This has been a prominent feature of gay men's health promotion work, where we have seen health messages that encourage condom use and monogamy to prevent AIDS and HIV used as a common strategy. But has this approach really tapped into the emerging changes to social and cultural traits well described in GBM health research? While there is research to support claims that some GBM engage in sexual promiscuity or risk taking (or both),[26, 27] this behavior is not common to all. It could be equally argued that many heterosexual men are known to engage in sexual promiscuity and risk-taking activities. Similarly, changing social norms associated with homophobia—for example, the inclusion of units on homosexuality in school curricula; openly gay representation in popular entertainment and social media; and increasing public support for same-sex marriage—all have the potential to change the health promotion investment targeted toward GBM.

In this chapter we use the experiences of gay men with prostate cancer to explain what the main issues are, and we provide suggestions about how these issues are best addressed. We begin by drawing on some past empirical research we conducted as the basis for this discussion. Because of the general silence surrounding gay men's, and their partners', experiences of prostate cancer, and their potentially unique concerns, this in-depth, qualitative exploration examines their experiences, frustrations, and perspectives.

THE EXPLORATORY PROCESS AND DOMINANT THEMES FROM THE DATA

The intent of this exploration was to gain an initial perspective on prostate cancer from the vantage point of gay men affected by the disease. Therefore, large numbers of men were not required. What was required was high-quality, illuminating information. Taking a case-study approach offered the opportunity to focus on the depth of information provided by participants, rather than attaining a large sample size.[28] This methodology is consistent with contemporary research literature that supports the power and utility of conducting small-N, qualitative research when carrying out interview-based research with subpopulations of gay men (in this case, $N = 3$).[29]

Participants were recruited through announcements at a local center for gay men's health, announcements through the state cancer council, and a small article in a local gay newspaper. Three dominant themes emerged from the data: (1) relationship changes, (2) gay sex and prostate cancer, and (3) heteronormativity and healthcare.

RELATIONSHIP CHANGES: "WE'RE NOT PREPARED FOR A DIAGNOSIS OF CANCER"

Both the patients and their partners noted that they experienced strains and changes in their romantic relationships, and relationships with other gay men, as a result of the diagnosis of prostate cancer. Part of this changed relationship dynamic, particularly for those men with partners, related to the ambiguous role of the partners in treatment and recovery.

This trend is best represented by the partner of a man with prostate cancer who claimed:

We both had a gut feeling something was wrong, and when he went to have these tests done, interestingly I was in denial about it all until . . . As all these tests were going forward, part of me denied it, thinking it's not cancer, it's just something that's, you know . . . easily fixed, no problem. And, of course, when he did tell me, I was devastated. We're not prepared for a diagnosis of cancer, whether it's yourself or your partner. And it took me a long time to come to terms with it. I went to have counseling, mainly because I wanted to be supportive to [my partner]. I have a lot of difficulty coping in stressful situations, and I didn't want to be a burden to [my partner], I didn't want my . . . difficulties in coping to impact on [my partner's] recovery.

Clearly, then, prostate cancer affects not just patients, but also their partners who love them. Comprehensive treatment should, therefore, not only attend to the concerns of the patient but also provide support for the partner. Of course, for this to happen, the healthcare system must recognize that the gay partner has concern and interest in the well-being of his sick partner.

However, it is not just partnered men who experience changes to their relationships. An unpartnered man expressed differences in the manner in which he related to other gay men, particularly in a sexual context:

> You've got scars on your abdomen where the robot, the Da Vinci robot, actually did the surgery. . . . Like, you wanted to go on the beach and wear your bathers on the beach, or go to the sauna, that could be very, um . . . I mean, I didn't really feel confident about going to a swimming pool or going to the beach for quite a few months after the operation. . . . For me, it was all about confidence approaching other gay men for sex, that was really sort of the thing, because of all that sort of emphasis on the body and not having an erection and all that sort of thing.

It is clear from these reflections that prostate cancer has a profound influence on these gay men's sense of self and body image and their ability and desire to relate to other gay men.[30] Recognition of these factors is critical to an understanding of gay men's experiences of prostate cancer, especially given the centrality of sex and sexuality to many gay men's lives. That difference was explicitly stated by one patient who said, "For gay men, you know, there's a different culture about sex." It is that difference, and the differences in sexuality enacted by prostate cancer treatment, that informs the second theme.

GAY SEX AND PROSTATE CANCER:
"I ALWAYS SAW MY PROSTATE AS A PLEASURE CENTER"
The patients in our study cited distinct changes to their libidos as a result of prostate cancer treatment. One patient said:

> The truth is that my libido has just vanished. You know, I don't have very much sexual urge at all anymore. You know, and every now and then I think I must do something out of, you know, out of

habit. You know, I don't really have any urge anymore, and . . . when I do have any sort of sexual activity, whether it's masturbation or sex with my partner, it's uh, it's become . . . more of, well I mean it's not entirely without pleasure, but it's, it's, become a bit of a bother actually. It's sort of, it's not something I lust for anymore, you know, which is a major thing. And I mean, . . . I was not expecting that, I didn't, I wasn't prepared for that.

In addition to those changes related to libido and sexual interest, prostate cancer is perceived as having a unique effect on gay men: "Well, I always saw my prostate as a pleasure center. And I knew from sexual experiences that, you know, massaging a prostate gland . . . could increase the pleasure of sexual intercourse enormously. And, to me, the prostate gland is a sort of major part of the male sexual experience."

Quite simply then, prostate cancer, by the very nature of the organ it afflicts, carries a unique significance to gay men and their sense of sexuality.[30, 31] Therefore, any clinical discussion about prostate cancer should recognize the meaning of the prostate gland in gay men's lives. It is noteworthy that this recognition did not appear to exist when the patients discussed their sexuality with their health service providers. The partner explained: "Certainly, my partner's doctor did give him information, primarily about symptoms and what to expect, but it didn't give that specialized information about being gay and how does that impact on relationships."

Similarly, health service providers did not seem to appreciate the reality that many gay men either are not coupled or engage in sex outside the primary relationship. This issue was identified by the single patient who claimed: "Because a lot of gay men don't have that kind of intimate kind of sexual contact. That sometimes it's more like meeting in saunas or things like that, or beats, or something like that. Where, um, an erection is kind of like a very important part of the whole kind of social ritual."

Frank and open discussion about postoperative sexuality is uncommon.[32] One patient described the information provided regarding postoperative sexuality as "disingenuous" and "coy," whereas another described it as "Victorian." Indeed, specific discussions regarding sex did not occur, and the literature provided to patients was not in the least informative, nor did it specifically address gay sex. However, a lack of frank information about sex was just one aspect of a range of concerns the men faced in terms of the healthcare system and their sexuality.

HETERONORMATIVITY AND HEALTHCARE:
"HE JUST ASSUMED I WAS HETEROSEXUAL"

Not only did the men in our study report a lack of discussion regarding the effect of prostate cancer on their sex lives, but they also reported a sense of not belonging in certain healthcare contexts, given their homosexual status, as detailed by other contributions to this book (chapters 6 and 8). A common frustration among the men was the assumption by most healthcare providers that their patients are married heterosexuals. One of the men described such an experience of assumed heterosexuality: "I felt they quite blatantly assumed I was heterosexual. My urologist is a lovely guy, [name of doctor], and I have no criticism of him in terms of his professional practice and medical practices. But, um, he just assumed I was heterosexual, and you know, he said, 'Would you like to bring your wife, or . . . to these meetings?' I mean (A) Was I married? Didn't ask. (B) Was I heterosexual? Didn't ask."

Despite these assumptions of heterosexuality, the men did not correct their providers by disclosing their own sexuality. This "closetedness" may have been due to the perception of homophobia in the healthcare system. One man said: "As far as like my experience of the whole going in and being told that you've actually got prostate cancer and all that, I felt very, um, I don't know. I suppose I see a hospital as a sort of heterosexual kind of place." Another man concurred: "You fear, you're frightened of the judgmental attitude of the doctor. You're frightened that he might not have your best interest at heart. Better to be silent about it all, and not create waves."

It is thus understandable that gay men would not want to place themselves in a vulnerable position by disclosing their sexuality. It is, therefore, the responsibility of healthcare providers to adopt accepting or, at the very least, tolerant discourse and attitudes toward gay men, gay sexual practices, and gay relationships in the context of prostate cancer. It is only through such open and compassionate dialogue that hospitals and other healthcare facilities may no longer be seen as "sort of heterosexual" places.[32]

LEGAL, ETHICAL, AND HEALTH PROMOTION IMPLICATIONS

INCLUDING PARTNERS: LEGALIZING SAME-SEX MARRIAGE

Within the context of gay rights, one of the greatest legal changes over the past decade has been many jurisdictions' recognition of same-sex marriages. The largest English-speaking jurisdiction to legalize same-sex marriage is the United States. In the groundbreaking decision *Obergefell v. Hodges,* the U.S. Supreme Court ruled that the right to marry one's same-sex partner was protected by the equal protection clause and the privacy penumbra of the U.S. Constitution. Justice Anthony Kennedy, writing for the Court, explained: "Same-sex couples [have been] consigned to an instability that opposite-sex couples would deem intolerable in their own lives. . . . It demeans gays and lesbians for the State to lock them out of a central institution of the Nation's society. Same-sex couples, too, may aspire to the transcendent purposes of marriage and seek fulfillment in its highest meaning."

With regard to the issues raised in our case study, these legal developments are profound. In jurisdictions where same-sex marriage has been recognized, no longer are partners relegated to the sidelines during treatment and care—a situation that would be, in the words of Justice Kennedy, "intolerable" to a heterosexual couple. We recall vividly the sense of frustration one of our participants expressed at his exclusion from the treatment and care of his long-term partner, merely because he was not a legal husband. His anger is a natural response to the systematic denial of access experienced by many LGBTQI non-spouse partners in the healthcare system.[33-35] For too long LGBTQI partners have been relegated to a secondary role in healthcare. Same-sex marriage may begin to alter that role.

In those jurisdictions with legal same-sex marriage, spouses now have the legal right to be present during consultation and treatment (with their partner's consent). In the United States, that right is reiterated by two federal regulations, 42 C.F.R. §§ 482.13(h) and 485.635(f).*

---

* These regulations allow a patient to designate those visitors whom he or she wishes to receive. A hospital may not restrict these visitors on the basis of a number of factors, including sexual orientation or gender identity. On April 15, 2010, President Obama signed an Executive Order reiterating his expectation that all hospitals comply with these regulations. President Trump later removed this order from the White House website.

The presence of one's spouse during treatment is critical. Not only is spousal presence obviously soothing, but treatment adherence increases when one's spouse is involved in consultation and care.[35] Moreover, recognition as a legal spouse is vital for a number of other reasons under U.S. law. For instance, the U.S. federal Family and Medical Leave Act (FMLA) allows spouses and immediate family members to take off up to 12 weeks from work to care for a family member with a serious medical condition.[33, 36] This protection is triggered for a legal spouse but not a "life partner," which could be a potentially critical distinction when caring for a loved one recovering from treatment for prostate cancer. Such an effect of the legal status of one's partner is demonstrative of a host of other legal benefits that are afforded to spouses but not partners. Simply stated, being a husband matters, and it is incumbent on jurisdictions to allow all men to become the husbands of their loved ones. The health and well-being of those loved ones could depend on it.

In the context of prostate cancer, spousal presence and support may be essential owing to the sexuality changes that prostate cancer may engender (see chapter 5). Open communication between partners during prostate cancer treatment has been linked to enhanced relationship quality and intimacy for prostate cancer survivors.[37] Similarly, both perceived and actual spousal support during prostate cancer treatment has been linked to better relationship quality and better erectile function after treatment.[38] Thus, the ability to be present during treatment and the capability to take time off from work immediately after treatment have the capacity to generate better treatment results for prostate cancer survivors. Hence, the law can help render treatment more effective.

RECOGNIZING SINGLE GAY MEN: DEMONSTRATING THE NEED FOR CULTURAL COMPETENCY

Though Justice Kennedy's language is to be lauded for its attempt to include LGBTQI Americans, it must also be criticized for the manner in which it does so. It places an enormous emphasis on the importance of marriage, suggesting it allows people to "seek fulfillment in its highest meaning." Perhaps that emphasis on marriage is to be expected in a case about same-sex marriage. Yet the reality remains that many gay men—especially *older* gay men—remain single.[39] Indeed, to this point, for a variety of social and economic reasons, it has mostly been younger gay men who have taken advantage of the newfound rights garnered by *Obergefell*.[39] That means that older gay men—those currently most likely to be affected by prostate cancer—are also those most likely to be single. This was the case for one of our participants, a single man in his fifties. His concerns pertaining to prostate cancer were related not to partner access, but to whether he would be able to attract a casual sexual partner (see chapter 2).

What is needed in the context of prostate cancer, then, is better cultural competency among clinicians.[34] Such competency would promote an understanding of gay men's lives and would, for example, encourage clinicians to understand that many older gay men remain unpartnered, even though same-sex marriage is legal in some jurisdictions. As Travis Chance has discussed, the law provides an excellent starting place for such a change in attitudes.[34] In the United States, for example, federal funding to medical schools and research hospitals can be made contingent on those institutions including units about sexual orientation and gender diversity in their curricula and research programs. Noncomplying institutions would lose federal funding, which would be a devastating result for many schools and hospitals, virtually guaranteeing compliance. U.S. states can tie physician registration and reregistration to completion of continuing education hours, some of which must include discussions of gender and sexual diversity. With such training, clinicians can come to discuss issues of sexuality and gender more honestly, competently, and compassionately with their clients, and begin to confront the heterosexism that has marred many gay men's encounters with the healthcare system. The law, then, far from being a foreign observer of prostate cancer, might be the starting point for the changes necessary to improve gay men's interactions with the healthcare system.

CONCLUSION

We have attempted to highlight the barriers and concerns that face gay men with respect to the physical, emotional, and social issues associated with prostate cancer. Within primary healthcare settings it is clear that clinicians who treat gay men with prostate cancer have the capacity to counteract heteronormative practice by becoming more inclusive. However, the wide-reaching and endemic nature of the problem requires more than a simple change in clinical practice. Changes at the policy and broader social and cultural levels are required to create long-term sustainable change. Such change will occur only when governments are prepared to acknowledge LGBTQI rights and relationships.

Currently in Australia, and many other places throughout the world, this is not the case. At the very least we need to begin working with primary healthcare workers to help them understand the rights and relationship status of gay men and the need to bring partners into the discussion about treatment and recovery processes. This will be an important step in helping gay men who are living with prostate cancer navigate the enormous changes that occur with prostate cancer diagnosis.

REFERENCES

1. Robertson S, Galdas PM, McCreary DR, et al. Men's health promotion in Canada: Current context and future direction. *Health Education Journal.* 2009; 68 (4): 266–272.

2. Robertson S, Baker P. Men and health promotion in the United Kingdom: 20 years further forward? *Health Education Journal.* 2017; 76 (1): 102–113.

3. Smith JA. Beyond masculine stereotypes: Moving men's health promotion forward in Australia. *Health Promotion Journal of Australia.* 2007; 18 (1): 20–25.

4. Smith JA, Robertson S. Men's health promotion: A new frontier in Australia and the UK? *Health Promotion International.* 2008; 23 (3): 283–289.

5. Cordier R, Wilson NJ. Community-based Men's Sheds: Promoting male health, wellbeing and social inclusion in an international context. *Health Promotion International.* 2014; 29 (3): 483–493.

6. Linnell S. Involving men in targeted primary health care: Men's health MOTs. *Community Practitioner.* 2010; 83 (5): 31.

7. Moffatt J, Hossain D. *Pit Stop at FarmFest 2010: Evaluation: Is Pit Stop effective?* Brisbane: GP Connections, University of Queensland; 2010.

8. Robinson M, Robertson S. The application of social marketing to promoting men's health: A brief critique. *International Journal of Men's Health.* 2010; 9 (1): 50.

9. Russell N, Harding C, Chamberlain C, Johnston L. Implementing a "Men's Health Pitstop" in the Riverina, South-west New South Wales. *Australian Journal of Rural Health.* 2006; 14 (3): 129–131.

10. Wilson NJ, Cordier R, Doma K, et al. Men's Sheds function and philosophy: Towards a framework for future research and men's health promotion. *Health Promotion Journal of Australia.* 2015; 26 (2): 133–141.

11. Courtenay WH. Constructions of masculinity and their influence on men's well-being: A theory of gender and health. *Social Science & Medicine.* 2000; 50 (10): 1385–1401.

12. Courtenay WH. Behavioral factors associated with disease, injury, and death among men: Evidence and implications for prevention. *Journal of Men's Studies.* 2000; 9 (1): 81–142.

13. Australian Institute of Health and Welfare (AIHW). *The health of Australia's males.* Canberra: AIHW; 2011.

14. Gough B, Robertson S. Promoting "masculinity" over health: A critical analysis of men's health promotion with particular reference to an obesity reduction manual. *In* Gough B, Robertson S, eds. *Men, masculinities & health: Critical perspectives.* New York: Palgrave Macmillan; 2010: 125–142.

15. Creighton G, Oliffe JL. Theorising masculinities and men's health: A brief history with a view to practice. *Health Sociology Review.* 2010; 19 (4): 409–418.

16. Evans J, Frank B, Oliffe JL, Gregory D. Health, illness, men and masculinities (HIMM): A theoretical framework for understanding men and their health. *Journal of Men's Health.* 2011; 8 (1): 7–15.

17. Robertson S, Williams B, Oliffe J. The case for retaining a focus on "masculinities" in men's health research. *International Journal of Men's Health.* 2016; 15 (1): 52–67.

18. White A, de Sousa B, de Visser R, et al. *The state of men's health in Europe: Extended report.* European Commission. 2011; http://ec.europa.eu/health/population_groups/docs/men_health_extended_en.pdf2011.

19. Australian Government, Department of Health and Ageing. *National male health policy: Building on the strengths of Australian males.* Canberra, 2010.

20. Smith JA, Robertson S, Richardson N. Letter: Understanding gender equity in the context of men's health policy development. *Health Promotion Journal of Australia.* 2010; 21 (1): 76.

21. Department of Health. *National Men's Health Action Plan Healthy Ireland: Working with men in Ireland to achieve optimum health and wellbeing.* Dublin: Department of Health; 2016.

22. Macdonald J. Building on the strengths of Australian males. *International Journal of Men's Health.* 2011; 10 (1): 82.

23. MacDonald J. A different framework for looking at men's health. *International Journal of Men's Health.* 2016; 15 (3): 283.

24. Pedrana A, Hellard M, Gold J, et al. Queer as F** k: Reaching and engaging gay men in sexual health promotion through social networking sites. *Journal of Medical Internet Research.* 2013; 15 (2): e25.

25. Crossley ML. The "Armistead" project: An exploration of gay men, sexual practices, community health promotion and issues of empowerment. *Journal of Community & Applied Social Psychology.* 2001; 11 (2): 111–123.

26. Crossley ML. Making sense of "barebacking": Gay men's narratives, unsafe sex and the "resistance habitus." *British Journal of Social Psychology.* 2004; 43 (2): 225–244.

27. Bancroft J, Janssen E, Strong D, et al. Sexual risk-taking in gay men: The relevance of sexual arousability, mood, and sensation seeking. *Archives of Sexual Behavior.* 2003; 32 (6): 555–572.

28. Patton M. *Qualitative research and evaluation methods.* Thousand Oaks, Calif.: Sage; 2002.

29. Filiault SM, Drummond MJ. Athletes and body image: Interviews with gay

sportsmen. *Qualitative Research in Psychology.* 2008; 5 (4): 311–333.

30. Ussher JM, Perz J, Rose D, et al. Threat of sexual disqualification: The consequences of erectile dysfunction and other sexual changes for gay and bisexual men with prostate cancer. *Archives of Sexual Behavior.* 2017: 46 (7) 2043–2057.

31. Filiault SM, Drummond MJN, Smith JA. Gay men and prostate cancer: Voicing the concerns of a hidden population. *Journal of Men's Health.* 2008; 5 (4): 327–332.

32. Rose D, Ussher JM, Perz J. Let's talk about gay sex: Gay and bisexual men's sexual communication with healthcare professionals after prostate cancer. *European Journal of Cancer Care.* 2017; 26(1).

33. Belt R. Disability: The last marriage equality frontier. *Stanford Public Law Working Paper No 2653117.* 2015; http://dx.doi.org/10.2139/ssrn.2653117.

34. Chance TF. "Going to pieces" over LGBT health disparities: How an amended Affordable Care Act could cure the discrimination that ails the LGBT community. *Journal of Health Care Law & Policy.* 2013; 16 (2): 375–402.

35. Kamen C, Mustian K, Johnson MO, Boehmer U. Same-sex couples matter in cancer care. *Journal of Oncology Practice.* 2015; 11 (2): e212–e215.

36. Perone AK. Health implications of the Supreme Court's *Obergefell vs. Hodges* marriage equality decision. *LGBT Health.* 2015; 2 (3): 196–199.

37. Manne S, Badr H, Zaider T, et al.. Cancer-related communication, relationship intimacy, and psychological distress among couples coping with localized prostate cancer. *Research and Practice.* 2010; 4 (1): 74–85.

38. Knoll N, Burkert S, Kramer J, et al.. Relationship satisfaction and erectile functions in men receiving laparoscopic radical prostatectomy: Effects of provision and receipt of spousal social support. *Journal of Sexual Medicine.* 2009; 6 (5): 1438–1450.

39. Goldsen J, Bryan AE, Kim H-J, et al. Who says I do: The changing context of marriage and health and quality of life for LGBT older adults. *Gerontologist.* 2017; 57 (suppl. 1): S50–S62.

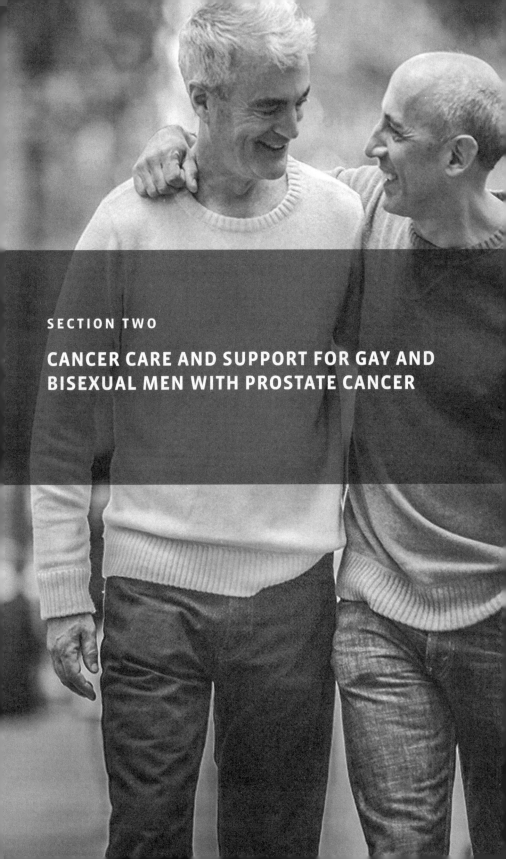

SECTION TWO

**CANCER CARE AND SUPPORT FOR GAY AND
BISEXUAL MEN WITH PROSTATE CANCER**

CHAPTER 8

Lack of Information and Unmet Needs

Gay and Bisexual Men's Sexual Communication with Healthcare Professionals about Sex after Prostate Cancer

Duncan Rose, Jane M. Ussher, and Janette Perz

CHAPTER SUMMARY

Although sexual changes after prostate cancer have specific meanings and consequences for gay and bisexual men (GBM), little is known about how GBM navigate sexual well-being support. We surveyed 124 GBM with prostate cancer and 21 male partners, and interviewed a subsample of 46 GBM and 7 male partners, to examine GBM's experiences of sexual communication with healthcare professionals after the onset of prostate cancer. GBM perceived a number of deficits in healthcare professional communication: heterosexuality of GBM patients was often assumed; sexual orientation disclosure was problematic; and GBM perceived rejection or lack of interest and knowledge from a majority of healthcare professionals with regard to gay sexuality and the effect of prostate cancer on GBM. Facilitators of communication were an acknowledgment of sexual orientation and exploration of the effect of prostate cancer on GBM. To improve support for GBM with prostate cancer, we conclude that healthcare professionals need to address issues of heterocentrism within prostate cancer care by improving facilitation of sexual orientation disclosure, recognizing that GBM with prostate cancer may have specific sexual and relational needs, and increasing knowledge and comfort discussing gay sexuality and gay sexual practices.

Ussher, Jane M., Perz, Janette, Rosser, B. R. Simon, eds., *Gay & Bisexual Men Living with Prostate Cancer*
dx.doi.org/10.17312/harringtonparkpress/2018.06.gbmlpc.008
© 2018 Harrington Park Press

communication with healthcare professionals; gay and bisexual men, prostate cancer, psychological, sexual identity disclosure, sexuality

INTRODUCTION

Healthcare professionals are increasingly recognizing sexual concerns following cancer treatment as an important issue to discuss with patients.[1, 2] Despite this recognition, a number of barriers to clinical discussions of cancer and sexuality have been identified, including deficits in healthcare professionals' knowledge, comfort, and confidence when talking about sex,[2] as well as structural constraints, such as education, privacy concerns, and lack of time.[3, 4] Although discussions of sexuality with healthcare professionals have been found to be more common in the context of prostate cancer compared to other cancer types,[5] sexual well-being support for men with prostate cancer has widely and consistently been reported as inadequate.[6]

Gay and bisexual men (GBM) with prostate cancer report higher dissatisfaction with prostate cancer treatment than heterosexual men, one that is associated with lower quality of life.[7, 8] One explanation for this dissatisfaction is that GBM-specific issues and concerns are often unaddressed by healthcare professionals.[9] Healthcare professionals working with cancer patients have reported that the sexual concerns of LGBT patients are less likely to be addressed, owing to practitioners' lack of confidence and knowledge of LGBT sexuality and relationships.[2, 10] However, research on communication between GBM with prostate cancer and healthcare professionals is scant, addressed only within two small-scale qualitative studies.[11, 12] In these studies, GBM perceived prostate cancer support as heteronormative: healthcare professionals often failed to discuss the physical and psychological effects of treatment on gay men and their partners and often assumed gay patients were heterosexual. In addition, communication by healthcare professionals when discussing gay sexuality was described as "disingenuous," "coy," and "Victorian."[11]

Research on lesbians with breast cancer,[13, 14] and wider LGBT health research,[15, 16] suggests that patients frequently perceive interactions with healthcare professionals as heterocentric and at times homophobic and discriminatory. Disclosure of sexual orientation, in order to receive targeted information and support, can be difficult. Although disclosing sexual orientation to healthcare professionals is associated with positive mental health outcomes[17] and greater satisfaction with care,[18] there is evidence that when sexual minority patients do disclose, responses from healthcare professionals range from accepting to ignoring;[19] and some healthcare professionals are reticent to discuss sexuality or provide relevant sexual information in response to disclosure.[20, 21] It has been suggested that these responses result from healthcare professionals' lack of knowledge and training regarding the sexual practices of sexual minorities[22] and their concern about appropriate use of language.[2, 23] Nondisclosure by sexual-minority patients has been associated with fear of mistreatment, privacy concerns, and uncertainty about whether sexual orientation is important to medical care.[13, 24] This chapter examines GBM's experience of communication with healthcare professionals after the onset of prostate cancer, focusing on issues related to sexuality and changes in sexual well-being.

STUDY DESCRIPTION

One hundred and twenty-four GBM who currently have, or have had, prostate cancer, and 21 male partners of men with prostate cancer, completed an online or postal survey, part of a larger program of mixed-methods research examining sexual well-being and quality of life after prostate cancer.[25–28] Full demographic details are presented elsewhere in this book (see chapter 2).[29] Open-ended survey questions asked participants about their experiences of sexual identity disclosure and discussing sexual well-being with healthcare professionals, satisfaction with such discussions, and interest in information about sexual changes after prostate cancer treatment. At the end of the survey, 62% of participants volunteered to take part in one-on-one semistructured interviews, lasting approximately one hour. Of these, we interviewed 46 GBM and 7 partners to further examine the subjective experiences of sexual communication and perceived support from healthcare professionals.

RESULTS

Of 118 participants who answered a question on whether they had spoken to anyone about sexual well-being, 95 (80.5%) responded that they had, and 23 (19.5%) responded they had not. Participants who had spoken to someone about their sexual well-being in relation to prostate cancer were asked whom they spoke to and how satisfied they were with the discussion (table 8.1). These participants reported most frequently speaking to social networks (89%), medical practitioners (86%), allied health professionals (41%), other supports (35%), and nursing

TABLE 8.1

Communication about Sexuality with Healthcare Professionals and Social Networks

	% of sample (*N*)	Satisfied with discussion % (*N*)
Social Network	**89.25 (83)**	
Partner	46 (57)	71.9 (41)
Friend	56.5 (70)	67.1 (47)
Family member/relative	31.5 (39)	46.2 (18)
Medical HCP	**85.95 (79)**	
General practitioner (GP)	50 (62)	51.6 (32)
Oncologist	18.5 (23)	60.9 (14)
Urologist	41.9 (52)	42.3 (22)
Radiologist	12.9 (16)	56.3 (9)
Surgeon	32.3 (40)	45 (18)
Nursing HCP	**24.73 (23)**	
Urological nurse	7.3 (9)	66.7 (6)
Prostate cancer nurse	10.5 (13)	53.8 (7)
Allied HCP	**40.86 (38)**	
Physiotherapist	9.7 (12)	50 (6)
Occupational therapist	1.6 (2)	0 (0)
Sex therapist	10.5 (13)	53.8 (7)
Social worker	1.6 (2)	100 (2)
Counselor	7.3 (9)	33.3 (3)
Psychologist	12.9 (16)	62.5 (10)
Other Support	**35.48 (33)**	
Support group	24.2 (30)	66.7 (20)
Prostate cancer support helpline	7.3 (9)	33.3 (3)
Religious group	3.2 (4)	25 (1)

health professionals (25%) about sexual well-being in relation to prostate cancer. Participants who had not spoken to anyone about their sexual well-being in relation to prostate cancer were asked why they had not spoken to anyone and whom they would like to speak to. In order of frequency, reasons for not speaking to anyone about sexual well-being were "I don't know how anyone could help" (52%), "embarrassment"

(35%), "I can cope on my own" (35%), "my sexual well-being and sexuality is a private matter" (22%), "I don't know who to talk to" (22%), "I don't know how to begin the discussion" (22%), "I plan to talk to somebody in the future" (13%), "I look up information on the Internet" (13%), and "the changes are not significant" (9%). Participants who had not spoken to anyone about sexual well-being most frequently reported wishing to speak to an allied health professional (74%), followed equally by social networks, specialists, general practitioners, and other supports (35% each), and nursing professionals (9%).

All participants were also asked when issues relating to prostate cancer and sexuality should be discussed with healthcare professionals and how they would like to receive more information about prostate cancer and sexuality. Of the 114 participants who responded to the question on timing of discussions on sexuality and prostate cancer, 15% selected "at the time of diagnosis," 15% "at the time of discussing treatments," 3% "post-treatment and during recovery," 57% "at all of these stages," and 2% "never." All 124 participants selected options for receiving more information on prostate cancer and sexuality, and websites were reported as the most desired medium of communication (61%), followed by newsletter (48%), book or leaflet (42%), group or information session (40%), social media (21%), telephone helpline (19%), and some other medium (5%).

Levels of satisfaction with the discussion were higher for personal networks than for other groups, varying across professional and social context (see table 8.1). Satisfaction was relatively high for discussion with partners (72%), which has implications for GBM's well-being because communication between partners during prostate cancer treatment has been linked to enhanced relationship quality and intimacy for prostate cancer survivors[30] (see chapter 7). For health professionals, satisfaction ranged from 67% for urological nurses to 33% for counselors, confirming previous findings of low rates of patient satisfaction with healthcare practitioner (HCP) discussion of sexual concerns after cancer treatment.[31-33] The analysis of open-ended survey responses and interviews, conducted using thematic analysis,[34] provides insight into the causes of dissatisfaction.

HEALTHCARE PROFESSIONALS ASSUME HETEROSEXUALITY: "IT'S AS THOUGH WE'RE INVISIBLE"

When sexual well-being was addressed by healthcare professionals, participants described it as a "one-size-fits-all approach" that was "geared up for straight men" and offered little, if any, psychosexual support to cope with the effects of prostate cancer on gay sexuality and relationships. As a result, our sample described being marginalized from support because of the fact that their prostate cancer care was not only cancer-centric, but also heterocentric. For example, Euan (gay, 66) said, "There was a whole lot of stuff that . . . does mean a lot to a gay man that wasn't fully explained," and Scott (gay, 59) told us there was "no real questioning or trying to understand my position as a gay male." Within this "heterosexual world of discussion," Henry (gay, 59) observed: "It's as though we're invisible. We're usually not considered, the assumption always seems to be that the man with prostate cancer sitting in front of them or on the end of the phone must be straight." This assumption was evident in several accounts of healthcare professionals referring to sexual partners as women. For example, Drew (gay, 65) told us, "Most of them [HCPs] cater to how you are adjusting with your wife," and Barry (gay, 61) recounted the following conversation, which he had in the hospital with two nurses, in the presence of his urologist: "I said 'Is it safe to share a bed with my partner?' And they said, 'Well, unless she's pregnant or very young, it should be fine.' And I said, 'That's my partner behind me.' They looked [laughter] dumbfounded and he looked very embarrassed."

Participant reports of the assumption of heterosexuality in clinical discussions were also reflected in printed material received from healthcare professionals, as Tristan (gay, 62) stated, "When you've been diagnosed with cancer, being presented with questions and forms that assume you to be heterosexual is very distressing." Andy (gay, 61) told us: "All the literature is about having sex with your wife when you come out of hospital, and doing this and doing that. . . . I just adjust the reading to make it more inclusive, but I shouldn't have to do that." Men who openly identify as heterosexual may be engaging in sex with men, and these men also experience marginalization of their sexual needs. Euan (gay, 66) commented: "With this generation you go to the sauna and—and almost I'd say half to three-quarters of the men there would be married and don't identify as gay. So the initial question of 'Do you want to go to the gay group or the straight group' might—might terrify them as well. You're—you're talking tricky negotiation."

NAVIGATING SEXUAL ORIENTATION DISCLOSURE

The perceived heterocentric nature of prostate cancer care necessitated GBM's disclosing their sexual orientation to healthcare professionals if they wanted to receive gay-specific sexual information or acknowledgment of their relationship context. Of the survey respondents, 80% indicated that they had disclosed sexual orientation to at least one HCP since the onset of prostate cancer. To gain deeper insight into sexual orientation disclosure in the context of prostate cancer, we asked interviewees about their experiences of disclosing or not disclosing. They reported three different approaches to disclosure: avoidance, hesitance, and forthrightness, as outlined below.

Avoidance: "Why go down that track if you can avoid it?" A minority (approximately one-fifth) of interviewees reported that they avoided disclosure of sexual orientation with healthcare professionals. A few participants said nondisclosure was a product of limitations within clinical settings, that "there didn't seem to be an appropriate time" and "the consultations are always very short and rushed." For a number of other men, disclosure was seen as a risk. Avoiding disclosure was a more deliberate choice motivated by "fear of rejection," "reservations as to whether healthcare professionals are accepting or not," not wanting "to be lectured," "privacy," and being "too embarrassed." For example, Tony (gay, 74) remarked: "I have some reservations as to whether some professionals are accepting or not. Why go down that track if you can avoid it? . . . They may be less likely to be as assisting as I would like them to be. I just don't want to take that risk." Some participants also told us they "did not see the need to disclose" and "it didn't seem relevant" during initial contact with healthcare professionals; however, the decision not to disclose often led to regret at a later stage when gay-specific sexual concerns arose. As Graham (gay, 74) stated: "I should have just taken the bull by the horn and said it straight out, that I'm a gay man. I [then] wouldn't have to complain about their lack of communication on that subject."

Given the discomfort, perceived risk, and doubt associated with avoidance of disclosure, many participants frequently indicated that healthcare professionals need to take greater responsibility to ask patients how they self-identify in terms of sexual orientation. For example, Jack (gay, 59) stated, "It would almost take the medical profession or the treatment people to open up that avenue of conversation," and Michael (gay, 69) said it is "important for all healthcare professionals" to take the initiative in ensuring targeted information is made available to GBM who may not be aware of the potential significance of prostate cancer on gay sexuality.

Hesitance: "It's a bit confronting, even after you've done it a thousand times." The majority of interviewees (approximately three-fifths) adopted a hesitant stance to disclosure, indicating that disclosure of sexual orientation to healthcare professionals was to some degree "difficult" or "uncomfortable"; the men described themselves as "a little bit hesitant" and grappling with their "duty of disclosure." As Steve (gay, 65) stated: "You have to, sort of, basically come out to people all the time, each time you meet somebody. You have to explain, and sometimes some people aren't really with it. Some people don't understand what it entails, and so sometimes it's a bit confronting, even after you've done it a thousand times."

As a result of the "confronting" nature of disclosure, several participants reported relying on an "unspoken awareness" of sexual orientation, disclosing indirectly to healthcare professionals by bringing a male partner or gay friend to an appointment, by using humor, or dropping hints. For example, Colin (gay, 68) said: "I haven't just come right out and said, 'Hi, doctor. I'm gay,' but when [my partner] shows up with me I make inappropriate jokes, and that's one of the strange ways I think that a lot of people deal with this is with a sense of humor."

Some healthcare professionals responded positively to such indirect disclosures. As Alan (partner, gay, 67) said, "I went into an appointment with Derek to see a beautiful doctor, she's just been amazing, and her assumption was that we were gay." Others reported that some healthcare professionals "would rather not deal with it, but will deal with it if they have to" (Alex, gay, 69), indicating that indirect disclosure can often fail to lead to desired discussions about sexuality. Louis (gay, 56) observed: "My consultant and specialist nurse are very helpful . . . but they don't touch the particular issues involving men who have sex with men . . . very odd, I give them the clues and they lead with them without any particular comment related to orientation. . . . I feel just like a general case." Such accounts suggest that men who adopt a hesitant stance might be to some extent reliant on how receptive healthcare professionals are to indirect disclosure of a patient's GB status.

Forthrightness: "I'm as comfortable as a train." A further minority (approximately one-fifth) of interviewees adopted a forthright stance, describing themselves as undeterred by anticipated reactions to disclosure and actively revealing their sexual orientation as a matter of course. For example, participants told us, "I've been absolutely open about my sexual orientation with every single health professional I've ever encountered" (Bruce, gay, 61), and "I have no hesitation to let them know I'm gay" (Gary, gay, 52). Participants who were forthright indicated it was the professional responsibility of healthcare professionals to be open to discussing health issues specific to GBM. For example, Vincent (partner, gay, 62) stated: "I'm as comfortable as a train . . . and I don't have any problems at all talking about my sexuality or whatever with health professionals. If they get embarrassed, they shouldn't be in the bloody trade, for God's sake. They need to be able to cover the breadth of human health." Additionally, some men who were forthright told us it was a strategic move that enabled them to gauge the level of knowledge and comfort of their HCP in discussing gay sexual practices and relationships. For example, Rick (gay, 59) told us, "It [disclosure] also gives them [HCPs] an opportunity, if they're not comfortable for any reason, well I prefer not to be there." Rick employs a high level of agency as a patient who engages only with healthcare professionals who are "comfortable" in incorporating his sexuality into their care.

By implication, healthcare professionals who are not "confident" in "understanding the different issues for GBM," or who have "baggage" or "limits" on what they will discuss, may find some forthright GBM with prostate cancer no longer seeking their care.

HEALTHCARE PROFESSIONAL RESPONSES TO DISCLOSURE AND REQUESTS FOR GAY-SPECIFIC SEXUAL INFORMATION

The reciprocal nature of healthcare professional and patient discussions of sexuality following prostate cancer was apparent in open-ended survey and interview responses. Tailored information and support were described as highly contingent on healthcare professional responses to sexual orientation disclosure and requests for gay-specific information.

Responses were described as rejecting, lacking interest or knowledge, or positive, as discussed below.

Rejecting responses: "I don't want to know anything about your sex life." Several men recounted rejection of discussion of gay sexuality by healthcare professionals following sexual identity disclosure and requests for gay-specific information. For example, Scott (gay, 59), after disclosing he was gay, recalled his urologist's response: "Let's just stick to what we're dealing with here, which is the prostate cancer." When Colin (gay, 68) asked a urologist about anal sex after prostatectomy, he said the urologist "looked as if I had maybe hit him in the face with a lemon meringue pie or that we were both in church and I had just broken wind and pointed at him." Rick (gay, 59) told us that in a discussion with his oncologist, "we started talking about anal intercourse and he said, 'Look, I can't go there,'" which left Rick feeling "is he thinking it's dirty, and he obviously thinks it's not normal, because I'm sure he doesn't stop heterosexual men from talking about having intercourse with their wives." Participants told us such responses from healthcare professionals made them "feel uncomfortable," "annoyed," "not natural," or "not safe." Zachary (partner, 59) stated that perceived discomfort from healthcare professionals also reinforces social constructions of "gay sexuality portrayed as the sort of, a bit smelly and on the sidelines . . . like a distasteful topic [laughs]." Additionally, experiences of rejection could result in a number of GBM avoiding future disclosure; Colin (gay, 68) observed, "It is because of occurrences like that [perceived rejection] that I think a lot of gay men are very guarded," adding, "What help is it if they [HCPs] know, but you don't feel safe in talking?"

Lack of knowledge or interest: "I could have said it to the wall." The majority of participants viewed healthcare professionals as "lacking interest" in discussing the specific needs of GBM in relation to prostate cancer, and HCP knowledge of gay sexuality was perceived as "very sketchy." For example, participants made comments such as "I could have said it [disclosed] to the wall, he had no reaction whatsoever, he wasn't remotely interested" (Jerry, gay, 66), and "Every doctor you meet is a straight man, and I don't think they have any idea. I don't think straight people have any idea about gay sex" (Mason, gay, 58). A number of men stated that healthcare professionals' lack of knowledge and interest left them without answers to requests for gay-specific information, as this account illustrates: "Nobody has ever been able to tell me, however, how long one should wait after being the receptive partner before having a PSA test. There seems to be an alarming ignorance in the profession on this issue and other issues affecting men who have sex with men" (Barry, gay, 61).

A number of men described how unanswered requests for gay-specific information led to their undertaking their own "voyage of discovery" or having to "make the primary connection" with referral sources for tailored support, which left them feeling "anxious" and "frustrated." Others felt "deflated" or "disappointed" by still not having the answers: "Is to be a bottom going to be dangerous, you know, for somebody who's been a top because you've had to have your prostate removed? All these sort of things I don't know, and I still don't know, but he [the urologist] sort of wasn't going there" (Euan, gay, 66). Such accounts highlight the potential psychological consequences for GBM when their sexual well-being needs are not acknowledged or followed up by primary care healthcare professionals. One bisexual man suggested that healthcare professionals were even less supportive of bisexual men: "People just don't understand what it's like to be bi, married, and not out. People understand gay and straight, but bi guys don't fit, so we seem to be ignored. It tears you apart internally and we get no help" (Cameron, bisexual, 65).

As a consequence of unmet sexual and emotional needs, some participants stated they sought out gay or "gay-friendly" healthcare professionals: "It should be with a male who is preferably gay" (Elijah, gay, 79); "I probably would have felt more comfortable if I saw a gay urologist" (Scott, gay, 59). However, the need for all healthcare professionals to be able to support GBM was also emphasized, owing to issues of access — "I live in a rural area so it is very difficult even to see a gay-friendly health professional" (Andy, gay, 61) — and the need for increased cultural competency about gay sexual needs.

Acknowledgment and positive support: "I found that quite comforting." Several participants stated that some healthcare professionals were responsive to sexual orientation disclosure and to requests for gay-specific information, openly and candidly discussing gay sexuality. For example, participants commented, "She was very interested in knowing about how gay men deal with this sort of thing and their sexual encounters" (David, gay, 64); "She sort of wanted me to talk to her so that she had a better perspective of where I was coming from" (Clive, gay, 70); "Both my GP and specialist are open to frank discussions" (Timothy, gay, 65). These men reported that although some healthcare professionals lacked the necessary knowledge and awareness to easily answer requests for gay-specific information, they were interested in understanding GBM's concerns and sought information and resources to support them, as this account illustrates: "I have been fortunate in having a very caring professional who has gone the extra distance to improve his knowledge of how prostate cancer affects gay men and their relationships. He is shocked at the lack of resources and support available to gay men. He has ordered a number of resources for myself and my partner from overseas to help" (Rick, gay, 59).

Healthcare professionals' efforts to explore the influence of prostate cancer on gay male sexuality were reported to have a positive effect on psychological adjustment and feelings of "comfort" after cancer treatment, as Mason's account shows: "Part of the process should be that there is someone who deals with your psychological and emotional side of what's going to happen to you, just as much as the physical. They've been very interested to try and find information that is specific to gay people. They've been very interested in listening to my story the whole way through. And I found that quite comforting" (Mason, gay, 68). Mason's experience suggests that positive responses to sexual orientation disclosure, and provision of sexual information targeted to GBM, have implications beyond the sexual domain.

DISCUSSION

Previous qualitative research investigating communication between sexual-minority patients and healthcare professionals found that cancer care was positioned as heterocentric or dismissed the relevance of sexual orientation to care, which resulted in reduced psychosocial support for sexual minorities.[2, 12, 35] It has been reported that healthcare professionals working in cancer often remark, "I treat all my patients the same," a stance that potentially reifies heterocentrism by assuming all patients are heterosexual.[36] This assumption can lead to the negation of the needs of GBM with prostate cancer, and it supports assertions that GBM with prostate cancer are an "invisible diversity"[9] or "hidden population."[11] For healthcare professionals to provide equitable care to GBM with prostate cancer, they need to acknowledge that a proportion of the patients they see are GBM whose needs and concerns might differ from those of heterosexual men because of the effect of prostate cancer on gay sexual practices, gay relationships, and gay identities.[8, 12] However, the success of bringing GBM's concerns into clinical discussions rests heavily on healthcare professionals' motivation to become culturally competent with regard to sexual orientation disclosure and discussion of gay sexual concerns.

Rates of disclosure by GBM in the present study were similar to those in other sexual-minority and health studies.[21, 37] The finding that some GBM used disclosure as a tool to gauge HCP confidence and comfort discussing gay sexuality reflects earlier research in which GBM reported changing urologists if theirs was not "gay-friendly."[12] GBM's reasons for avoiding or hesitating to disclose support previous research in which difficulties disclosing were associated with anticipation of disapproval on the bases of past experiences of discrimination, concerns about medical mistreatment or privacy, and patient beliefs that disclosure is irrelevant to care.[13, 38, 39] The hesitant stance to disclosure adopted by the majority of the sample supports earlier sexual orientation disclosure research drawing on self-presentation theory,[40] which posits that individuals, wishing to present themselves favorably, often gauge the probability of a negative reaction before disclosing a potentially stigmatizing characteristic.

A key aspect of culturally competent care to ameliorate these difficulties is HCP facilitation of sexual orientation disclosure.[41] Such disclosure has a number of benefits: HCP-led facilitation of disclosure has been shown to allay fears of disapproval and improve care;[38] sexual minorities dislike it when healthcare providers presume that they are heterosexual, even if they are too fearful to disclose; and incidents of disclosure are purported to foster greater self-acceptance[42] while reducing the negative health outcomes of internalized homophobia and concealment.[17, 43] Additionally, if healthcare professionals were to demonstrate GB cultural competency by explicitly acknowledging sexual orientation, they could resolve patient uncertainty about the relevance of sexual orientation to prostate cancer care and begin discussing the potential effects of prostate cancer on GBM patients. Previous research has suggested that discussions of sexuality are often absent in cancer care because some patients "trust in the expert," believing healthcare professionals will talk about sexuality if it is important.[4] This finding further reinforces the need for healthcare professionals to take responsibility for educating GBM on the relevance of sexual orientation to prostate cancer to bring relevant concerns to the attention of patients. In addition to verbal facilitation of disclosure, healthcare professionals can support disclosure by fostering an inclusive clinical environment with "gay-friendly" visual cues such as posters, brochures, and information,[41] such as the information kits recently developed for GBM prostate cancer patients and their healthcare professionals.[44, 45] Such practices, if adopted by healthcare professionals in the context of prostate cancer, may offset GBM's perceptions that healthcare professionals are unaware of or uninterested in GBM issues and thereby lead to increased discussion of GBM's sexual concerns.

A key aspect of culturally competent clinician-patient communication is an overtly nonjudgmental, affirming attitude to sexual minorities,[41] which in this study was perceived to be adopted by only a minority of healthcare professionals: levels of satisfaction with HCP discussions were below 50% on average. GBM with prostate cancer perceived many healthcare professionals as lacking the skills, comfort, interest, and knowledge to communicate about gay sexuality. This finding supports earlier research estimates that when healthcare professionals know the sexual orientation of their sexual-minority patients, fewer than 20% of them provide medical information relevant to their patients' sexual behaviors.[21] Although limitations to discussing sex within clinical settings, such as time restraints, were perceived by patients, primary care physicians serve as an ongoing contact throughout prostate cancer care. Education and training of healthcare professionals regarding how to communicate about gay sexuality is essential, and healthcare professionals need either to ensure that they have the resources to provide relevant information regarding GBM and prostate cancer, or to seek out answers to GBM's concerns as they arise rather than ignoring them. HCP education on the significance of prostate cancer to GBM could increase HCP confidence in discussing such issues, which would in turn reduce perceptions that healthcare professionals possess insufficient knowledge, interest, or comfort to discuss gay sexuality in the context of prostate cancer.

ACKNOWLEDGMENTS

This study was funded by the Prostate Cancer Foundation of Australia (PCFA) in the form of new concept grant no. NCG 0512, in partnership with the Australian and New Zealand Urogenital and Prostate Cancer Trials Group (ANZUP). This chapter draws on a previously published paper, Rose D, Ussher JM, Perz J. Let's talk about gay sex: Gay and bisexual men's sexual communication with healthcare professionals after prostate cancer. *European Journal of Cancer Care.* 2017; 26 (1).

REFERENCES

1. Lindau ST, Surawska H, Paice J, Baron SR. Communication about sexuality and intimacy in couples affected by lung cancer and their clinical care providers. *Psycho-Oncology.* 2011; 20 (2): 179–185.

2. Ussher JM, Perz J, Gilbert E, et al. Talking about sex after cancer: A discourse analytic study of health care professional accounts of sexual communication with patients. *Psychology and Health.* 2013; 28 (12): 1370–1390.

3. Hautamaki K, Miettinen M, Kellokumpu-Lehtinen PL, et al. Opening communication with cancer patients about sexuality-related issues. *Cancer Nursing.* 2007; 30 (5): 399–404.

4. Hordern AJ, Street AF. Constructions of sexuality and intimacy after cancer: Patient and health professional perspectives. *Social Science and Medicine.* 2007; 64 (8): 1704–1718.

5. Hawkins Y, Ussher JM, Gilbert E, et al. Changes in sexuality and intimacy after the diagnosis and treatment of cancer: The experience of partners in a sexual relationship with a person with cancer. *Cancer Nursing.* 2009; 32 (4): 271–280.

6. King AJ, Evans M, Moore TH, et al. Prostate cancer and supportive care: A systematic review and qualitative synthesis of men's experiences and unmet needs. *European Journal of Cancer Care.* 2015.

7. Torbit LA, Albiani JJ, Crangle CJ, et al. Fear of recurrence: The importance of self-efficacy and satisfaction with care in gay men with prostate cancer. *Psycho-Oncology.* 2014; 24 (6): 691–698.

8. Ussher JM, Perz J, Rose D, et al. Threat of sexual disqualification: The consequences of erectile dysfunction and other sexual changes for gay and bisexual men with prostate cancer. *Archives of Sexual Behavior.* 2017: 46 (7) 2043–2057.

9. Blank TO. Gay men and prostate cancer: Invisible diversity. *Journal of Clinical Oncology.* 2005; 23 (12): 2593–2596.

10. Perz J, Ussher JM, Gilbert E. Constructions of sex and intimacy after cancer: Q methodology study of people with cancer, their partners, and health professionals. *BMC Cancer.* 2013; 13 (1): 270.

11. Filiault SM, Drummond MJN, Smith JA. Gay men and prostate cancer: Voicing the concerns of a hidden population. *Journal of Men's Health.* 2008; 5 (4): 327–332.

12. Thomas C, Wootten A, Robinson P. The experiences of gay and bisexual men diagnosed with prostate cancer: Results from an online focus group. *European Journal of Cancer Care.* 2013; 22 (4): 522–529.

13. Boehmer U, Case P. Physicians don't ask, sometimes patients tell: Disclosure of sexual orientation among women with breast carcinoma. *Cancer.* 2004; 101 (8): 1882–1889.

14. DeHart DD. Breast health behavior among lesbians: The role of health beliefs, heterosexism, and homophobia. *Women & Health*. 2008; 48 (4): 409–427.

15. Semp D. A public silence: The discursive construction of heteronormativity in public mental health services and the implications for clients. *Gay & Lesbian Issues and Psychology Review*. 2008; 4 (2): 94–107.

16. Rounds K, McGrath BB, Walsh E. Perspectives on provider behaviors: A qualitative study of sexual and gender minorities regarding quality of care. *Contemporary Nurse*. 2013; 44 (1): 99–110.

17. Durso LE, Meyer IH. Patterns and predictors of disclosure of sexual orientation to healthcare providers among lesbians, gay men, and bisexuals. *Sexual Research and Social Policy*. 2013; 10 (1): 35–42.

18. O'Hanlan KA, Cabaj RP, Schatz B, et al. A review of the medical consequences of homophobia with suggestions for resolution. *Journal of the Gay and Lesbian Medical Association*. 1997; 1 (1): 25–39.

19. Katz A. Gay and lesbian patients with cancer. *Cancer and Sexual Health*. 2011; 397–403.

20. Nusbaum MR, Hamilton CD. The proactive sexual health history. *American Family Physician*. 2002; 66 (9): 1705–1712.

21. Labig CE Jr., Peterson TO. Sexual minorities and selection of a primary care physician in a midwestern U.S. city. *Journal of Homosexuality*. 2006; 51 (3): 1–5.

22. Stott DB. The training needs of general practitioners in the exploration of sexual health matters and providing sexual healthcare to lesbian, gay and bisexual patients. *Medical Teaching*. 2013; 35 (9): 752–759.

23. Hinchliff S, Gott M, Galena E. "I daresay I might find it embarrassing": General practitioners' perspectives on discussing sexual health issues with lesbian and gay patients. *Health and Social Care in the Community*. 2005; 13 (4): 345–353.

24. St. Pierre M. Under what conditions do lesbians disclose their sexual orientation to primary healthcare providers? A review of the literature. *Journal of Lesbian Studies*. 2012; 16 (2): 199–219.

25. Ussher JM, Perz J, Kellett A, et al. Health-related quality of life, psychological distress, and sexual changes following prostate cancer: A comparison of gay and bisexual men with heterosexual men. *Journal of Sexual Medicine*. 2016; 13 (3): 425–434.

26. Ussher JM, Perz J, Rose D, et al. Threat of sexual disqualification: The consequences of erectile dysfunction and other sexual changes for gay and bisexual men with prostate cancer. *Archives of Sexual Behavior*. 2017: 46 (7) 2043–2057.

27. Rose D, Ussher JM, Perz J. Let's talk about gay sex: Gay and bisexual men's sexual communication with healthcare professionals after prostate cancer. *European Journal of Cancer Care*. 2017; 26 (1).

28. Ussher JM, Rose D, Perz J. Mastery, isolation, or acceptance: Gay and bisexual men's construction of aging in the context of sexual embodiment after prostate cancer. *Journal of Sex Research*. 2017; 54 (6): 802–812.

29. Ussher JM, Perz J, Kellett A, et al. Health-related quality of life, psychological distress, and sexual changes following prostate cancer: A comparison of gay and bisexual men with heterosexual men. *Journal of Sexual Medicine.* 2016; 13 (3): 425–434.

30. Manne S, Badr H, Zaider T, et al. Cancer-related communication, relationship intimacy, and psychological distress among couples coping with localized prostate cancer. *Research and Practice.* 2010; 4 (1): 74–85.

31. Gilbert E, Perz J, Ussher JM. Talking about sex with health professionals: The experience of people with cancer and their partners. *European Journal of Cancer Care.* 2016; 25: 280–293.

32. Ussher JM, Perz J, Gilbert E. Information needs associated with changes to sexual well-being after breast cancer. *Journal of Advanced Nursing.* 2013; 69 (3): 327–337.

33. Hordern AJ, Street AF. Communicating about patient sexuality and intimacy after cancer: Mismatched expectations and unmet needs. *Medical Journal of Australia.* 2007; 186 (5): 224–227.

34. Braun V, Clarke B. Using thematic analysis in psychology. *Qualitative Research in Psychology.* 2006; 3 (2): 77–101.

35. Sinding C, Barnoff L, Grassau P. Homophobia and heterosexism in cancer care: The experiences of lesbians. *Journal of Cancer Nursing Research.* 2004; 36 (4): 170–188.

36. Quinn GP, Schabath MB, Sanchez JA, et al. The importance of disclosure: Lesbian, gay, bisexual, transgender/transsexual, queer/questioning, and intersex individuals and the cancer continuum. *Cancer.* 2014; 121 (8): 1160–1163.

37. Petroll AE, Mosack KE. Physician awareness of sexual orientation and preventive health recommendations to men who have sex with men. *Sexually Transmitted Disease.* 2011; 38 (1): 63–67.

38. Stein GL, Bonuck KA. Physician-patient relationships among the lesbian and gay community. *Journal of the Gay and Lesbian Medical Association.* 2001; 5 (3): 87–93.

39. Neville S, Henrickson M. Perceptions of lesbian, gay and bisexual people of primary healthcare services. *Journal of Advanced Nursing.* 2006; 55 (4): 407–415.

40. Barbara A, Quandt S, Anderson R. Experiences of lesbians in the health care environment. *Women and Health.* 2001; 34: 45–62.

41. McNair RP, Hegarty K. Guidelines for the primary care of lesbian, gay, and bisexual people: A systematic review. *Annals of Family Medicine.* 2010; 8 (6): 533–541.

42. Schrimshaw EW, Siegel K, Downing MJ, Parsons JT. Disclosure and concealment of sexual orientation and the mental health of non-gay-identified, behaviorally bisexual men. *Journal of Consulting and Clinical Psychology.* 2013; 81 (1): 141–153.

43. Pachankis JE. The psychological implications of concealing a stigma: A cognitive-affective-behavioral model. *Psychological Bulletin.* 2007; 133 (2): 328–345.

44. Prostate Cancer Foundation of Australia. Prostate cancer pack: Information for gay and bisexual men. 2014; www.prostate.org.au/awareness/for-recently-dia nosed-men-and-their-families/gay-and-bisexual-men/download-information/.

45. Prostate Cancer UK. Prostate facts for gay and bisexual men. 2014; http://pros tatecanceruk.org/prostate-information/our-publications/publicationsprostate-facts-for-gay-and-bisexual-men.

CHAPTER 9

Prostate Cancer Treatment Decision-Making and Survivorship Considerations among Gay and Bisexual Men

Implications for Sexual Roles and Functioning

Gwendolyn P. Quinn, Matthew B. Schabath, and Clement K. Gwede

CHAPTER SUMMARY

A man who identifies as a gay or bisexual man (GBM), or as a man who has sex with men (MSM), and who is diagnosed with prostate cancer may experience survivorship and sexual roles and functioning differently from a man who identifies as heterosexual or straight. Whether actual treatment decisions differ between gay or bisexual men and straight or heterosexual men is not known. The effects and consequences of prostate cancer treatment are typically experienced by all men, regardless of sexual orientation, but the concern and bother of treatment side effects in survivorship may have different manifestations. Partnered men of all sexual orientations may have improved survivorship over men not in relationships. Younger men, particularly younger GBM, may have poorer quality of life in cancer survivorship. Healthcare providers are encouraged to create safe and accepting environments for patients to disclose sexual orientation and gender identity and to make the appropriate clinical decisions based on this information with knowledgeable recommendations and strategies during treatment decision making and survivorship. In this chapter we review the published literature about GBM with prostate cancer, decision making when considering treatment options, symptom burden, and sexual roles and functioning in survivorship. Interspersed throughout the chapter are qualitative comments collected by our group from a series of surveys conducted among the LGBT community about their experiences with receiving general healthcare.

Ussher, Jane M., Perz, Janette, Rosser, B. R. Simon, eds., *Gay & Bisexual Men Living with Prostate Cancer*
dx.doi.org/10.17312/harringtonparkpress/2018.06.gbmlpc.009
© 2018 Harrington Park Press

gay and bisexual men, prostate cancer, quality of life, treatment decision making

INTRODUCTION

Among 1,000 LGBT respondents who answered a survey in Florida about their experiences with receiving general healthcare, 12 respondents identified as GBM who had experienced prostate cancer. One gay respondent characterized his experience: "So they sent me to a psychiatrist because I said I would rather die of this cancer and be able to have sex than live a few more years and be impotent. Maybe if I had a steady partner it would be different, but I'm a single gay man and I'm not getting any younger. I'm not ashamed of my life, but these doctors seem to be. Maybe it's not what they would choose, but it is what I chose for me" (67-year-old gay prostate cancer patient).

As is discussed elsewhere in this book, prostate cancer is the most frequently diagnosed cancer in men and the second-leading cause of cancer-related death. In 2017 approximately 161,360 new cases of prostate cancer and 26,730 prostate cancer–related deaths were predicted in the United States.[1] Estimates suggest approximately 4%[2] of men in the United States have had sex with another man and, among those, approximately 50% are in committed same-sex relationships.[3] Although all men are at risk for prostate disease, as outlined in chapter 1, there are limited data on the effect of prostate disease among gay and bisexual men (GBM) and other men who have sex with men (MSM) and almost no data on transgender women.

In 2016 Rosser and colleagues estimated that approximately 100,000 GBM are living with a prostate cancer diagnosis, and there are 50,000 or more gay or bisexual prostate cancer survivors in the United States.[4] However, there are no data to support the view that MSM are at greater risk for prostate cancer. On the contrary, Boehmer and colleagues examined results from 51,233 men from the California Health Interview Survey and found gay men had a significantly lower prevalence estimate for prostate cancer (5.3%) than heterosexual men (16.5%) and bisexual men (14.3%).[4] Advanced age, African ancestry, a family history of prostate cancer, and geographical locale are well-established risk factors for prostate cancer.[5] According to the American Cancer Society, prostate cancer is the most common cancer diagnosis among men in North America, northwestern Europe, Australia, and the Caribbean islands.[6] It is less common in Asia, Africa, and Central and South America, which may be a reflection of differences in risk factors and socioeconomic status. Risk factors associated with prostate cancer are age greater than 65 years, race or ethnicity, family history, and diet, and there is some evidence that active cigarette smoking is significantly associated with prostate cancer incidence[7] and mortality.[8, 9] Clearly, not all gay or bisexual men are HIV-positive; however, there is also evidence that men with HIV are at lower risk of prostate cancer than men in the general population.[10]

Other factors may intersect with GBM's identity beyond sexual orientation, and these may influence treatment decision making or have implications for survivorship. Racial and ethnic or cultural background, HIV status, and substance use are all important factors in identity and have implications for communication, patient-centered care, and shared decision making. The confluence of multiple minority statuses (e.g., gay, Hispanic, smoker) may create a synergistic negativity when a patient is seeking healthcare. Providers may have unconscious biases or stereotypes of patients with these identities and make assumptions about treatment decisions, compliance,[11] and outcomes. However, having dual minority status is also a gateway into multiple cultures, and such persons may be effective change agents to improve institutional cultural competency and patient-physician communication.[12, 13] Understanding how race, sexual orientation, and gender identity can simultaneously influence clinical interactions and shared decision making is an important step in addressing health disparities among these populations.[14]

TREATMENT OPTIONS, SYMPTOM BURDEN, AND TREATMENT DECISION MAKING

Men diagnosed with early prostate cancer (localized or locally advanced) have many treatment options, which are largely dependent on stage of disease, life expectancy, performance status (a measure of how well a person is able to carry on ordinary daily activities while living with cancer), and patient preferences.[15–17] Treatment options for localized or early-stage prostate cancer include definitive active treatment with surgery, different radiation treatments alone or in combination with hormone therapy, and active surveillance and monitoring whereby initial treatment is deferred (but with a plan for active treatment to be initiated if the disease begins to progress or when the patient requests treatment).[15–17] These treatment options can result in a number of acute and chronic side effects that often require significant considerations and shared decision making during treatment selection. Depending on the treatment selected, the most common and bothersome side effects include sexual dysfunction (e.g., erectile dysfunction or impotence, loss of sexual libido); urinary incontinence or irritation; rectal toxicity, including irritation or pain or reduced sexual sensitivity; hormone-related changes such as gynecomastia (enlargement in male breasts often associated with pain or discomfort and body image concerns); changes in quality of life; and psychosocial distress and relationship adjustments,[17, 18] as outlined in chapters 1–7. The severity and bother of these symptoms vary among individuals by treatment type or dose, by age, and possibly by sexual orientation. For example, in one study by Ussher and colleagues in which GBM diagnosed with prostate cancer were compared to heterosexual men with prostate cancer, GBM reported significantly lower sexual functioning and quality of life, increased psychosocial distress, and distruptive dyadic sexual communication.[19] However, the GBM in that study were younger than the heterosexual men, less likely to be in an ongoing relationship, and more likely to report casual sexual partners; thus, their concern with preserving sexual function and maintaining erectile and ejaculatory function, and their reported distress and concerns about relationships and sexual encounters, may have been a function of age rather than sexual orientation.

Treatment-related symptoms and toxicities are important considerations in informed treatment and shared decision making, as these aspects of quality of life may be associated with post-treatment regret.[15, 20] Christie and colleagues conducted a systematic review examining decisional regret in prostate cancer treatment, without consideration of sexual orientation.[21] Among the 28 publications with relevant data, the most commonly identified factors associated with decisional regret included toxicity factors related to sexual and urinary function, older age, and longer time since treatment. Patients who selected radical prostatectomy were more associated with regret than those who chose external beam radiotherapy or brachytherapy. A survey of 934 prostate cancer survivors[20] (without consideration of sexual orientation) across six states in the United States examined decisional regret at six months after treatment and again 15 years later. The findings suggest regret occurred infrequently (14.6% of respondents had regret at 15 years) and was most likely to occur among men who had surgery or radiotherapy. Regret was strongly correlated with moderate to large sexual function bother (39.0%), moderate to large bowel function bother (7.7%), and PSA concern (> 1.01 change). Men who felt they made an informed treatment decision or were older at diagnosis were less likely to report regret.

Treatment decisions made through shared decision-making aids or values clarification tools between a healthcare provider and the patient and perhaps a partner, friend, or family member are less likely to be associated with regret.[22–24] Men who identify as GBM may have different quality-of-life considerations related to sexual functioning and prostate cancer treatment options than men who identify as heterosexual. In making treatment decisions, GBM may weigh sexual and psychosocial changes after prostate cancer treatment differently from heterosexual men,[19, 25, 26] as we discuss below.

There are limited published studies examining differences in treatment outcomes and quality of life by sexual orientation, and none we are aware of compare prostate cancer treatment decision making between GBM and heterosexual men (see chapter 1, tables 1.1 and 1.2). Boehmer and colleagues examined cancer survivors' self-reported health among pooled data from the California Health Interview Survey, finding no differences in self-reported health among gay versus straight men.[5] Several studies report worse outcomes and decreased quality of life among GBM with prostate cancer compared to published norms on heterosexual men.[19, 25–29] In a cross-sectional survey of gay prostate cancer survivors in the United States, men ages 50 to 74 reported lower masculine self-esteem than survivors older than 75 years.[27] Wassersug and colleagues conducted an international study among heterosexual ($N = 460$) and nonheterosexual men ($N = 96$) and identified no differences in incidence of urinary incontinence, bone pain, or erectile dysfunction. In both populations, only 20–25% of survivors reported the ability to achieve an erection during sex. Of those who attempted penetration, 38% reported never or almost never feeling satisfied with their ability to achieve orgasms. However, nonheterosexual men reported significantly worse bother about difficulty ejaculating after any type of prostate cancer treatment,[19, 30] as illustrated in the following account: "My husband and I have been together a long time. Maybe that makes a difference? I decided I would take the treatment five years ago, even though it meant potential incontinence and loss of erection. My husband said the most important thing was that I stay alive. And yes, I have those and other side effects but I'm old, I might have had them anyway" (75-year-old gay prostate cancer survivor).

The effects of prostate cancer intersect with several physical, social, and emotional domains that probably influence treatment decisions and quality of life in survivorship.[19, 25, 26] Sexual (e.g., erectile dysfunction), urinary, and bowel (e.g., irritation, incontinence, tenesmus) treatment-related side effects can have substantial and long-lasting effects on quality of life among prostate cancer patients and survivors, regardless of sexual orientation,[31, 32] as Ussher and colleagues (chapter 2) and Wibowo and Wassersug (chapter 10) outline. The majority of qualitative studies that include or are focused on gay prostate cancer survivors conclude that the cancer experience significantly affected their lives;[33] however, that finding is probably not unique to gay men or prostate cancer. The type of cancer treatment chosen by or offered to GBM may influence future sexual behaviors and thus has implications for survivorship. The effect of poorer sexual functioning for GBM should be considered in light of sexual behavior, such as preferences for anal intercourse that may require a firmer erection than vaginal insertive sex, as well as potential anal discomfort associated with treatment.[28, 34]

For example, a study of 15 GBM with prostate cancer reported that within the group of those receiving surgery who previously had insertive ($N = 4$) and receptive ($N = 3$) anal intercourse roles, only one person from the insertive intercourse group maintained this role after surgery. Additionally, 14% reported no change in sexual practice, 28% reported increased activity in mutual stimulation, and 57% reported increased self-stimulation. Within the group receiving radiation therapy ($N = 7$), survivors who had either an insertive or receptive role ($N = 2$) in anal intercourse maintained those roles.[28] In another study of 36 GBM prostate cancer survivors who participated in focus groups, a common theme was the repercussions of side effects in relation to sexual practices.[35] Men who practiced anal receptive sex were less bothered by erectile dysfunction than those men who practiced insertive anal sex. Another concern felt by all the men in the study was the gay community's reaction to weight gain from hormone treatments and the pressure of being "unable to perform sexually in a sexually charged community." Another qualitative study from Canada conducted among three gay couple dyads found that as sexual roles changed and couples made novel accommodations in roles and boundaries, their perception of sexual functioning improved.[36]

Individuals experiencing significant rectal toxicity may need to make post-treatment receptive sexual role adjustments to avoid pain and discomfort. Hart and colleagues examined changes in sexual roles among gay prostate cancer survivors. These men reported better sexual functioning than heterosexual men in published norms, which suggests that effective post-treatment sexual adjustments can be achieved and quality of life can be preserved,[23] as outlined in chapters 10 and 11 in this book. These adjustments may not occur easily or without relationship disruption or substantial distress about sexual inadequacy.[19, 28] Further, treatments that include hormonal therapy may result in substantive body image concerns related to hot flashes, enlarged breasts, perceived changes in masculinity, and sexual performance issues such as reduction in penis size and firmness that could affect penetrative sex (see chapters 2 and 6).[19] Despite the availability of medical and psychosocial management modalities to address some, but not all, treatment-related toxicities, communication challenges still remain and substantively preclude the effective assessment, deliberation, and implementation of supportive solutions to promote quality of life and positive adjustment after prostate cancer treatment. These communication challenges include failure of the provider or the healthcare system to inquire about sexual orientation and failure of GBM to disclose sexual orientation (see chapters 7 and 8). Without an open discussion between patients and providers about sexual orientation and behaviors, GBM may not be able to participate effectively in shared decision making and to make informed choices about prostate cancer treatment.

Another important aspect is the potential role of racial disparities in the decision-making process of prostate cancer treatment. Gordon and colleagues found that 74% of black men with intermediate- or high-risk cancer considered the effect that treatment would have on their daily activities to be very important.[37] However, only 58% of white men rated that factor as very important. Black men were also significantly more concerned about recovery time (81% versus 50%), and there were significant racial differences when it came to cost concerns (66% of blacks versus 32% of whites). Whether these racial disparities persist among GBM is currently unknown.

Communication is also an important issue in one's circle of support—partners, family, and friends. GBM often face intersectional issues that are compounded by lack of social support, poor communication, and stressful clinical interactions with providers regarding treatment-related concerns or insufficient help to navigate sexual well-being after treatment,[19, 26] as outlined in chapter 8 in this book. Consider the following observation from a 58-year-old gay prostate cancer survivor:

"I have a great group of friends and surprisingly supportive adult children. Their support means everything to me. One day I hope to find a doctor who understands what it's like to be a gay man with prostate cancer, but in the meantime, I'm thankful for the friends and family."

Social support can affect quality-of-life survivorship in men with prostate cancer.[38] Though previous studies have predominantly focused on heterosexual men married at the time of diagnosis and treatment, recent studies are recognizing the significant role of social support among same-sex couples.[39, 40] Kamen and colleagues note that "couple-hood," perhaps particularly in same-sex couples, may reduce psychological distress in cancer patients and survivors,[40] as chapter 4 of this book discusses. Further, being in a coupled relationship has also been shown to improve adherence to medication use.[41]

The chronic stress experienced by some GBM may be somewhat alleviated by couplehood or supportive social networks. Men with prostate cancer who are single generally report poorer quality of life, greater unmet needs,[42, 43] and poorer survival outcomes[44, 45] than men with prostate cancer who are partnered. Partners, friends, family, and social networks of men with prostate cancer can play a vital role in providing emotional and practical support.[46] Thus, unpartnered GBM with prostate cancer are a potentially vulnerable group. GBM with prostate cancer have been shown to have different concerns after their cancer treatment from heterosexual men, such as desire to maintain sexual functioning over longevity, lack of social support, and greater bother from side effects such as weight gain and gynecomastia.[19, 33] In addition, there is evidence that older gay or bisexual men may be particularly isolated socially and may report issues with their healthcare such as heterosexism, as well as difficulties disclosing their sexual identity to providers,[47] as chapter 8 of this book discusses.[25]

Future observational and intervention studies will need to address the effect of social support with a consideration of support from sources other than a spouse or partner, including friends or the LGBT community more broadly.[34] In addition, the sources and extent of social support may be limited for GBM who are not open about their sexual orientation. Finally, given the ongoing treatment-related side effects that persist for at least a decade after treatment,[31] it is important for oncologists, urologists, and primary care providers to discuss all these issues during treatment decision making and in post-treatment clinical interactions (table 9.1).

IMPLICATIONS, CONCLUSIONS, AND RECOMMENDATIONS

Perhaps one first step is to create inclusive atmospheres in the oncology healthcare setting. If sexual orientation information is collected at intake and safe spaces are created within the clinical setting, GBM may be more willing to provide this information. It is incumbent on the healthcare provider to explain why knowing a patient's sexual orientation is important and to incorporate this knowledge into shared decision making about treatment and survivorship care. Specifically, video vignettes that show these patients' unique communication needs (conversations about treatment preferences, concerns about treatment and survivorship) could give providers concrete examples of how to initiate, probe, and respond during conversations at intake, during treatment, and during survivorship care.[6, 48]

Greater awareness by providers and attention to opening lines of communication that elicit the concerns and needs of GBM during treatment, as well as engaging in informed shared decision making about treatment, during treatment, and after treatment, are needed. For a patient to disclose his sexual-minority status and hear his provider say, "I treat all my patients the same,"[49] may elicit a very hollow feeling. Few quality care standards and culturally relevant approaches to address unmet supportive care and treatment decision-making needs of GBM in this context have been developed.[50] However, some recent clinician guidelines to improve cancer care of LGBT people[50] must be integrated into national best practices, and care guidelines must recognize that sexual and gender minorities face unique challenges related to cancer risk, discrimination, and other psychosocial issues. The American Society of Clinical Oncology (ASCO) recently released guidelines recommending strategies to create safe and high-quality healthcare environments for sexual and gender minorities (SGM). These strategies address patient-, provider-, institution-, and policy-level characteristics to address the needs of SGM communities during treatment and into survivorship (table 9.1).

The ASCO strategies highlight and reinforce the idea that the solutions lie in multiple constituencies and domains, including patients, providers, institutions, and policies. For example, patients need tools and education that support effective disclosure of their sexual orientation, gender identity, and related values and priorities for cancer treatment and outcomes without fear of discrimination and stigma. Institutions

TABLE 9.1

American Society of Clinical Oncology Strategies for Reducing Cancer Health Disparities among Sexual and Gender Minorities

Patient Education and Support	Providers	Institutions	Policy
Enhance patient navigation and care coordination	Expand and promote cultural competency training	Collect and use SGM-relevant data for quality improvement	Create and enforce policies ensuring access to culturally competent, equitable cancer care
Expand education for SGM patients with cancer and survivors	Incorporate SGM training into training curricula, training requirements, and certification exam content	Ensure prompt follow-up and continuity of care	Ensure adequate insurance coverage to meet the needs of SGM individuals affected by cancer
Increase patient access to culturally competent support services	Foster safe environments for SGM staff and providers		Ensure policies prohibiting discrimination
Create safe spaces for SGM patients	Integrate a focus on SGM physicians in oncology workforce diversity efforts		
Increase cancer prevention education for SGM individuals			

Source: Adapted from Jennifer Griggs, Shail Maingi, Victoria Blinder, et al., American Society of Clinical Oncology Position Statement: Strategies for Reducing Cancer Health Disparities among Sexual and Gender Minority Populations. *Journal of Clinical Oncology.* 2017; 35 (19): 2203–2208.

and licensing bodies should incorporate best practices for oncology care standards for SGM into training curricula, training requirements, and certification exam content to ensure quality shared decision making, timely care, and prompt follow-up and continuity of care for LGBT people in general and for GBM with prostate cancer specifically. Policies ensuring adequate insurance coverage and prohibiting discrimination are likely to help secure access and delivery of quality cancer care for LGBT people in general and GBM with prostate cancer. This chapter outlines important and unique treatment and survivorship-related concerns of GBM and transgender and transsexual patients with prostate cancer and identifies strategies the oncology community can adopt to improve the quality of care and institutional changes that could be made to improve cancer care for these patients. The ASCO guidelines are quite recent (2017); thus, it is important to monitor and assess whether these strategies produce equity and improve quality in cancer care among sexual and gender minorities.

REFERENCES

1. American Cancer Society. *Cancer facts & figures 2017*. Atlanta: American Cancer Society; 2017.

2. Purcell DW, Johnson CH, Lansky A, et al. Estimating the population size of men who have sex with men in the United States to obtain HIV and syphilis rates. *Open AIDS Journal.* 2012; 6: 98–107.

3. Kurdek LA. Are gay and lesbian cohabitating couples really different from heterosexual married couples? *Journal of Marriage and Family.* 2004; 66 (4): 880–900.

4. Boehmer U, Miao X, Ozonoff A. Cancer survivorship and sexual orientation. *Cancer.* 2011; 117 (16): 3796–3804.

5. Klassen AC, Platz EA. What can geography tell us about prostate cancer? *American Journal of Preventive Medicine.* 2006; 30 (2 Suppl.): S7–S15.

6. American Cancer Society. Prostate cancer risk factors. 2016; https://www.cancer.org/cancer/prostate-cancer/causes-risks-prevention/risk-factors.html#written_by. Accessed June 26, 2017.

7. Ho T, Howard LE, Vidal AC, et al. Smoking and risk of low- and high-grade prostate cancer: Results from the REDUCE study. *Clinical Cancer Research.* 2014; 20 (20): 5331–5338.

8. Huncharek M, Haddock KS, Reid R, Kupelnick B. Smoking as a risk factor for prostate cancer: A meta-analysis of 24 prospective cohort studies. *American Journal of Public Health.* 2010; 100 (4): 693–701.

9. Moreira DM, Aronson WJ, Terris MK, et al. Cigarette smoking is associated with an increased risk of biochemical disease recurrence, metastasis, castration-resistant prostate cancer, and mortality after radical prostatectomy: Results from the SEARCH database. *Cancer.* 2014; 120 (2): 197–204.

10. Shiels MS, Goedert JJ, Moore RD, et al. Reduced risk of prostate cancer in US men with AIDS. *Cancer Epidemiology, Biomarkers & Prevention.* 2010; 19 (11): 2910–2915.

11. Williams DR, Kontos EZ, Viswanath K, et al. Integrating multiple social statuses in health disparities research: The case of lung cancer. *Health Services Research.* 2012; 47 (3): 1255–1277.

12. Tan JY, Xu LJ, Lopez FY, et al. Shared decision making among clinicians and

Asian American and Pacific Islander sexual and gender minorities: An intersectional approach to address a critical care gap. *LGBT Health.* 2016; 3 (5): 327–334.

13. Schneider JA, Zhou AN, Laumann EO. A new HIV prevention network approach: Sociometric peer change agent selection. *Social Science and Medicine.* 2015; 125: 192–202.

14. Peek ME, Lopez FY, Williams HS, et al. Development of a conceptual framework for understanding shared decision making among African-American LGBT patients and their clinicians. *Journal of General Internal Medicine.* 2016; 31 (6): 677–687.

15. Gwede CK, Pow-Sang J, Seigne J, et al. Treatment decision-making strategies and influences in patients with localized prostate cancer. *Cancer.* 2005; 104 (7): 1381–1390.

16. Johnson DC, Mueller DE, Deal AM, et al. Integrating patient preference into treatment decisions for men with prostate cancer at the point of care. *Journal of Urology.* 2016; 196 (6): 1640–1644.

17. Barocas DA, Alvarez J, Resnick MJ, et al. Association between radiation therapy, surgery, or observation for localized prostate cancer and patient reported outcomes after 3 years. *Journal of the American Medical Association.* 2017; 317 (11): 1126–1140.

18. Chen RC, Basak R, Meyer AM, et al. Association between choice of radical prostatectomy, external beam radiotherapy, brachytherapy, or active surveillance and patient-reported quality of life among men with localized prostate cancer. *Journal of the American Medical Association.* 2017; 317 (11): 1141–1150.

19. Ussher JM, Perz J, Kellett A, et al. Health-related quality of life, psychological distress, and sexual changes following prostate cancer: A comparison of gay and bisexual men with heterosexual men. *Journal of Sexual Medicine.* 2016; 13 (3): 425–434.

20. Hoffman RM, Lo M, Clark JA, et al. Treatment decision regret among long-term survivors of localized prostate cancer: Results from the Prostate Cancer Outcomes Study. *Journal of Clinical Oncology.* 2017; 35 (20): 2306–2314.

21. Christie DR, Sharpley CF, Bitsika V. Why do patients regret their prostate cancer treatment? A systematic review of regret after treatment for localized prostate cancer. *Psycho-Oncology.* 2015; 24 (9): 1002–1011.

22. Davison BJ, So AI, Goldenberg SL. Quality of life, sexual function and decisional regret at 1 year after surgical treatment for localized prostate cancer. *BJU International.* 2007; 100 (4): 780–785.

23. Diefenbach M, Mohamed NE, Horwitz E, Pollack A. Longitudinal associations among quality of life and its predictors in patients treated for prostate cancer: The moderating role of age. *Psychology, Health and Medicine.* 2008; 13 (2): 146–161.

24. Hu JC, Kwan L, Krupski TL, et al. Determinants of treatment regret in low-income, uninsured men with prostate cancer. *Urology.* 2008; 72 (6): 1274–1275.

25. Rose D, Ussher JM, Perz J. Let's talk about gay sex: Gay and bisexual men's sexual communication with healthcare professionals after prostate cancer. *European Journal of Cancer Care.* 2017; 26 (1).

26. Torbit LA, Albiani JJ, Crangle CJ, et al. Fear of recurrence: The importance of self-efficacy and satisfaction with care in gay men with prostate cancer. *Psycho-Oncology.* 2015; 24 (6): 691–698.

27. Allensworth-Davies D, Talcott JA, Heeren T, et al. Health effects of masculine self-esteem following treatment for localized prostate cancer among gay men. *LGBT Health.* 2016; 3 (1): 49–56.

28. Lee TK, Breau RH, Eapen L. Pilot study on quality of life and sexual function in men-who-have-sex-with-men treated for prostate cancer. *Journal of Sexual Medicine.* 2013; 10 (8): 2094–2100.

29. Motofei IG, Rowland DL, Popa F, et al. Preliminary study with bicalutamide in heterosexual and homosexual patients with prostate cancer: A possible implication of androgens in male homosexual arousal. *BJU International.* 2011; 108 (1): 110–115.

30. Wassersug RJ, Lyons A, Duncan D, et al. Diagnostic and outcome differences between heterosexual and non-heterosexual men treated for prostate cancer. *Urology.* 2013; 82 (3): 565–571.

31. Chen RC, Chang P, Vetter RJ, et al. Recommended patient-reported core set of symptoms to measure in prostate cancer treatment trials. *Journal of the National Cancer Institute.* 2014; 106 (7): dju32.

32. Davis KM, Kelly SP, Luta G, et al. The association of long-term treatment-related side effects with cancer-specific and general quality of life among prostate cancer survivors. *Urology.* 2014; 84 (2): 300–306.

33. Thomas C, Wootten A, Robinson P. The experiences of gay and bisexual men diagnosed with prostate cancer: Results from an online focus group. *European Journal of Cancer Care.* 2013; 22 (4): 522–529.

34. Blank TO. Gay men and prostate cancer: Invisible diversity. *Journal of Clinical Oncology.* 2005; 23 (12): 2593–2596.

35. Asencio M, Blank T, Descartes L, Crawford A. The prospect of prostate cancer: A challenge for gay men's sexualities as they age. *Sexuality Research and Social Policy Journal of NSRC.* 2009; 6 (4): 38–51.

36. Hartman ME, Irvine J, Currie KL, et al. Exploring gay couples' experience with sexual dysfunction after radical prostatectomy: A qualitative study. *Journal of Sex and Marital Therapy.* 2014; 40 (3): 233–253.

37. Gordon BBE, Basak R, Usinger DS, et al. Factors influencing prostate cancer treatment decisions for African American (AA) and Caucasian (CA) men. *Journal of Clinical Oncology.* 2017; 35 (15 suppl.): 6517.

38. Paterson C, Jones M, Rattray J, Lauder W. Exploring the relationship between coping, social support and health-related quality of life for prostate cancer sur-

vivors: A review of the literature *European Journal of Oncology Nursing* 2013; 17 (6): 750–759.

39. Capistrant BD, Torres B, Merengwa E, et al. Caregiving and social support for gay and bisexual men with prostate cancer. *Psycho-Oncology.* 2016; 25 (11): 1329–1336.

40. Kamen C, Mustian K, Johnson MO, Boehmer U. Same-sex couples matter in cancer care. *Journal of Oncology Practice.* 2015; 11 (2): 212–215.

41. Johnson MO, Dilworth SE, Taylor JM, et al. Primary relationships, HIV treatment adhereance and virologic control. *AIDS and Behavior.* 2012; 16 (6): 1511–1521.

42. Dieperink KB, Hansen S, Wagner L, et al. Living alone, obesity and smoking: Important factors for quality of life after radiotherapy and androgen deprivation therapy for prostate cancer. *Acta Oncologica.* 2012; 51 (6): 722–729.

43. McSorley O, McCaughan E, Prue G, et al. A longitudinal study of coping strategies in men receiving radiotherapy and neo-adjuvant deprivation for prostate cancer: A quantitative and qualitative study. *Journal of Advanced Nursing.* 2014; 70 (3): 625–638.

44. Krongrad A, Lai H, Burke MA, et al. Marriage and mortality in prostate cancer. *Journal of Urology.* 1996; 156 (5): 1696–1700.

45. Matheson L, Watson EK, Nayoan J, et al. A qualitative metasynthesis exploring the impact of prostate cancer and its management on younger, unpartnered and gay men. *European Journal of Cancer Care.* 2017; doi: 10.1111/ecc.12676.

46. Harden JK, Northouse LL, Mood DW. Qualitative analysis of couples' experience with prostate cancer by age cohort. *Cancer Nursing.* 2006; 29 (5): 367–377.

47. Fenge LA, Hicks C. Hidden lives: The importance of recognising the needs and experiences of older lesbians and gay men within healthcare practice. *Diversity in Health & Care.* 2011; 8 (3): 147–154.

48. Lim FA, Brown DV Jr., Justin Kim SM. Addressing health care disparities in the lesbian, gay, bisexual, and transgender population: A review of best practices. *American Journal of Nursing.* 2014; 114 (6): 24–34.

49. Shetty G, Sanchez JA, Lancaster JM, et al. Oncology healthcare providers' knowledge, attitudes and practice behaviors regarding LGBT health. *Patient Education and Counseling.* 2016; 99 (10): 1676–1684.

50. Margolies L. *LGBT patient-centered outcomes: Cancer survivors teach us how to improve care for all.* National LGBT Cancer Network. 2013; www.cancer-network.org/patient_centered_outcomes.

CHAPTER 10

Sexual Aids for Gay and Bisexual Men and Transgender Women after Prostate Cancer Treatments

Erik Wibowo and Richard Wassersug

CHAPTER SUMMARY

Prostate cancer treatments can affect the sexual experience of individuals regardless of sexual orientation. While the absence of orgasm is a common result of most treatments for prostate cancer, some patients have reported experiencing multiple, more intense, or diffuse orgasm after prostate cancer treatment. Interestingly, many transgender women also claim similar orgasmic changes after sexual reassignment. In this chapter we discuss how some products that are marketed as sex aids or "toys" may facilitate sexual recovery after prostate cancer treatments. These products include external penile prostheses, penile sleeves, and penile support devices. We stress the relevance of having a partner or partners for satisfactory sexual recovery. This includes the importance of involving partners in selecting sexual aids and using the aids in a way that develops an erotic association between the aids and the partner. Statistically, gay men are more likely than heterosexual men to be unpartnered. Being single may be a contributing, but under-investigated, factor in the higher level of distress experienced by gay prostate cancer patients in contrast to their heterosexual counterparts.

KEY TERMS

multiple orgasms, penile sleeve, penis support device, sex aids, sex toys, sexual partner, strap-on dildo, vacuum erection device, vibrators

INTRODUCTION

The majority of patients experience erectile dysfunction (ED) after primary prostate cancer treatments such as surgery or radiotherapy.[1, 2] Most

Ussher, Jane M., Perz, Janette, Rosser, B. R. Simon, eds., *Gay & Bisexual Men Living with Prostate Cancer*
dx.doi.org/10.17312/harringtonparkpress/2018.06.gbmlpc.010
© 2018 Harrington Park Press

patients who are on androgen deprivation therapy (ADT) will experience substantial depression of their libido as well.[3, 4] In this chapter we summarize how prostate cancer treatments affect the sexual life of gay and bisexual men (GBM) and transgender women (TGW). We also discuss sexual aids that could potentially be incorporated into sex practices to recover rewarding sex after prostate cancer treatment.[5] While the evidence of effectiveness for these aids has been mostly anecdotal (see chapter 11), GBM and TGW prostate cancer patients may consider trying them as a pathway to sexual recovery. Discussion of the role partners can play in sexual recovery for GBM and TGW prostate cancer patients is also included.

CHANGES IN SEXUAL FUNCTION AFTER PROSTATE CANCER TREATMENTS

Changes in erection, libido, and ejaculation are discussed in chapters 1–7. Here we focus on how prostate cancer treatment may affect genital skin sensitivity and orgasms.

HORMONE STATUS AND IMPLICATIONS FOR SKIN SENSITIVITY

The influence of prostate cancer treatment, most notably ADT, on genital skin sensitivity may be relevant for some men. Currently, how ADT affects genital skin sensitivity has not been explored in prostate cancer patients, but the loss of androgens reduces the receptive field size of the nerves and the physiology of the mechanoreceptors in the perineal skin of male rodents.[6] We have not found any study reporting a change in genital sensitivity after men receive ADT. However, if the change is gradual, the patients themselves may not consciously notice the changes. A cross-sectional quantitative study on patients, comparing the experiences of those who are on ADT with those who are not, is warranted to determine if genital skin sensitivity is altered. If ADT indeed reduces skin sensitivity in the anogenital region for prostate cancer patients, that change may affect the ease of reaching orgasms from tactile genital stimulation (hand job) or the sexual pleasure one receives from oral sex, for example, fellatio (blow job) or anilingus (rimming). Furthermore, with a loss of erection, more pressure may be needed to sufficiently stimulate mechanoreceptors in the genital skin because the corpora cavernosa tissue is flaccid rather than tumescent and less able to resist compression.

It remains to be established whether prostate cancer patients who are on estrogen therapy have better genital skin sensitivity than those who are androgen-suppressed and not receiving supplemental estrogen. In ovariectomized rodents, exogenous estrogens can increase the sensory field of genital skin.[7] If estrogen can increase genital skin sensitivity in prostate cancer patients on ADT, sexual arousal from tactile stimulation may also potentially be improved. Whether supplemental estrogen may help improve sexual pleasure during genital stimulation for prostate cancer patients with reduced erectile function or depressed libido remains to be investigated. Even if estrogen treatment is found not to alter skin sensitivity, estrogen may still benefit androgen-deprived patients by helping maintain libido.[8, 9] Such a study will have clinical relevance for prostate cancer patients overall, but even more for TGW with prostate cancer because they are commonly on estrogen therapy.

ORGASMIC CHANGES

Many men experience impaired orgasms that become painful or reduced in frequency and intensity after prostate cancer treatments[10, 11] regardless of their sexual orientation. However, a small number of men report experiencing more intense orgasm after prostate cancer treatment (1.2 – 9% for post-prostatectomy patients).[12] There are also case reports of patients experiencing multiple orgasms after receiving prostatectomy, radiation therapy, and ADT.[13] Previously, we pointed out that the loss of ejaculation may contribute to multiorgasmic capability after a prostatectomy because, in the absence of ejaculation, a refractory period no longer occurs.[11] Following normal ejaculation, a refractory period occurs during which the likelihood of having another ejaculation or orgasm is dampened.[11] However, after prostate cancer treatment, the reduced ejaculate volume results in a decreased internal pressure in the posterior urethra at the emission stage. Thus, with no ejaculation, there is no refractory period, allowing in theory for additional orgasms to occur over a short period — that is, multi-orgasmia.

How orgasm changes after prostate cancer treatment for GBM or TGW has not been specifically investigated. In one survey study of 558 patients, the frequency of orgasm after treatment did not appear to differ between heterosexual and GBM patients, but that study did not compare the men's orgasmic intensity or multiorgasmic capability after prostate cancer treatment.[14] Previously, we pointed out that some men are capable of having multiple orgasms using sex toys.[11] Sex aid or toy use is generally more prevalent among GBM than heterosexual men,[15] so if more GBM are open to using such sex aids after prostate cancer treatment than heterosexual men, their orgasmic experience after treatment may differ as well.

To our knowledge, no studies have explored how TGW experience changes in their orgasms after prostate cancer treatment, or how often sex aids or toys are used in their sexual practices to help compensate for iatrogenic sexual dysfunction. A major limitation for conducting such a study is the low number of TGW who are treated for prostate cancer (table 10.1).[16] Comparing the orgasmic experience of TGW and non-TGW* prostate cancer patients would help determine the effect of gonadal steroids on orgasmic function. Estrogen treatment may potentially influence orgasms because estrogen receptors are present in the perineal muscles[17] that are involved in orgasm. In previous studies, about 30–40% of TGW reported being multiorgasmic, and 56% claimed to experience intensified orgasms after sex reassignment surgery, which consequently reduces ejaculation.[11] It is thus possible that some TGW who have not gone through full sexual reassignment may also experience multiple or intensified orgasms after prostate cancer treatment.

ADJUSTING SEXUAL PRACTICES AFTER PROSTATE CANCER TREATMENT

Patients who are sexually active before prostate cancer treatment may need to adjust their sexual practices when faced with sexual dysfunction following prostate cancer treatments (see chapters 1–3). Overcoming sexual dysfunction is often at the expense of spontaneous sex[32,33] because most ED treatments (including oral medications) require some planning and preparation. For both patients and their partners, the loss of spontaneous sex may be bothersome, and the problem can be exacerbated when there is reduced libido as a result, for example, of ADT. If patients have regular partners, their partners may need to take the initiative in sexual activity, and such a change can be challenging if the patient was the one who initiated sex more frequently before prostate cancer treatment. Furthermore, if the patient needs an erectile aid, such as intracavernous injection (ICI) or the vacuum erection device (VED), the patient or the patient's partner may be uncomfortable with

---

* Many TGW have been on long-term cross-sex hormone therapy and surgically castrated by the time of their prostate cancer diagnosis. Thus, prostate cancer is extremely rare among transgender women; the estimated prevalence is approximately 13 cases in 5,000, or 0.26%.

TABLE 10.1

Characteristics of Transgender Women with Prostate Cancer

Study	Sample Size	Age	Duration of Cross-Sex Hormone (Years)	Surgically Castrated?
Markland [18]	1	54	6	Yes
Thurston [19]	1	64	12	Not indicated
van Kesteren et al. [20]	0 out of 9	Mean age = 60.2	15.8	Yes
van Kesteren et al. [21]	1	64	12	Yes
van Haarst et al. [22]	1	63	10	Yes
Miksad et al. [23] and Molokwu et al. [24]	1	60	41	Yes
Dorff et al. [25]	1	78	27	Yes
Asscheman et al. [26]	1 out of 966	Mean age = 31.4	Overall sample = 19.4	Not indicated
Wierckx et al. [27]	0 out of 50	Mean age = 43.0	Started at an average age of 36.7	Yes
Turo et al. [28]	1	75	30	Yes
Gooren and Morgentaler [16]	1 out of 2,307	Mean age = 29.3 Prostate cancer patient = 63	Overall sample = 21.4 Prostate cancer patient = 10	Yes
Brown and Jones [29]	0 out of 1,579	Mean age = 55.65	7.6 for 80% of study participants	Not indicated
Ellent and Matrana [30]	1	65	35	After prostate cancer diagnosis
Krakowsky et al. [31]	1	Not specified	< 1	Yes
Sharif et al. [59]	1	56	20	No
Deebel et al. [60]	1	65	20	No

Note: Three papers (20, 27, 29) explored whether any transgender women had prostate cancer but found none. We included these papers to be comprehensive. These studies of TGW did not find any prostate cancer, confirming the rarity of prostate cancer in this population. For papers 20 and 27, the last column says "Yes" because the studies focused solely on TGW who were already surgically castrated.

the complexity of its use. Couples in this circumstance could manage the situation by scheduling sexual activity[34] or incorporating the sexual aid in foreplay.[35] Whether GBM and TGW patients are more bothered by loss of spontaneity than heterosexual patients is not known.

The effect of prostate cancer treatment on men may also differ depending on the patients' preferred sexual practices — for example, whether they have male or female partners, or both, and their preference for being the receptive or insertive partner (see chapters 1–4 and 7). Pelvic pain or rectal bleeding may occur during receptive anal sex after certain prostate cancer treatments, and some patients may be distressed by these conditions.[36–38] For TGW with a neovagina, it is not known whether receptive vaginal sex is associated with increased discomfort following any prostate cancer treatment. Goldstone suggested that GBM prostate cancer patients who prefer a receptive role try inserting a lubricated small dildo in the anus and gradually increasing the dildo size before penile penetration.[36] That suggestion can also be applied to TGW with prostate cancer — that is, by inserting the dildo into their anus if they practice anal receptive sex. TGW are also normally counseled to use vaginal dilators after surgery to construct a neovagina.

Phosphodiesterase type-5 inhibitors (PDE5i) remain the first treatment prescribed to patients with ED[39] partly because patients typically prefer to start with the least invasive option.[40] If PDE5i drugs are not effective, patients may elect other treatments, such as ICI, VED, or penile implants. However, all these ED treatments have a major problem: specifically, poor long-term adherence.[35] The main reasons that patients stop ED treatment are treatment ineffectiveness, partner's lack of interest, concerns about side effects from pharmacological agents,[41] mechanical failure of penile implants,[42] and inconvenience or discomfort associated with using ICI or the VED.[43]

Non-pharmacological and nonsurgical sexual aids can be incorporated into sexual activities, including activities that do not depend on the patient's having a residual erection.[5] Some authors recommend that patients with ED accept noncoital sexual practices, such as oral sex and mutual masturbation, as an alternative to penetrative sex.[44] However, the use of the devices discussed below may offer a pathway to rewarding sex, even with unresolved ED, because they allow the comfort of the full embrace and body contact that is experienced during normal copulatory postures.

Little is known about how often healthcare providers discuss non-pharmacological and nonsurgical sexual aids with patients, regardless of sexual orientation (see chapter 8). Admittedly, the efficacy of these products is not well investigated, and published data remain largely anecdotal.[5] Considering that GBM are more open to using sex aids and toys than heterosexual men,[15, 45] GBM patients might be more willing to explore these options than heterosexual patients, as Ussher and colleagues report in chapter 11. In the following section we discuss some of these non-pharmacological and noninvasive strategies for patients with ED.

EXTERNAL PENILE PROSTHESIS

An external penile prosthesis has the common name of "strap-on dildo."[5] In a case study, a prostate cancer patient with severe ED reported that he had satisfying orgasmic sex with a female partner using such a prosthesis.[13] Coitus was dildo-vaginal rather than penile-vaginal, and the partner provided direct manual stimulation to the man's flaccid penis. The patient reported that their coital posture and body movements so closely matched that of regular penile-vaginal intercourse that the sensation readily led to orgasm. The neurobiology of how this is possible is discussed in detail in Wassersug and Wibowo.[5] The patient further reported that, during prosthesis-vaginal intercourse, he experienced multiple orgasms, which he had never experienced before his prostate cancer treatments. Though no similar cases have been reported in the research literature for GBM or TGW prostate cancer patients, there is no reason to presume that this strategy for sexual recovery would not work for them.

A wide variety of external penile prostheses are available on the market. Dildos and harnesses come in different sizes, colors, and shapes. Furthermore, personalizing a dildo so it matches one's penis is now possible by using penis-casting products, provided they are used before ED develops, or with an erection achieved with aids such as ICI. Some of these products can be found online at CloneAWilly.com, CopyMe Kits.com, and CreateaMate.com. For the harnesses, the Deuce from SpareParts (www.myspare.com/product/deuce) has been specifically designed for men. Other products like the Zoro or Armour Knight from PerfectFitBrand.com have a dildo coupled to the harness, but those dildos cannot be customized.

PENILE SLEEVE AND VIBRATORS

A penile sleeve can be placed on the penis for rigidity, even when the penis itself is not firm enough for penetrative sex. The device can then be used as a masturbatory aid or for penetrative sex. Like external penile prostheses, various types of penile sleeves are available, including those with an opening at the end for exposing the glans, those with protrusions to enhance stimulation, and those coupled to vibrators. Others can be attached to a harness, resembling the external penile prosthesis just described, and used in penetrative sex (for example, those from RxSleeve, www.rxsleeve.com).

A vibrator, either as a separate item or attached to a penile sleeve, may provide tactile stimulation for both patients and partners.[5] Some examples of vibrators that can be used as masturbatory aids include Cobra Libre from funfactory.com, Pulse from hotoctopuss.com, or the Viberect,[5] which is a medical-grade product with adjustable vibration frequency and intensity. Though these vibrators are not intended to be used in penetrative sex, the first two can be placed between a couple's genitalia during sexual activity. That is, the patient's penis is inserted into the device while the device is directly in contact with his partner's genitals.

Penile sleeves can allow a man with ED to continue to be the insertive partner in penetrative intercourse. How effective they can be in providing satisfactory sex will depend on a number of parameters, however, such as the size, shape, and thickness of the device. It is important to choose the right luminal sleeve size. For example, a lumen that is too large can result in the penis easily sliding out of the sleeve.

At least one company (RxSleeve) has a product that can be customized to one's penis size. This product has three different hardness options: Firm, Average, and Soft. Patients who want to use the RxSleeve for anal penetration may need to choose the Firm or Average hardness, depending on their residual erection. In choosing the Firm option, patients must accurately measure their penile length and circumference for the model to fit them properly because the Firm sleeve does not allow stretching inside the internal lumen. Those choosing the Average firmness would require some residual erection. The Average sleeve has a wall thickness of one-quarter inch (0.6 cm) to maintain the sleeve's rigidity and can stretch around the semierect penis.

All sleeves are, to some extent, a physical barrier between the skin of the penis and the tissue of the receptive partner. However, unlike external penile prostheses, penile sleeves permit penile-penetrative sex. It is not yet known which patients would have greater sexual satisfaction—those wearing an external penile prosthesis or those wearing a penile sleeve.

EXTERNAL PENILE SUPPORT DEVICE

An external penile support device called the Elator (see TheElator.com) has been developed for men with ED. The device braces the penile shaft and concurrently stretches the penile shaft while pulling the glans away from the base of the penis. An instructional video on how to use the Elator can be found at www.youtube.com/watch?v=AokWVYxpzY4. Like the other two categories of devices just discussed, penile support devices can work without any residual erection. In addition, a penile support device may provide direct contact between the patient's penis and the patient's partner's vaginal or anal/rectal mucosa. However, published data on the effectiveness of the Elator in helping men have satisfactory coitus or achieve orgasms are lacking for both GBM and non-GBM.

ANEROS

There is also the Aneros (www.aneros.com), which is a sex toy that can be inserted into the anus or the neovagina. People can then use the muscles of their perineum to move the device. While the Aneros is not used as an erectile device, anecdotally some men who use the Aneros achieve multiple orgasms,[11] both before and after prostate cancer treatment (see discussion on www.aneros.com/forum). Physiological research to confirm the reports of multiple orgasms with the Aneros has not yet been undertaken.

VACUUM ERECTION DEVICE

The VED is the first non-pharmacological treatment commonly recommended to patients with ED.[46] Although the VED is popular and is offered to patients as a noninvasive aid for maintaining penis size, it has poor long-term compliance.[47, 48] Some patients may find pumping a VED an inconvenient step in achieving an erection; others may have difficulty in getting a good vacuum seal. Any negative experience when using a VED may dampen a person's sexual arousal. In addition, despite the VED's being able to produce penile tumescence, the erections they produce may not be ideal. Indeed, the VED draws blood only to the penile shaft, but not into the roots of the penis within the perineum. The result is the "hinging" of the penile shaft on the body wall,[46] which may subsequently affect penetration angle. Without the penis pointing upward at the proper angle, the penis is at risk of sliding out of the anus or vagina during pelvic thrusting.[5] If the penis slides out during anal or vaginal sex, the unanticipated disruption can frustrate one or both partners, negatively affecting the sexual experience. This problem may be worse during anal sex because repenetrating an anus is more challenging than repenetrating a vagina.

With a hinged erection, postural adjustment may be necessary by the patient and partner to maintain intercourse to orgasm. One possible adaptation is for the patient's partner to be on top, because in such a position the partner can better control the movement of the penis during sex.

CHALLENGES IN BEING A SINGLE PROSTATE CANCER PATIENT

Sexual practices and relationships are generally more diverse in the nonheterosexual than the heterosexual population. GBM and TGW may be in open or closed relationships, have regular or casual partners, and have more than one regular partner (see chapters 2 and 6). However, they may not have a partner committed to work with them to aid in their sexual recovery. Single individuals with sexual dysfunction may face difficulty in finding new partners, and this may also be true for GBM and TGW prostate cancer patients.[49] Sexual dysfunction may lower men's self-esteem and confidence in starting a relationship because of the fear of rejection by new social contacts. There can be genuine anxiety about what one might do, or should say, if one enters the dating scene and that leads to sexual interest from someone else. Dating or even just meeting new people can become overwhelmingly scary. Many prostate cancer patients with ED declare—whether GBM or straight men—their sex life as over when afflicted with iatrogenic ED.[38, 49, 50] Whether meeting in a club, a bar, or online, they face a dilemma on when, where, and how to disclose their cancer diagnosis or sexual dysfunction.

GBM who do not have a regular partner may engage in casual sex. However, if having erections is a definition of being a man, then losing erections may "disqualify" a man from the GBM sexual world.[38] This disqualification represents an enormous obstacle to GBM with iatrogenic ED seeking new sex partners. Those who already have one or more casual partners before prostate cancer may continue to receive support (sexual or otherwise) from those partners. However, those who are not in any relationship may be at increased risk of social isolation and loneliness.

THE VALUE OF PARTNERS IN SEXUAL RECOVERY

Several publications have stressed the importance of having a partner in ED management[10, 51, 52] (see chapters 3 and 4) and that simply recovering the ability to get an erection does not ensure satisfactory sex with a partner.[53] Having a supportive partner is important in renegotiating sexual practices, especially when sexual dysfunction happens abruptly, as it generally does after prostate cancer surgery. Undoubtedly, for patients who were sexually active with a committed partner or partners before treatment, the loss of erectile function or libido (or both) in the patients can indirectly affect their partners' quality of life, as chapters 3 and 4 outline.

Many clinical psychologists and sex therapists now encourage patients to engage their partners in the treatment of sexual dysfunction. However, when presented with ED treatment options, partners and patients may hold divergent views about the best course of action;[51] that is, the patient's or partner's interest in trying novel treatments may not always be the same. Thus, selecting treatments that both patients and partners are enthusiastic about is important in avoiding failure and subsequent regret. What is also important to consider is the partner's health status. If the partner has a preexisting medical condition that affects sexual function (e.g., ED in a male partner or postmenopausal vaginal dryness in a female partner), that may also influence how much sexual activity a couple could have post–prostate cancer treatment.

The partner's engagement can influence the effectiveness of the treatment itself, such as by eroticizing any sexual aids the patient might use. Kukula and colleagues suggested that all ED treatments can potentially be eroticized—for example, by involving a partner in assisting the patient in getting an erection during foreplay—and linked to the sexual pleasure provided by the partner.[35] Such eroticization may be best achieved when there is partner involvement in selecting the aid and the partner is enthusiastic from the start in trying the aid. This is also true when a clinician recommends sex aids or products (e.g., vibrator, lubricants): the patients and their partners may benefit from being encouraged to select and purchase the products together.

Involving partners in the management of ED after prostate cancer treatment recognizes that ED hinders the sexual life of patients and their partners.[54] The perception of how bothersome ED is may differ, though, between patients and partners.[51] The libido and functional status of partners can influence the patient's bother from ED, as well as his interest in and adherence to ED treatment. How sexually intimate a couple is before treatment may contribute to ED bother for both patients and partners; for example, an elderly couple that is close and supportive yet have been sexually inactive for a long period may be little bothered by ED.[55] Undoubtedly, the dynamic of a couple's sexual relationship before cancer diagnosis may contribute to how successful sexual recovery is after prostate cancer treatment.[51]

CONCLUSIONS

Sexual problems commonly occur after prostate cancer treatments, regardless of sexual orientation. However, there are major knowledge gaps on how prostate cancer treatments affect GBM and TGW populations sexually and how to provide the best care for each patient.

As chapter 8 discusses,[56] the issues of heteronormativity and homonegativity by healthcare providers often prevent GBM prostate cancer patients getting high-quality, personalized healthcare.[32, 57, 58] In the past, GBM and TGW prostate cancer patients might have been reluctant to talk about their sexuality with healthcare providers because of such fears. In countries that provide legal protections against discrimination on the basis of sexual orientation (e.g., the United Kingdom, Canada, South Africa, and New Zealand), this situation has presumably improved. It is also possible that the legalization of same-sex marriages has had a positive effect (e.g., in Canada, the United Kingdom, New Zealand, Australia, and the United States) (see chapter 4). We are optimistic that concerns about discrimination will diminish as more countries accept diversity in sexual orientation and practice. Healthcare providers, nevertheless, still need to know how to provide care that best preserves prostate cancer patients' sexual quality of life, which will be specific to the needs and desires of individual prostate cancer patients. To do so, they need to be aware of the diversity of sexual practices in the GBM and TGW communities and take into consideration the patients' preferred sexual activities.

ACKNOWLEDGMENTS

We thank Tsz Kin (Bernard) Lee, Gary Dowsett, and Meghan McInnis for critical feedback on our draft article, as well as RxSleeve and the Elator for the discussion on the use of their products for anal intercourse.

REFERENCES

1. Samplaski MK, Lo KC. Erectile dysfunction in the setting of prostate cancer. *In* Lipshultz LI, Pastuszak AW, Goldstein AT, et al, eds. *Management of sexual dysfunction in men and women.* New York: Springer; 2016: 73–86.

2. McConkey R. Effect of erectile dysfunction following prostate cancer treatment. *Nursing Standard.* 2015; 30 (12): 38–44.

3. Wassersug RJ. Maintaining intimacy for prostate cancer patients on androgen deprivation therapy. *Current Opinion in Supportive and Palliative Care.* 2016; 10 (1): 55–65.

4. Cheung AS, de Rooy C, Hoermann R, et al. Quality of life decrements in men with prostate cancer undergoing androgen deprivation therapy. *Clinical Endocrinology.* 2016; 86 (3): 388–394.

5. Wassersug R, Wibowo E. Non-pharmacological and non-surgical strategies to promote sexual recovery for men with erectile dysfunction. *Translational Andrology and Urology.* 2017; 6 (Suppl. 5): S776–794.

6. Johnson RD, Murray FT. Androgen dependent penile mechanoreceptors in the rat. *Anatomia, Histologia Embryologia.* 1990; 19 (1): 86.

7. Kow LM, Pfaff DW. Effects of estrogen treatment on the size of receptive field and response threshold of pudendal nerve in the female rat. *Neuroendocrinology.* 1973; 13 (4): 299–313.

8. Wibowo E, Wassersug RJ. The effect of estrogen on the sexual interest of castrated males: Implications to prostate cancer patients on androgen-deprivation therapy. *Critical Reviews in Oncology/Hematology.* 2013; 87 (3): 224–238.

9. Gilbert DC, Duong T, Kynaston HG, et al. Quality-of-life outcomes from the Prostate Adenocarcinoma: TransCutaneous Hormones (PATCH) trial evaluating luteinising hormone-releasing hormone agonists versus transdermal oestradiol for androgen suppression in advanced prostate cancer. *BJU International.* 2016; 119 (5): 667–675.

10. Fode M, Serefoglu EC, Albersen M, Sonksen J. Sexuality following radical prostatectomy: Is restoration of erectile function enough? *Sexual Medicine Reviews.* 2017; 5 (1): 110–119.

11. Wibowo E, Wassersug RJ. Multiple orgasms in men—what we know so far. *Sexual Medicine Reviews.* 2016; 4 (2): 136–148.

12. Frey A, Sonksen J, Jakobsen H, Fode M. Prevalence and predicting factors for commonly neglected sexual side effects to radical prostatectomies: Results from a cross-sectional questionnaire-based study. *Journal of Sexual Medicine.* 2014; 11 (9): 2318–2326.

13. Warkentin KM, Gray RE, Wassersug RJ. Restoration of satisfying sex for a castrated cancer patient with complete impotence: A case study. *Journal of Sex and Marital Therapy.* 2006; 32 (5): 389–399.

14. Wassersug RJ, Lyons A, Duncan D, et al. Diagnostic and outcome differences

between heterosexual and nonheterosexual men treated for prostate cancer. *Urology*. 2013; 82 (3): 565–571.

15. Rosenberger JG, Schick V, Herbenick D, et al. Sex toy use by gay and bisexual men in the United States. *Archives of Sexual Behavior*. 2012; 41 (2): 449–458.

16. Gooren L, Morgentaler A. Prostate cancer incidence in orchidectomised male-to-female transsexual persons treated with oestrogens. *Andrologia*. 2014; 46 (10): 1156–1160.

17. Wibowo E, Calich HJ, Currie RW, Wassersug RJ. Prolonged androgen deprivation may influence the autoregulation of estrogen receptors in the brain and pelvic floor muscles of male rats. *Behavioural Brain Research*. 2015; 286 (2015): 128–135.

18. Markland C. Transexual surgery. *Obstetrics and Gynecology Annual*. 1975; 4: 309–330.

19. Thurston AV. Carcinoma of the prostate in a transsexual. *British Journal of Urology*. 1994; 73 (2): 217.

20. van Kesteren P, Meinhardt W, van der Valk P, et al. Effects of estrogens only on the prostates of aging men. *Journal of Urology*. 1996; 156 (4): 1349–1353.

21. van Kesteren PJ, Asscheman H, Megens JA, Gooren LJ. Mortality and morbidity in transsexual subjects treated with cross-sex hormones. *Clinical Endocrinology*. 1997; 47 (3): 337–342.

22. van Haarst EP, Newling DW, Gooren LJ, et al. Metastatic prostatic carcinoma in a male-to-female transsexual. *British Journal of Urology*. 1998; 81 (5): 776.

23. Miksad RA, Bubley G, Church P, et al. Prostate cancer in a transgender woman 41 years after initiation of feminization. *JAMA*. 2006; 296 (19): 2316–2317.

24. Molokwu CN, Appelbaum JS, Miksad RA. Detection of prostate cancer following gender reassignment. *BJU International*. 2008; 101 (2): 259; author reply, 259–260.

25. Dorff TB, Shazer RL, Nepomuceno EM, Tucker SJ. Successful treatment of meta-static androgen-independent prostate carcinoma in a transsexual patient. *Clinical Genitourinary Cancer*. 2007; 5 (5): 344–346.

26. Asscheman H, Giltay EJ, Megens JA, et al. A long-term follow-up study of mortality in transsexuals receiving treatment with cross-sex hormones. *European Journal of Endocrinology*. 2011; 164 (4): 635–642.

27. Wierckx K, Mueller S, Weyers S, et al. Long-term evaluation of cross-sex hormone treatment in transsexual persons. *Journal of Sexual Medicine*. 2012; 9 (10): 2641–2651.

28. Turo R, Jallad S, Prescott S, Cross WR. Metastatic prostate cancer in transsexual diagnosed after three decades of estrogen therapy. *Canadian Urological Association Journal*. 2013; 7 (7–8): E544–546.

29. Brown GR, Jones KT. Incidence of breast cancer in a cohort of 5,135 transgender veterans. *Breast Cancer Research and Treatment*. 2015; 149 (1): 191–198.

30. Ellent E, Matrana MR. Metastatic prostate cancer 35 years after sex reassignment surgery. *Clinical Genitourinary Cancer*. 2016; 14 (2): e207–209.

31. Krakowsky Y, Ferrara S, Kulkarni G, Grober E. Active surveillance for low risk prostate cancer in a trans female—A case study and knowledge gap. *Journal of Sexual Medicine.* 14 (2): e92.

32. Thomas C, Wootten A, Robinson P. The experiences of gay and bisexual men diagnosed with prostate cancer: Results from an online focus group. *European Journal of Cancer Care.* 2013; 22 (4): 522–529.

33. Arrington MI. Sexuality, society, and senior citizens: An analysis of sex talk among prostate cancer support group members. *Sexuality & Culture.* 2000; 4 (4): 45–74.

34. Walker LM, Robinson JW. A description of heterosexual couples' sexual adjustment to androgen deprivation therapy for prostate cancer. *Psycho-Oncology.* 2011; 20 (8): 880–888.

35. Kukula KC, Jackowich RA, Wassersug RJ. Eroticization as a factor influencing erectile dysfunction treatment effectiveness. *International Journal of Impotence Research.* 2014; 26 (1): 1–6.

36. Goldstone SE. The ups and downs of gay sex after prostate cancer treatment. *Journal of Gay and Lesbian Psychotherapy.* 2005; 9 (1 & 2): 43–55.

37. Lee TK, Handy AB, Kwan W, et al. Impact of prostate cancer treatment on the sexual quality of life for men-who-have-sex-with-men. *Journal of Sexual Medicine.* 2015; 12 (12): 2378–2386.

38. Ussher JM, Perz J, Rose D, et al. Threat of sexual disqualification: The consequences of erectile dysfunction and other sexual changes for gay and bisexual men with prostate cancer. *Archives of Sexual Behavior.* 2017; 46 (7): 2043–2057.

39. Chen L, Staubli SE, Schneider MP, et al. Phosphodiesterase 5 inhibitors for the treatment of erectile dysfunction: A trade-off network meta-analysis. *European Urology.* 2015; 68 (4): 674–680.

40. Jarow JP, Nana-Sinkam P, Sabbagh M, Eskew A. Outcome analysis of goal directed therapy for impotence. *Journal of Urology.* 1996; 155 (5): 1609–1612.

41. Corona G, Rastrelli G, Burri A, et al. First-generation phosphodiesterase type 5 inhibitors dropout: A comprehensive review and meta-analysis. *Andrology.* 2016; 4 (6): 1002–1009.

42. Chung E, Van CT, Wilson I, Cartmill RA. Penile prosthesis implantation for the treatment for male erectile dysfunction: Clinical outcomes and lessons learnt after 955 procedures. *World Journal of Urology.* 2013; 31 (3): 591–595.

43. Lewis RW, Witherington R. External vacuum therapy for erectile dysfunction: Use and results. *World Journal of Urology.* 1997; 15 (1): 78–82.

44. Ussher JM, Perz J, Gilbert E, et al. Renegotiating sex and intimacy after cancer: Resisting the coital imperative. *Cancer Nursing.* 2013; 36 (6): 454–462.

45. Reece M, Rosenberger JG, Schick V, et al. Characteristics of vibrator use by gay and bisexually identified men in the United States. *Journal of Sexual Medicine.* 2010; 7 (10): 3467–3476.

46. Trost LW, Munarriz R, Wang R, et al. External mechanical devices and vascular surgery for erectile dysfunction. *Journal of Sexual Medicine.* 2016; 13 (11): 1579–1617.

47. Raina R, Pahlajani G, Agarwal A, et al. Long-term potency after early use of a vacuum erection device following radical prostatectomy. *BJU International.* 2010; 106 (11): 1719–1722.

48. Baniel J, Israilov S, Segenreich E, Livne PM. Comparative evaluation of treatments for erectile dysfunction in patients with prostate cancer after radical retropubic prostatectomy. *BJU International.* 2001; 88 (1): 58–62.

49. Matheson L, Watson EK, Nayoan J, et al. A qualitative metasynthesis exploring the impact of prostate cancer and its management on younger, unpartnered and gay men. *European Journal of Cancer Care.* 2017; doi: 10.1111/ecc.12676.

50. Wassersug RJ, Westle A, Dowsett GW. Men's sexual and relational adaptations to erectile dysfunction after prostate cancer treatment. *International Journal of Sexual Health.* 2016; 29 (1): 69–79.

51. Li H, Gao T, Wang R. The role of the sexual partner in managing erectile dysfunction. *Nature Reviews Urology.* 2016; 13 (3): 168–177.

52. Dorey G. Partners' perspective of erectile dysfunction: Literature review. *British Journal of Nursing.* 2001; 10 (3): 187–195.

53. Althof SE. When an erection alone is not enough: Biopsychosocial obstacles to lovemaking. *International Journal of Impotence Research.* 2002; 14 (Suppl. 1): S99–S104.

54. Movsas TZ, Yechieli R, Movsas B, Darwish-Yassine M. Partner's perspective on long-term sexual dysfunction after prostate cancer treatment. *American Journal of Clinical Oncology.* 2016; 39 (3): 276–279.

55. Tsang V, Skead C, Palmer-Hague J, Wassersug RJ. Impact of prostate cancer treatments on men's sense of manhood: Implications for understanding masculinity. In preparation.

56. Rose D, Ussher JM, Perz J. Let's talk about gay sex: Gay and bisexual men's sexual communication with healthcare professionals after prostate cancer. *European Journal of Cancer Care.* 2017; 26 (1).

57. Kelly D, Sakellariou D, Fry S, Vougioukalou S. Heteronormativity and prostate cancer: A discursive paper. *Journal of Clinical Nursing.* 2017; 27 (1–2): 461–467.

58. Blank TO. Gay men and prostate cancer: Invisible diversity. *Journal of Clinical Oncology.* 2005; 23 (12): 2593–2596.

59. Sharif A, Malhotra NR, Acosta AM, et al. The development of prostate adenocarcinoma in a transgender male to female patient: Could estrogen therapy have played a role? *Prostate.* 2017; 77 (8): 824–828.

60. Deebel NA, Morin JP, Autorino R, et al. Prostate cancer in transgender women: Incidence, etiopathogenesis, and management challenges. *Urology.* 2017; 110: 166–171.

CHAPTER 11

Experiences of Sexual Rehabilitation after Prostate Cancer

A Comparison of Gay and Bisexual Men with Heterosexual Men

Jane M. Ussher, Duncan Rose, Janette Perz, Gary W. Dowsett, and Andrew Kellett

CHAPTER SUMMARY

In a study of sexual rehabilitation after prostate cancer, gay and bisexual men (GBM) were more likely than heterosexual men (79% versus 56%) to report having tried medical or other aids to address erectile dysfunction. GBM were also more likely to have tried more than one medical aid (GBM $M = 1.65$ aids, heterosexual men $M = 0.83$ aids), including medication, penile injection, penile implant, and vacuum pump, and to have sought information about sexual rehabilitation after prostate cancer on the Internet, through counseling, or through a support group. There were no differences between the groups in satisfaction with the use of sexual aids. Accounts of satisfaction described medical and sexual aids as indispensable in maintaining sexual functioning and relationships. However, the majority of men in the study described hindrances, both physical and social, associated with using medical or sexual aids, which resulted in discontinued use of such aids. These barriers were the perceived artificiality of medical and other sexual aids; loss of sexual spontaneity and necessity to plan for sex; physical side effects; failure to achieve erectile response; financial cost; and lack of access to sexual rehabilitation information and support.

KEY TERMS

erectile dysfunction, medical aids, penile implant, sexual aids, sexual rehabilitation, vacuum pump

Ussher, Jane M., Perz, Janette, Rosser, B. R. Simon, eds., *Gay & Bisexual Men Living with Prostate Cancer*
dx.doi.org/10.17312/harringtonparkpress/2018.06.gbmlpc.011
© 2018 Harrington Park Press

INTRODUCTION

In the context of erectile and other sexual changes experienced by gay and bisexual men (GBM) and other men who have sex with men (MSM) after prostate cancer,[1, 2] researchers and clinicians have identified a need to help individuals and couples reestablish their sexual lives.[1, 3–6] Some attention has been paid to "renegotiation"[2] or "reframing"[5] of sexual activities, such as the development of "flexibility"[7] in relation to sexual practices.[5] In comparison with heterosexual couples coping with prostate cancer, gay couples are more likely to engage in novel practices to deal with sexual challenges following treatment, such as engaging in concurrent sexual relationships[8] or a change in sexual mode or position from insertive to receptive.[7] However, little is known about differences between gay and heterosexual men in adoption of medical or sexual aids for sexual rehabilitation following erectile difficulties.[5]

Sexual rehabilitation after prostate cancer has most often focused on regaining erectile function to improve sexual satisfaction and penile health.[5] Common biomedical interventions for erectile dysfunction or penile rehabilitation include PDE5 inhibitor drugs (e.g., Cialis, Viagra, and Levitra), penile injection therapy, penile implant (i.e., surgical prosthesis), and vacuum pump erection devices (see chapter 10). Approximately half of prostate cancer patients report using a medical aid for penile rehabilitation after prostate cancer treatment.[9, 10] However, despite reports of gains in penile rigidity, up to 73% of patients discontinue using these aids within the first year.[5] Little is known about why couples abandon the use of aids; there is a need for more research in this area.[11] It has been suggested that reasons for discontinuation include difficulties achieving erectile firmness that is equivalent to that experienced before treatment or that required for penetrative sex;[12] a mismatch between treatment effectiveness and patient's expectations for recovery;[13] a sense that use of aids results in unnatural and obligatory intercourse;[14] limited motivation from some partners regarding sexual recovery;[15] and lack of ongoing information and support across the disease pathway to address difficulties with rehabilitation when they arise.[16] However, many of the published accounts of patient experience of sexual rehabilitation after prostate cancer are based on clinical vignettes, and there is a lack of literature reporting on men's subjective experiences of sexual rehabilitation to support treatment recommendations and delivery of care.[11]

Sexual rehabilitation research and recommendations also focus almost entirely on heterosexual samples and vaginal intercourse, neglecting anal intercourse and the sexual rehabilitation needs and experiences of GBM with prostate cancer.[3, 17] As just one example, it has been suggested that first-line oral therapies may be less effective for GBM adopting an insertive role during anal intercourse because firmer erections are required for anal sex than for vaginal sex.[18] To date, however, there is no published research on how many GBM, in comparison to heterosexual men, adopt medical or other aids for sexual rehabilitation, and there has been only one study examining GBM's experiences of sexual aids after prostate cancer.[19] This chapter presents the findings of a study that compared GBM and heterosexual men with respect to the use of medical and other sexual aids after prostate cancer.

THE STUDY

One-hundred and twenty-four GBM and 225 heterosexual men who currently have, or have had, prostate cancer participated in an online survey, and 73 took part in semistructured interviews (53 GBM and 20 heterosexual men), part of a larger program of mixed-methods research examining sexual well-being and quality of life after prostate cancer.[2, 20–22] The GBM were significantly younger than the heterosexual men (GB 64.25 years; heterosexual 71.54 years), less likely to be partnered (GB 50%; heterosexual 86%), less likely to report a current relationship of over two-year duration if partnered (GB 81%; heterosexual 93%), and more likely to have casual sexual partners (GB 40%; heterosexual 4%). Prostate cancer had been diagnosed 5.9 years previously for GBM and 7.7 years previously for heterosexual men; diagnosis resulted in a range of treatments, and the majority of participants were at the time of the survey being monitored after treatment.[20] Participants were primarily recruited in Australia (71%), and a minority were recruited from the United States (21%) and the United Kingdom (8%).

GBM were significantly more likely to report having tried medical or other aids to address sexual dysfunction than heterosexual men (73.4% GBM, 51.1% heterosexual men) (table 11.1) and having tried more than one aid (GBM $M = 1.65$ aids, heterosexual men $M = 0.83$ aids), including medication, penile injection, penile implant, vacuum pump, and other aids (e.g. cock ring, dildo, vibrator). GBM were also significantly more likely to have sought information about sexual rehabilitation after prostate cancer on the Internet, through counseling, or through a support group. There were no differences between the groups in satisfaction with the use of sexual aids and no differences between partnered and unpartnered men in the use of aids.

In the accounts below, we examine descriptions of successful and unsuccessful sexual rehabilitation, drawing on open-ended survey responses and interviews, analyzed through thematic analysis.[23]

SUCCESSFUL SEXUAL REHABILITATION: "THERE IS NO WAY I WOULD HAVE FUNCTION WITHOUT IT"

A minority of both heterosexual men and GBM reported satisfaction with using one or more medical aids after prostate cancer (table 11.1). Positive accounts focused on increased erectile function and improved penile form. For example, participants said: "It [Cialis] has been 100% effective. . . . There appeared to be no way I would have been able to have any function without it" (Billy, gay, partnered, 72); "It [Cialis] restored some of the feelings that I had. . . . The penis was stuffed but it was working" (Brad, heterosexual, partnered, 75); "I've used that [vacuum pump] fairly regularly and that has made a difference, both to my satisfaction with penile length as well as the feeling of consistency in my penis" (Bruce, gay, partnered, 61).

Participants who used a combination of medical and sexual aids often described increased erectile response. For example, Connor (gay, partnered, 61) reported using a vacuum device and Cialis alongside penile vasoconstriction devices (colloquially described as "cock rings" and "lassoes"): "There was some healing happening. . . . There was no longer just a soft penis, kind of, struggling with that, there was actually sensation in the masturbation again and the penis was inflated enough to look like my penis." Positive responses to the use of medical aids included "pleasurable" and "intensely satisfying," and the use of such aids was often reported to lead to incorporation of additional aids to support pleasure during sex. For example, Elliot (heterosexual, partnered, 64) described using a vibrator for "extra help" to achieve an erection and to receive anal pleasure: "I think it just sort of increases the intensity of it. . . . You're trying to sort of generate pleasure from some part of your body, and that's an area that's quite sensitive and I was able to get something else out of." Harry (gay, partnered, 71) said, "We use toys a bit and the vibrator, which helps me a lot to get me going" to support pleasure during sex. Jonny (bisexual, partnered, 54) told us he had developed an interest in a variety of sexual aids, including erotic

TABLE 11.1

Nonheterosexual versus Heterosexual Men: Sex Aid Use and Satisfaction

Variable	Nonheterosexual N = 124		Heterosexual N = 225	
	M	*SD*	*M*	*SD*
Number of different aids tried	1.65	1.39	0.83	1.05
Types of Aids Tried	*n*	%	*n*	%
Oral medication***				
Yes	82	66.13	85	37.78
No	42	33.87	140	62.22
Penile injection**				
Yes	32	25.81	30	13.33
No	92	74.19	195	86.67
Penile implant*				
Yes	11	8.87	8	3.56
No	113	91.13	217	96.44
Vacuum pump***				
Yes	33	26.61	24	10.67
No	91	73.39	201	89.33
Other sex aids or "toys" (e.g., vibrator, dildo, cock ring)***				
Yes	44	35.48	36	16.00
No	80	64.52	189	84.00

TABLE 11.1

Nonheterosexual versus Heterosexual Men: Sex Aid Use and Satisfaction

	Nonheterosexual		Heterosexual	
	N = 124		**N = 225**	
Variable	**M**	**SD**	**M**	**SD**
Number of different aids tried	1.65	1.39	0.83	1.05
Sexual Aids Satisfaction	**n**	**%**	**n**	**%**
Oral medication satisfaction				
Dissatisfied	31	47.69	41	64.06
Neither satisfied nor dissatisfied	12	18.46	4	6.25
Satisfied	22	33.85	19	29.69
Penile injection satisfaction				
Dissatisfied	13	41.94	19	70.37
Neither satisfied nor dissatisfied	2	6.45	1	3.70
Satisfied	16	51.61	7	25.93
Penile implant satisfaction				
Dissatisfied	3	33.33	2	50.00
Neither satisfied nor dissatisfied	5	55.56	—	—
Satisfied	1	11.11	2	50.00
Vacuum pump satisfaction				
Dissatisfied	13	46.43	10	50.000
Neither satisfied nor dissatisfied	10	35.71	3	15.00
Satisfied	5	17.86	7	35.00

(continued)

TABLE 11.1 *(continued)*

Nonheterosexual versus Heterosexual Men: Sex Aid Use and Satisfaction

	Nonheterosexual		Heterosexual	
	N = 124		*N* = 225	
Variable	*M*	*SD*	*M*	*SD*
Number of different aids tried	1.65	1.39	0.83	1.05
Support from Formal or Informal Sources	*n*	%	*n*	%
Internet***				
Yes	46	37.10	28	12.44
No	78	62.90	197	87.56
Psychotherapy/counseling***				
Yes	17	13.71	4	1.78
No	107	86.29	221	98.22
Support groups***				
Yes	31	25.00	14	6.22
No	93	75.00	211	93.78

Significance level of difference between groups, chi squared: *p < .05; **p < .01; ***p < .001

electrostimulation, a vibrating vacuum pump, an anal plug, and latex accessories used in bondage: "I've taken quite an interest in trying out different things," including "e-stim," "milking machines," "butt plugs," and "vac-racks." The use of sexual aids appears to serve multiple functions, including increase of pleasure, taking the focus away from the penis, supporting or enhancing arousal, and facilitating sex. Paradoxically, the loss of erectile function may have led men to broaden their exploration of sexual pleasure though aids that stimulate multiple sites of the body, an exploration that might not have come about without loss of penile function and form.

The utility of medical and other aids was most often described in terms of whether they made intercourse possible, increased sexual confidence, and facilitated sex with regular partners. For example, Rick (gay, partnered, 59), as a result of using Cialis, Viagra, and a cock ring, said, "I have been able to have penetrative sex with my partner, which has been great for him and for me." Darryl (heterosexual, partnered, 65) observed: "When you're having sex, you can go as long as you like. . . . It [the penile implant] works perfectly every time. . . . It's given me a lot more confidence and it's meant that we've been able to be much more intimate."

A number of participants, particularly GBM, also reported that medical and other aids enabled them to pursue casual sexual encounters. For example, Michael (gay, single, 69), who took Cialis and used a cock ring, said, "I just disappear into the toilet and give myself an injection, and then I have got an erection for about an hour or an hour and a half, and that can be rather good." The downside was that Michael had to take along his "gear" when going out: "Let's say I met somebody and I didn't have my gear with me, then it becomes much more difficult." Use of oral medication was more straightforward in terms of planning, as Oliver (gay, single, 66) said: "It works wonderfully well [laughs] for me. That's all I need—half a Viagra—when I'm going out, to have a good time." Mark (gay, single, 45) described how the consistent erection he achieved through his penile implant supported his inclusion within a gay sexual community: "I think the disqualification [from a gay sexual community], historically, was much worse. That's been replaced, you know, because I can function sexually with the pump [penile implant]." Graham (gay, single, 74) described being "proud" of his penile implant, which enabled him to go to saunas "where a man with an erection is sought after and highly valued, and I go there, because I can do it." Graham had been given the nickname "Robocock," and he associated openness and lack of embarrassment with a positive outcome in relation to casual sexual partners: "One of the differences between gay sex and straight sex is it is much more up-front and personal and close. I mean, a man will either just grab you by the balls and he will feel this horrible thing and just go and run screaming into the night. But, if I talk about it first, and I defuse that, then they become intrigued by it and very understanding." Graham's comment about "defusing" potential negative reactions from partners illustrates the importance of confidence and a positive attitude toward medical and sexual aids, particularly in the context of casual sexual interactions.

ARTIFICIALITY, FAILURE, COST, AND SIDE EFFECTS: NEGATIVE EXPERIENCES OF MEDICAL AND OTHER SEXUAL AIDS

While some men reported success and satisfaction using aids, most men experienced hindrances, both physical and social, associated with using medical or other sexual aids. As a consequence of these hindrances, many participants described discontinuing use of such aids. These hindrances were the perceived artificiality of medical and other sexual aids; loss of sexual spontaneity and necessity to plan for sex; physical side effects; failure to achieve erectile response; financial cost; and lack of access to sexual rehabilitation information and support.

The artificiality of an assisted erection. The description of medical and other sexual aids as artificial was evident in both heterosexual men's and GBM's accounts. Achieving erectile functioning through penile implants or injections was described as "more mechanical" and "really artificial," where "the naturalness has gone." Comparisons were made that positioned nonassisted erections as superior and "real." For example, Graham (gay, single, 74) said: "I really miss that first flush of excitement when I was younger and I used to get turned on by something or other. . . . Now it's not natural, I just press a button and I'm turned on." Similarly, Scott (gay, single, 59) said his erection is "something that I've lost" and described the difficulty of injecting at sex-on-premises venues among other men who have an erection: "I've got the hand on the container and the swab and the lights and the toilet and when I'm sort of just sitting around waiting for something to happen, you start watching other guys going backwards and forwards, the thought bubble says, 'Boys, you have no idea how lucky you are to have your own hard-on.'" Scott, who stated he no longer perceived his erection to be his own, described a qualitative difference in the type of erection experienced. The external assistance he received produced a poor "imitation" of an erection, one he described as "not real" and feeling "artificial" to him.

For some men, the reliance on sexual aids to achieve an erection challenged their sense of being a man. For example, Darryl (heterosexual, partnered, 65) said, "You lose some of your manhood somewhere along the way. You feel less of a bloke because you can't get it up or you've got to rely on this artificial device." Billy (gay, single, 75) described himself as "damaged goods," and the experience as "cheap and nasty," when he "had to take a tablet" after a prospective partner said to him, "'Look, let us go. Let us have some fun.'" Neil (heterosexual, partnered, 68) said the experience of having to "make a conscious decision" to inject for an erection was inferior. He added: "Having an erection is not just signaling that I'm capable, it's actually a message to both of you, a subliminal message that everything is okay. I'm relaxed, I've got an erection. It means I can have sex, it means I'm healthy, it means a lot of things. And what I realized is that the erection just isn't about being able to penetrate, it's about, it's about a bloke saying everything is okay, I'm right, I'm healthy, here I am."

These men, both heterosexual and gay or bisexual, here reveal that dealing with erection problems—the central and most frequent side effect of prostate cancer treatment—is a loss, a diminution of pleasures, and damage to a sexual sense of self. These problems are relentless and ongoing because, while medical and sexual aids offer some respite from those problems, they do not fix them. Lee and colleagues describe this feeling as one of being "compromised," and no amount of accommodation to the aids available to men will adequately replace what has been lost.[24]

Loss of sexual spontaneity. The accounts of artificiality frequently noted a loss of spontaneous sexual activity since treatment. Many men described their earlier "natural" or spontaneous erections as having instigated sexual encounters, the loss of which led to challenges initiating sex and to difficulties with sexual communication. Using medical aids during the sexual encounter was described as "a passion killer," "impersonal," and "clinical, not romantic" because "you had to plan ahead if you were going to have sex" or "stop in the middle of making love." Participants described this lack of spontaneity as an "interruption." For example, Sid (transgender, heterosexual, married, 64) said: "You've got to preprogram it all. Even with the injections, you get a bit amorous and what have you, you say let's have sex, hang on a moment, I need an injection, then you've lost it." Neil (heterosexual, partnered, 68) noted, "The lack of the spontaneous trigger or signal of an erection seems to reduce the ardor." As a result of loss of spontaneity and the need to plan sexual encounters, Jonny (bisexual, partnered, 54) said he no longer instigated sex: "I wait more for signals from my wife that she would like to have sex rather than springing a surprise on her and then find that it's just not a good time." In contrast, Billy (gay, partnered, 72) said, "It was always me that instigated it before because I was the one that was damaged goods. . . . He didn't know whether I was ready or not."

The loss of spontaneity associated with using specific medical aids was described as especially problematic for casual sexual encounters and for dating. Using penile injections was highlighted as particularly so. "The logistics of injecting in casual sex situations is a complete joke. I mean, it's abhorrent" (Mark, gay, single, 45). "It's not the easiest thing to do discreetly, you're puncturing your dick, which means you have an open wound, which means there's blood there, and that invites a certain extra level of risk" (Scott, gay, single, 59). "Having to use the injection therapy is a big hurdle. It's hard enough meeting people, especially females, and trying to establish a good, healthy friendship with them, which includes hopefully some sex, when you know that this hurdle's there" (Brian, heterosexual, single, 63). These reflections suggest that the flow of encounters well understood by these men is disrupted by the use of medical aids, particularly in casual sexual encounters, and may ruffle the expectations of partners: users of medical aids are on their own, having either to use aids discreetly to avoid this disruption, or to disclose to partners and hope for an accepting or patient response.

Physical side effects. The side effects and complications associated with use of medical aids were frequently reported. As a result of these side effects, participants described enduring or forgoing the use of medical aids.

PDE5 inhibitor tablets were reported by many participants to result in frequent headaches, nausea, and disorientation. For example, one man told us: "I took the full Viagra and I got so disorientated and I went to bed. And then I thought I'd better get up and have a shower and I got up and I vomited everywhere" (Drew, gay, partnered, 65). "I had all the three different types of pills . . . all it did was make me have these incredible hot flushes and everything would turn blue and I'd have thumping headaches" (Jim, heterosexual, partnered, 58). For these men, such side effects outweighed the benefits of using PDE5 inhibitors. Damon (gay, single, 52) ruminated: "Do I wanna take a tablet, and wait 45 minutes and have that, what I find sometimes rather unpleasant, flush to the head feeling, and then urinate, and then have a wank. . . . Sometimes I think, oh, you know what, can't be bothered."

Penile injections were described as causing physical pain during and following use, and prolonged use of penile injections was associated with penile curvature and deformity. For example, participants said that "the comedown from the injection was not very comfortable; it was quite painful" (Bruce, gay, partnered, 61); "Too much muscle in penis turned to gristle. Now can't continue with aid" (Alf, gay, single, 55). In addition, penile injections occasionally resulted in priapism for some men, including Darryl (heterosexual, partnered, 65), who described "finishing up in accident and emergency" and waiting "seven hours by the time they got it down." He added, "It's the most embarrassing thing in my life," after which he noticed he was "getting a bit of a bend in my penis when it was erect, and it had caused scarring." Drew (gay, partnered, 65) described his one experience of penile injection as "hopeless" because he had an "intense erection for about four hours," which left him thinking, "No, never again, and I certainly wouldn't recommend them to anyone." Other participants focused on the pain of the injection itself: "Penile injections hurt too much, feel that the pain was not worth the erections" (Henry, gay, single, 56); "I just find it's far too much pain to be actually bothered with it" (David, gay, partnered, 64).

The negative side effects of the penile implant were described by some men as penile shortening and difficulty reaching orgasm. For example, Darryl (heterosexual, partnered, 65) said: "The penile implants shorten your penis. . . . They knock about two, two and a half, three centimeters off the length, and that could be hard for a bloke to take, too." This is a matter of concern given that many men report worries about penis size after prostate cancer treatment and before using medical and other aids[2, 17] (see chapter 2). Mark (gay, single, 45) said, "Before the implant, I mean, with no erection at all I could still reach orgasm," whereas during the surgery for the procedure "that all got chopped out, that's all gone"; he added, "While I now technically have sexual functioning, I have considerably impaired sexual satisfaction."

In addition, the presence of a mechanical pump within the scrotum when using the penile implant often led to a negative response from partners. For example, Mark (gay, single, 45) told us: "[Casual sexual partners] do feel [the pump] in the scrotum, and you can see they do a very definite nonverbal pause. . . . A couple of people will then have stopped the sexual encounter. Other people have continued but seem wary of it." Darryl (heterosexual, partnered, 65) said, "[My wife] doesn't like the feel of it, because the pump's inside the scrotum. . . . Once upon a time she would have fondled me down there, she doesn't like it because it's all, all bumpy with this plumbing in it." An additional concern was also raised by Graham (gay, single, 74): "The implant doesn't cover the full length of my penis, so there is a bit of a droopy tip. So I always say it's a bit like a Concord taking off, you know, the sort of wobbly thing at the end which makes insertion a little bit harder . . . especially for a gay man and would probably be easier for a straight man." Graham's experience suggests that men may require further assistance or information to make effective use of the implant. For Graham, this was an unsupported process of trial and error: "At first it [insertion] was just really difficult," whereas later "I have learned how to deal with that, just by pulling back on the skin."

Medical aids do not work. Many participants reported that they tried using medical aids after prostate cancer treatment but found them ineffective. Participants reported attempting a range of medical aids with unsatisfactory results. There were several examples: "Oral medication, tried them all, nil results. Penile injections, tried 10 and 20 Caverject and 10/20 double injections, nil result" (Angelo, heterosexual, partnered, 64). "I'd used [PDE5 inhibitors] on and off over the years leading up to the cancer. It worked maybe 70 to 80% of the time. Now they don't work at all, the pills are useless" (Henry, gay, partnered, 59).

Other participants reported some effect from medical aids, but some, such as Jonny (bisexual, partnered, 54), noted that it was temporary: "The effectiveness [of the penile injection] is beginning to wear off so it's not giving as good erections now as it did initially, so I'm concerned long-term—am I going to even lose this opportunity of getting a decent erection?" After a lack of response from PDE5 inhibitors, Mark (gay, single, 45) said, "I got a climax injectable, and the first time I used it, it worked profoundly well. It was fantastic. I thought, God's gift, you know? And it never worked again after that." These accounts suggest that a number of men were prepared to experiment with a range of medical aids, but that in at least some cases, the effectiveness was temporary.

Cost of medical aids. Participants who described achieving a positive erectile response from medical aids often reported that the "mighty expense" of the aids was a barrier to continued use in contexts in which the costs were not covered by personal health insurance or national health support. For some Australian men, this expense was too difficult to meet: "Injection was extremely successful but is now too expensive" (Adam, gay, single, 60); "Cialis, that works and it worked well. . . . But then after I retired of course I didn't have quite the income that I had before, so I gave them away" (Hugh, heterosexual, partnered, 73). For other participants, use of medical aids was often a careful financial decision that involved a trade-off with other expenses. For example, Nick (bisexual, single, 66) told us, "I can afford them, but a couple of years down the track, who knows, I might want to direct that money into something else"; Robert (gay, partnered, 66) observed: "When I go onto Cialis for the whole month, it [erectile functioning] starts to approach where it used to be, but I've got to again find that money to actually do that. So that means I just go without doing something else to have that. Often I think I'd much rather go out and have dinner."

While Viagra is now off patent and much lower in price in many places, other PDE5i drugs are not. National health schemes and private or public health insurance plans sometimes cover some of the cost, but not in all countries or uniformly. The issue of cost and lack of subsidy for many men living with erectile difficulties after prostate cancer treatments is an ironic example of how "masculinity," often equated with erections in the prostate cancer field, does not seem to signify much to mostly male politicians and governments.

Absence of information and support. Across the sample, there were inconsistent accounts regarding the amount of information and support provided by health professionals for sexual rehabilitation, and specialist referrals were offered only to a minority of men. For example, Aaron (gay, single, 59) said he was referred to a sexual rehabilitation specialist before surgery and over a course of months was placed on "a program" of Cialis, Levitra, penile injections, and vacuum pumping: "I've almost done it like as if it's the therapy. It's like the doctor's orders. . . . I do it as a mechanical exercise . . . and I have to say there's been a slight improvement." As a consequence of "following this program," Aaron said, "that's why, psychologically, I haven't been depressed or anything."

Conversely, participants who did not engage with timely sexual rehabilitation often regretted missing opportunities to preserve sexual functioning: "The vacuum pump should be advised and used early after the operation, to help in the repair of the erection process. I may have left it too long, but that was the advice" (George, heterosexual, single 56); "I would've appreciated an immediate introduction to the notion of a penile rehabilitation program because I had to discover all that myself, after my surgery" (Bruce, gay, partnered, 61). Lack of sexual rehabilitation support was associated with lower prostate cancer treatment satisfaction by some participants. For example, Brian (heterosexual, single, 63) reported lack of interest from his urologist in addressing his sexual challenges following treatment: "I just got the impression that my bloke [urologist] didn't want to dig into that area much at all. Like, he'd done his job and he considered it was successful and he was not that keen to get involved with me there." Other men talked of distressing interactions with healthcare professionals when rehabilitation was offered. For example, Graham (gay, single, 74) described "feeling like an object" when his urologist demonstrated his penile implant to a "strange lady" without asking permission to do so: "When I was in hospital after the penile implant, I was just lying there in bed with my—my puffed-up penis, all wrapped up in bandages, and the doctor just walked in, the urologist walked in, with some strange lady that I had no idea who she was, and without saying anything, he just grabs my bandaged thing and undid it and demonstrated how you puff it up. And I was really put out by that."

Gareth (gay, single, 65) asked his doctor what he could do to address reduced penis size and was told "I don't want to know anything about your sex life." The lack of healthcare professional knowledge of the effect of prostate cancer on gay sex is a concern for many GBM, in relation to anal sex, reduction in penis size, the prostate as a site of pleasure, and absence of ejaculate, all mentioned as areas where rehabilitation information had been sought but was not forthcoming[21] (see also chapters 2, 3, and 6).

CONCLUSION

The findings of this study show the challenges and diverse reactions that heterosexual men and GBM experience in using medical and other sexual aids following prostate cancer treatment. GBM were more likely to try sexual aids, to use a range of aids, and to move from one aid to another if they were not satisfied with the results, regardless of relationship status. They are also more likely to seek information and support about sexual rehabilitation from informal and formal sources. This search for information may reflect the greater importance placed on sex and sexual functioning by GBM and their partners,[25, 26] their greater openness to using sex aids and toys,[27, 28] and the higher levels of distress and sexual bother associated with sexual dysfunction in gay and bisexual men following prostate cancer treatment[4, 20] in comparison to heterosexual men. Interest in and willingness to use sexual aids may also reflect GBM's greater openness to sexual experimentation,[29] and can lead to renegotiation of sexual activities in the context of cancer.[2, 7, 8] GBM may also have a greater willingness to communicate with their partners about sexual changes or difficulties,[2] and couple communication is key to achieving sexual functioning after cancer.[30] Further research is needed to examine couple communication about sexual rehabilitation in GBM and heterosexual men.

A substantial proportion of both heterosexual men and GBM reported dissatisfaction with medical and other sexual aids, which is consistent with previous reports on heterosexual men.[5, 31] There was a high degree of variability in dissatisfaction with specific aids, which suggests that individual differences need to be taken into account, regardless of sexual identity. These differences imply that support provided to help couples use assistive aids effectively and consistently needs to go beyond the mechanics of sexual aids, or the achievement of an erection, to incorporate the meaning of sex and sexual aids, along with individual coping strategies.[5] Schover and colleagues suggest there is a need for support in development of more timely and realistic expectations of the use of aids.[32] These expectations can be incorporated into sexual counseling, focusing on areas such as increasing communication and stimulation skills, ideally offered as part of the routine care offered to couples after prostate cancer treatment.[11] It has also been argued that the couple should be the focus of treatment, where possible, to enable shared ownership of the treatment and provide the potential for eroticization of the treatment itself.[5]

The specific needs and concerns of GBM associated with sexual functioning after prostate cancer should be taken on board by clinicians offering advice about rehabilitation.[17, 33] The eroticization of ejaculation for many gay men[2] suggests that treatment for prostate cancer may be inherently distressing because of the absence of ejaculate after treatment.[4] The likelihood that anal sex requires firmer erections than vaginal sex has led some researchers to propose that providers should educate GBM about the limitations of oral therapies for erectile dysfunction and consider more invasive treatments sooner.[4] Assessment and treatment of rectal damage after prostate cancer treatment is an important area of concern for GBM who adopt a receptive position during anal intercourse. This concern is often neglected in primary care, and until recently it was absent from rehabilitation research[17, 34] It has previously been reported that heterosexual men are more likely to try assistive aids if they are currently in a relationship, particularly if their partner has good sexual function and is younger.[32] Our findings suggest that there was no difference between partnered and unpartnered men in use of sexual aids. Many GBM are also using assistive aids in casual sexual encounters, which presents specific challenges associated with the practicalities and negotiation of use of such aids. Finally, because GBM are more likely to report difficulties in communicating with healthcare professionals about sex and sexual rehabilitation[21] (see chapters 3, 6, and 8), there are clearly unmet needs in this area.

Delaying the start of penile rehabilitation after radical prostatectomy is associated with poorer outcomes for erectile functioning,[35, 36] which suggests that information about medical and sexual aids should be provided at diagnosis, or at least before treatment.[5] Providing this information early may serve to increase satisfaction with and efficacy of medical sexual aids, with positive implications for psychological well-being and the maintenance of relationships after cancer (see chapters 2–6). However, medical and other aids should not be seen as the sole solution to sexual challenges after prostate cancer treatment. Sex therapists can help men who are open to changing their sexual repertoire to include new activities and substitute practices, and to experiment with alternative modes of positioning, improve communication with sexual partners, and negotiate role changes.[34] Because GBM are more likely to report sexual renegotiation or flexibility,[8] as well as the use of medical and sexual aids (see chapter 10),[27, 28] heterosexual men and their clinicians may have something positive to learn from GBM's experience in addressing the sexual challenges and recovery after prostate cancer treatment.

ACKNOWLEDGMENTS

This study was funded by the Prostate Cancer Foundation of Australia (PCFA), in the form of a new concept grant no. NCG 0512, in partnership with the Australian and New Zealand Urogenital and Prostate Cancer Trials Group (ANZUP).

REFERENCES

1. Rosser BRS, Merengwa E, Capistrant BD, et al. Prostate cancer in gay, bisexual, and other men who have sex with men: A review. *LGBT Health.* 2016; 3 (1): 32–41.

2. Ussher JM, Perz J, Rose D, et al. Threat of sexual disqualification: The consequences of erectile dysfunction and other sexual changes for gay and bisexual men with prostate cancer. *Archives of Sexual Behavior.* 2017; 46 (7): 2043–2057.

3. Latini DM, Hart SL, Coon DW, Knight SJ. Sexual rehabilitation after localized prostate cancer: Current interventions and future directions. *Cancer Journal.* 2009; 15 (1): 34.

4. Hart TL, Coon DW, Kowalkowski MA, et al. Changes in sexual roles and quality of life for gay men after prostate cancer: Challenges for sexual health providers. *Journal of Sexual Medicine.* 2014; 11 (9): 2308–2317.

5. Walker LM, Wassersug RJ, Robinson JW. Psychosocial perspectives on sexual recovery after prostate cancer treatment. *Nature Reviews Urology.* 2015; 12 (3): 167–176.

6. Wassersug RJ, Westle A, Dowsett GW. Men's sexual and relational adaptations to erectile dysfunction after prostate cancer treatment. *International Journal of Sexual Health.* 2017; 29 (1): 69–79.

7. Dowsett GW, Lyons A, Duncan D, Wassersug RJ. Flexibility in men's sexual practices in response to iatrogenic erectile dysfunction after prostate cancer treatment. *Sexual Medicine.* 2014; 2 (3): 115–120.

8. Hartman ME, Irvine J, Currie KL, et al. Exploring gay couples' experience with sexual dysfunction after radical prostatectomy: A qualitative study. *Journal of Sexual and Marital Therapy.* 2014; 40 (3): 233–253.

9. Bergman J, Gore JL, Penson DF, et al. Erectile aid use by men treated for localized prostate cancer. *Journal of Urology.* 2009; 182 (2): 649–654.

10. Schover LR, Fouladi RT, Warneke CL, et al. Seeking help for erectile dysfunction after treatment for prostate cancer. *Archives of Sexual Behavior.* 2004; 33 (5): 443–454.

11. Beck AM, Robinson JW, Carlson LE. Sexual intimacy in heterosexual couples after prostate cancer treatment: What we know and what we still need to learn. *Urologic Oncology: Seminars and Original Investigations.* 2009; 27 (2): 137–143.

12. Nelson CJ, Scardino PT, Eastham JA, Mulhall JP. Back to baseline: Erectile function recovery after radical prostatectomy from the patients' perspective. *Journal of Sexual Medicine.* 2013; 10 (6): 1636–1643.

13. Wittmann D, He C, Coelho M, et al. Patient preoperative expectations of urinary, bowel, hormonal and sexual functioning do not match actual outcomes 1 year after radical prostatectomy. *Journal of Urology.* 2011; 186 (2): 494–499.

14. Gray RE, Fitch MI, Phillips C, et al. Prostate cancer and erectile dysfunction: Men's experiences. *International Journal of Men's Health.* 2002; 1 (1): 15.

15. Neese LE, Schover LR, Klein EA, et al. Finding help for sexual problems after prostate cancer treatment: A phone survey of men's and women's perspectives. *Psycho-Oncology.* 2003; 12 (5): 463–473.

16. Sinfield P, Baker R, Camosso-Stefinovic J, et al. Men's and carers' experiences of care for prostate cancer: A narrative literature review. *Health Expectations.* 2009; 12 (3): 301–312.

17. Rosser BRS, Kohli N, Lesher L, et al. What gay and bisexual prostate cancer patients want in a sexual rehabilitation program: Results of the *Restore* needs assessment. *Urology Practice.* 2017.

18. Gebert S. Are penile prostheses a viable option to recommend for gay men? *International Journal of Urological Nursing.* 2014; 8 (3): 111–113.

19. Rosser BRS, Konety BR. What gay and bisexual men treated for prostate cancer are offered and attempt as sexual rehabilitation for prostate cancer: Quantitative results from the Restore study with implications for clinicians. *Urology Practice.* 2017.

20. Ussher JM, Perz J, Kellett A, et al. Health-related quality of life, psychological distress, and sexual changes following prostate cancer: A comparison of gay and bisexual men with heterosexual men. *Journal of Sexual Medicine.* 2016; 13 (3): 425–434.

21. Rose D, Ussher JM, Perz J. Let's talk about gay sex: Gay and bisexual men's sexual communication with healthcare professionals after prostate cancer. *European Journal of Cancer Care.* 2017; 26 (1).

22. Ussher JM, Rose D, Perz J. Mastery, isolation, or acceptance: Gay and bisexual men's construction of aging in the context of sexual embodiment after prostate cancer. *Journal of Sex Research.* 2017; 54 (6): 802–812.

23. Braun V, Clarke B. Using thematic analysis in psychology. *Qualitative Research in Psychology.* 2006; 3 (2): 77–101.

24. Lee TK, Handy AB, Kwan W, et al. Impact of prostate cancer treatment on the sexual quality of life for men-who-have-sex-with-men. *Journal of Sexual Medicine.* 2015; 12 (12): 2378–2386.

25. Bancroft J, Carnes L, Janssen E, et al. Erectile and ejaculatory problems in gay and heterosexual men. *Archives of Sexual Behavior.* 2005; 34 (3): 285–297.

26. Pitts M, Smith A, Mitchell A, Patel S. *Private lives: A report on the health and well-being of GLBTI Australians.* Melbourne: Australian Research Centre in Sex, Health and Society, La Trobe University; 2006.

27. Reece M, Herbenick D, Dodge B, et al. Vibrator use among heterosexual men varies by partnership status: Results from a nationally representative study in the United States. *Journal of Sex and Marital Therapy.* 2010; 36 (5): 389–407.

28. Rosenberger JG, Schick V, Herbenick D, et al. Sex toy use by gay and bisexual men in the United States. *Archives of Sexual Behavior.* 2012; 41 (2): 449–458.

29. Lyons A, Pitts M, Smith G, et al. Versatility and HIV vulnerability: Investigating the proportion of Australian gay men having both insertive and receptive anal intercourse. *Journal of Sexual Medicine.* 2011; 8 (8): 2164–2171.

30. Perz J, Ussher JM, Gilbert E. Feeling well and talking about sex: Psycho-social predictors of sexual functioning after cancer. *BMC Cancer.* 2014; 14 (1): 228–247; doi: 10.1186/1471-2407-14-228.

31. Rajpurkar A, Dhabuwala CB. Comparison of satisfaction rates and erectile function in patients treated with sildenafil, intracavernous prostaglandin E1 and penile implant surgery for erectile dysfunction in urology practice. *Journal of Urology.* 2003; 170 (1): 159–163.

32. Schover LR, Fouladi RT, Warneke CL, et al. The use of treatments for erectile dysfunction among survivors of prostate carcinoma. *Cancer.* 2002; 95 (11): 2397–2407.

33. Rosser BRS, Capistrant B, Torres B, et al. The effects of radical prostatectomy on gay and bisexual men's mental health, sexual identity and relationships: Qualitative results from the Restore study. *Sexual and Relationship Therapy.* 2016; 31 (4): 446–461.

34. Amiel GE, Goltz HH, Wenker EP, et al. Gay men and prostate cancer: Opportunities to improve HRQOL and access to care. *In* Boehmer U, Elk R, eds. *Cancer and the LGBT Community.* New York: Springer; 2015: 159–168.

35. Chung E, Gillman M. Prostate cancer survivorship: A review of erectile dysfunction and penile rehabilitation after prostate cancer therapy. *Medical Journal of Australia* 2014; 200 (10): 582–585.

36. Mulhall JP, Parker M, Waters BW, Flanigan R. The timing of penile rehabilitation after bilateral nerve-sparing radical prostatectomy affects the recovery of erectile function. *BJU International.* 2010; 105 (1): 37–41.

CHAPTER 12

Illness Intrusiveness and Social Support in Gay and Bisexual Men with Prostate Cancer

Tae L. Hart, Crystal Hare, and David M. Latini

CHAPTER SUMMARY

Although the literature on gay and bisexual men (GBM) living with prostate cancer has grown in recent years, little is known about the influence of social support and relationship status on illness adjustment in this group of men. The Illness Intrusiveness Theoretical Framework posits that the context of chronic illness, such as disease-related, treatment-related, and social factors, can either exacerbate or ameliorate the disruption of patients' valued life activities. Using this framework, our study examined the relationship between positive social support and three domains of illness intrusiveness (relationships and personal development, sex and intimacy, and instrumental areas such as health, employment, and active recreation). Additionally, we examined how the association between social support and illness intrusiveness was affected by relationship status (i.e., being partnered or unpartnered). This cross- sectional research project recruited 92 self-identified GBM from the online community and from local community centers that serve GBM. Participants completed a self-report packet of questionnaires online. Results showed that unpartnered (versus partnered) men reported less positive social support. We found that for unpartnered men, reporting greater positive social support was associated with less illness intrusiveness in two areas of their lives: relationships and personal development, as well as instrumental areas (health, finance, recreation). However, greater positive social support was not associated with reduced illness intrusiveness in partnered men. Although our findings cannot tell us whether positive support causes less illness intrusiveness, these data suggest that unpartnered GBM with prostate

Ussher, Jane M., Perz, Janette, Rosser, B. R. Simon, eds., *Gay & Bisexual Men Living with Prostate Cancer*
dx.doi.org/10.17312/harringtonparkpress/2018.06.gbmlpc.012
© 2018 Harrington Park Press

cancer seem to benefit from greater levels of positive social support. Healthcare providers need to assess the availability of instrumental and emotional support for unpartnered GBM, and they should be prepared to offer resources and to facilitate positive support.

KEY TERMS
illness intrusiveness, Illness Intrusiveness Theoretical Framework, positive social support, relationship status

INTRODUCTION
Until recently, little was known about health-related quality of life (HRQOL) in gay and bisexual men (GBM) with prostate cancer or how it might differ from that of their heterosexual counterparts. However, to establish a rationale for studying gay and bisexual men with prostate cancer, the first few published studies focused on HRQOL rather than the effect of prostate cancer on gay and bisexual men's relationships.[1-4] As we summarize the changes in HRQOL in the literature (see also chapter 1), several patterns emerge. In studies where comparisons were made with heterosexual men, GBM generally reported significantly worse urinary and bowel function.[1-5] The picture for sexual functioning and distress over poor sexual functioning (often described as "sexual bother") is more complex, possibly because of the use of different quality-of-life measures or differences in how patients were selected for studies. The results for ejaculatory function and distress over lack of ejaculation after treatment are clearer — all studies reported greater sexual bother for gay and bisexual men than for heterosexual men.[1,2]

Social support is an important predictor of quality of life and mental health after prostate cancer treatment. For heterosexual men, support frequently comes from a spouse or intimate female partner.[6] Some intervention studies conducted with heterosexual samples have examined support from healthcare professionals, but Huntley and colleagues suggest in their literature review that peer support is a more effective tool for men with prostate cancer.[7] GBM are less likely than heterosexual men to be in long-term monogamous relationships at the time of prostate cancer diagnosis, and they are less likely to have established social support systems in place.[8] Therefore, social support for GBM from other sources is important in the face of prostate cancer. In their review of the literature, Rosser and colleagues describe the limited amount we know about social support for GBM with prostate cancer.

Their review confirms that most GBM rely on family, friends, or others they connect with through prostate cancer support groups (chapter 1). In a recent qualitative study, respondents described the importance of gay-specific, cancer-related support. They indicated that such sources of support affirmed their gay identity or supported their coming out as gay.[9] In light of the lower frequency of primary partnerships among GBM and the reliance on primarily qualitative descriptions of social support for GBM with prostate cancer, we sought to describe social support among GBM with prostate cancer. We wondered how social support might vary on the basis of relationship status, as well as what the effect of social support and relationship status would be on lifestyle disruptions in the face of prostate cancer.

THEORETICAL FRAMEWORK AND RESEARCH MODEL

The study we present in this chapter is based on the Illness Intrusiveness Theoretical Framework (IITF), a model of intrapersonal, interpersonal, and sociocultural factors affecting the subjective well-being of persons living with a chronic disease.[10] This framework has been extensively tested across a variety of chronic diseases for more than 20 years.[10-18] Illness intrusiveness refers to both perceived illness disruption as well as treatment-related disruption and its influence on valued life activities.[10] Illness intrusiveness is conceptualized as "an intervening variable that links the circumstances of disease and treatment with subjective well-being and emotional distress."[19] Thus, the effects of intrusiveness stem from an illness preventing one from being able to participate in valued life activities (such as recreation or sexual activities, for example) and therefore not being able to derive pleasure or positive outcomes from those activities. In addition, not being able to participate in valued life activities then reduces one's sense of control over one's ability to obtain positive outcomes or avoid negative ones.

Studies examining the IITF document illness intrusiveness as a problem in several cancers, including prostate.[19] Although the IITF has primarily been applied to diseases other than cancer, it has particular relevance for prostate cancer survivors because of the chronic nature of treatment-related side effects. For example, many treated for prostate cancer feel distressed by symptoms such as urinary incontinence (see chapter 2).[5, 20] Men experiencing such problems feel less in control of their lives if their incontinence forces them to curtail work or social activities. In the IITF there is a relationship between treatment-related factors, such as being upset about physical symptoms (like urinary incontinence or erectile dysfunction), and illness intrusiveness. In addition, there is also a relationship between a lack of sense of control over one's cancer and more illness intrusiveness.

The sense of intrusion of prostate cancer in GBM's lives may be even greater owing to the smaller proportion who have a primary partner, compared to the heterosexual population. Single GBM also have the same challenges that single heterosexual men face after prostate cancer—not having a primary partner with whom they have long-established trust and affection.[21] As McCarthy has pointed out, resolving sexual dysfunction for single men is challenging because a new partner may be less forgiving of poor sexual performance than a long-standing one. For some GBM, sexual dysfunction after prostate cancer has substantive negative effects on body image and sense of self.[5] Lack of a supportive partner and changes in a man's sense of himself as a sexual being may exacerbate the physical changes caused by prostate cancer treatment (see chapters 3, 4, and 10). Importantly, the IITF shows that psychological and social factors provide a critical context that can moderate the effect of disease or treatment factors on illness intrusion. Using this framework, the study compared how having a primary partner or not affected illness intrusiveness in three areas: relationships and personal development; sex and intimacy; and instrumental areas such as health, finances, and active recreation.

STUDY DESCRIPTION

All 92 men who participated in the study were at least 18 years of age, diagnosed with prostate cancer within the preceding four years, self-identified as gay or bisexual, able to receive study materials by mail or complete an online questionnaire, and able to speak and understand English. Participants were recruited using a broad array of approaches that have been successful in our previous studies,[22-27] and each received $25 for completing the questionnaire. A full and complete description of participant recruitment, procedures, and demographic and medical characteristics is provided in our main study publication.[1]

The Illness Intrusiveness Ratings Scale (IIRS) was used to determine the extent to which prostate cancer interfered with three life domains: (a) interpersonal relationships and personal development, including family and other social interpersonal relations; self-expression and self-improvement; and religious, community, and civic activities;

(b) sex and intimacy, including intimate relationships and sex life; and (c) instrumental areas, including health, employment, and recreational activities.[28] For each of the three domains, higher scores indicated greater illness intrusiveness.

Social support was measured with a composite set of measures used in previous studies of older adults. Questions were derived from the Inventory of Socially Supportive Behaviors,[29] Lubben Social Network Index,[30] Satisfaction with Support, and Negative Interactions.[31, 32] Questions assessed (a) size and strength of social networks (e.g., family, friends, neighbors), frequency of contact, and how strongly participants feel they can rely on these people for emotional or instrumental support; (b) type and frequency of support received (e.g., emotional, tangible, and informational); (c) satisfaction with support; and (d) type and frequency of negative interactions (such as others being critical or one's feeling taken advantage of by other people in one's social network). A positive social support total score was calculated by adding all scores (and subtracting the negative interaction items), so that higher scores reflected greater positive support.

DATA ANALYSIS

First, partnered and unpartnered men were compared on a number of demographic variables (e.g., age, income) and medical variables (e.g., time since diagnosis) to determine if there were any significant differences between men who were in long-term relationships and those who were not. Next, we examined the relationship between positive social support and each of the three illness intrusiveness domains, and whether being partnered had any differential effect on these three relationships. This type of analysis is known as a moderation analysis, and it specifically addresses the question of whether relationship status affects the relationship between social support and illness intrusiveness differently. Each moderation analysis controlled for time since diagnosis, education, and income.

RESULTS

Sixty-four men (69.6%) reported that they were either married ($N = 42$), in a primary partnered relationship ($N = 16$), or dating one or more people ($N = 6$), whereas the remainder reported being single ($N = 28$; 30.4%). Over 90% of the sample self-identified as Caucasian; race did

TABLE 12.1

Demographic and Medical Information for Gay and Bisexual Men with Prostate Cancer

Variable	Partnered Men	Unpartnered Men	Significance
Age	M = 57.98, SD = 9.99	M = 57.50, SD = 6.9	0.82
Years since prostate cancer diagnosis	M = 1.88, SD = 1.44	M = 1.99, SD = 1.29	0.75
Education High school Some college University degree Graduate degree	7.8% 17.2% 31.3% 43.8%	0.0% 36.0% 28.0% 36.0%	0.28
Yearly income < $30,000 $30,000 – $50,000 $50,000 – $75,000 > $75,000	9.6% 20.6% 19.0% 50.8%	38.4% 23.1% 15.4% 23.1%	0.02
Gleason score	M = 4.14, SD = 1.59	M = 3.68, SD = 1.45	0.88
Positive social support	M = 31.80, SD = 7.12	M = 24.90, SD = 8.33	0.001
Illness intrusiveness: Instrumental	M = 2.54, SD = 1.81	M = 3.15, SD = 1.99	0.16
Illness intrusiveness: Relationships and personal development	M = 1.69, SD = 1.67	M = 2.22, SD = 1.82	0.12
Illness intrusiveness: Sex and intimacy	M = 3.51, SD = 1.92	M = 4.42, SD = 2.54	0.07

Note: *M* = mean. SD = standard deviation.

not differ on the basis of relationship status. Although we did not ask men to report whether they identified as gay or bisexual, the sample as a whole was largely "out" in terms of sexual identity. As we detailed in an earlier publication, these study participants were more out to family, friends, and coworkers than were other published samples of gay men.[1] As table 12.1 shows, partnered versus unpartnered men did not significantly differ on age, time since diagnosis, Gleason score, or education. However, partnered men reported higher income and significantly

TABLE 12.2

Correlation Matrix Showing the Relationships among the
Three Domains of Illness Intrusiveness with Positive Social
Support and Relationship Status

	Positive Social Support	Relationship Status
Illness intrusiveness: Relationships and personal development	$r = -.43^*$	$r = -.19$
Illness intrusiveness: Sex and intimacy	$r = -.36^*$	$r = -.18$
Illness intrusiveness: Instrumental	$r = -.38^*$	$r = -.14$

Note: r = Pearson correlation. $^*p < .01$, indicating statistical significance.

greater positive social support than unpartnered men. We did not see any significant differences on any of the three illness intrusiveness domains on the basis of whether men were partnered or not.

As table 12.2 shows, greater positive support was significantly associated with less illness intrusiveness in all three illness intrusiveness domains. However, relationship status (that is, being partnered or not) was not significantly associated with any of the three illness intrusiveness domains. Being in a relationship was significantly associated with greater positive support.

MODERATION ANALYSES

We examined the relationship between positive social support and each of the three illness intrusiveness domains (relationships and personal development scale, sex and intimacy, and instrumental) and the influence that being in a relationship had on these three associations.

First, we found that men who were more recently diagnosed with cancer and reported less positive social support had significantly more illness intrusiveness in the instrumental domain. As we expected, the moderation analysis showed a significant differential effect for those not in a relationship (compared to those who were in a relationship). Specifically, for men who were unpartnered, positive social support was found to be associated with significantly less illness intrusiveness. However, this relationship was not found for partnered men. Figure 12.1 shows the relationship between illness intrusiveness (vertical axis) and

FIGURE 12.1 Instrumental illness intrusiveness, relationship status, and social support

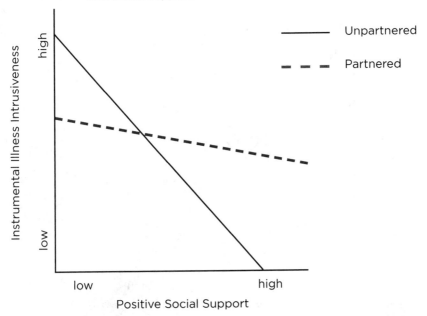

social support (horizontal axis) for partnered and unpartnered men: the slope of the line indicates the strength of the relationship. Men who are unpartnered (solid line) show a much steeper slope, indicating that as social support increases, this group shows a much greater decline in illness intrusiveness than partnered men (dashed line), who in general show lower levels of illness intrusiveness regardless of social support.

We found a similar pattern for illness intrusiveness in the relationships and personal development domain. Men who were more recently diagnosed with cancer and reported less positive social support had significantly more illness intrusiveness in this area. Again, the moderation analysis showed a significant differential effect for those not in a relationship (compared to those who were in a relationship). Specifically, for men who were unpartnered, positive social support was found to be associated with significantly less illness intrusiveness. However, this relationship was not found for partnered men. Figure 12.2 shows the different relationships between illness intrusiveness and positive social support for men who are partnered and those who are not. Once again, men who are unpartnered (solid line) show a much steeper slope, indicating that as social support increases, this group shows a

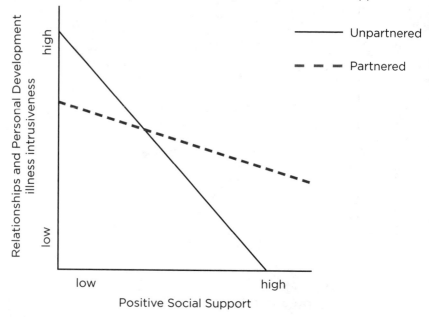

FIGURE 12.2 Relationships and personal development illness intrusiveness, relationship status, and social support

much greater decline in illness intrusiveness than partnered men (dashed line), who in general show lower levels of illness intrusiveness regardless of social support.

Finally, relationship status was not found to significantly differentially affect the relationship between positive social support and illness intrusiveness in the intimacy domain. Table 12.3 shows the full statistical findings of all moderation analyses for each of the three illness intrusiveness domains that we examined.

DISCUSSION

Our study examined positive social support and its association with how much gay men perceived that prostate cancer disrupted their valued life activities (i.e., illness intrusiveness). It also examined how the link between social support and illness intrusiveness was differentially affected by relationship status. Compared to partnered men, unpartnered men reported less perceived social support. Among the unpartnered men, having greater social support reduced their perception of illness intrusiveness. This finding suggests that for unpartnered men, having good social support was related to fewer disruptions from prostate cancer

TABLE 12.3

Moderation Analyses Predicting Domains of Illness Intrusiveness by Positive Social Support and Relationship Status

	Relationships and Personal Development		Sex and Intimacy		Instrumental	
	B	SE	B	SE	B	SE
Time since diagnosis	- 0.01***	0.01	- 0.01*	0.01	- 0.01*	0.01
Education	- 0.05	0.19	- 0.23	0.25	- 0.22	0.22
Income	- 0.21	0.12	- 0.03	0.17	- 0.22	0.15
Positive social support	-0.08***	0.02	- 0.10**	0.03	- 0.05	0.03
Relationship status	0.25	0.21	- 0.06	0.28	0.22	0.25
Social support by relationship status interaction	0.05*	0.03	- 0.01	0.03	0.06*	0.03

Note: B = B weight. SE = Standard error. Relationships and personal development $R^2 = 0.33$***; sex and intimacy $R^2 = 0.21$**; Instrumental $R^2 = 0.19$***. *$p < .05$; **$p < .01$; ***$p < .001$.

in their relationships as well as instrumental areas, such as health, employment, and active recreation. We did not observe this relationship for partnered men—that is, greater social support did not reduce illness intrusiveness. We know from earlier research that social support is important for cancer survivors.[33, 34] Our results suggest that this finding is even stronger for unpartnered gay men. Men who were unpartnered and managed to find social support from important others in their lives reported that their illness had less effect on their lives. Our data are consistent with findings from a qualitative metasynthesis that examined issues for unpartnered men (both gay and heterosexual) and found that unpartnered men with prostate cancer may be at risk of social isolation and fear social rejection from potential partners.[35] Indeed, all these factors fit into the contextual, psychological, or social variables that the IITF comprises.

Most previous studies on men with prostate cancer have not asked about sexual orientation. Thus, the studies we discuss below may have included some gay and bisexual men, but their numbers among other samples are unreported. However, it is still useful to compare our results to other studies of men who are probably heterosexual. Our findings are similar to those of Mehnert and colleagues, who found in a large sample of 511 men with prostate cancer that unmarried men reported lower positive support than married men.[36] Interestingly, we did not find significant differences in any of the three areas of illness intrusion between unpartnered and partnered men, which stands in contrast to other studies showing that single men have worse adjustment after prostate cancer diagnosis. For example, Gore and colleagues found in 291 low-income men with prostate cancer that unpartnered men reported lower mental HRQOL, more urinary function bother, more symptom distress, and less spirituality, even after controlling for age, ethnicity, disease stage, and treatment type.[37] However, Bergman and colleagues found that although unpartnered men with prostate cancer reported significantly more bowel bother and worse sexual functioning, relationship status was not associated with mental or physical HRQOL.[38]

As we expected, positive social support was significantly related to less illness intrusiveness in all three areas examined. Although the relationship between positive social support and illness intrusiveness has, to our knowledge, not been examined in prostate cancer, an ever-expanding literature supports a robust association between positive social support and better adjustment after prostate cancer diagnosis, albeit in studies that are probably composed of heterosexual men.[36, 39, 40] The IITF suggests that social resources and social factors lead to individual variability regarding the degree to which cancer disrupts one's life.[19] For example, a study of breast-cancer patients showed those with worsening illness intrusiveness over time reported significantly less positive social support than those with decreasing or consistently low levels of illness intrusiveness.[41] This finding shows the inverse relationship between illness intrusiveness and social support—as illness intrusiveness worsens, social support is perceived as lower. Earlier studies suggest that keeping social support strong or improving social support may be one way to help lessen the negative influence of cancer on patients' valued life activities.

What do these findings mean for GBM with prostate cancer? Adding to this literature, our study used validated, standardized measures of social support to show that positive social support may play a role in protecting unpartnered GBM with prostate cancer from illness intrusiveness, particularly for the instrumental and the relationships and personal development domains. This finding is consistent with the "buffering hypothesis," which posits that social support can mitigate the negative effects of stressful experiences, such as diagnosis and treatment of cancer.[42] For example, Benedict and colleagues found in advanced prostate cancer patients that men with more social support reported more positive mood, even when facing high levels of stress.[39] Similarly, in a sample of older adults diagnosed with multiple chronic illnesses, including cancer, positive social support provided a buffering effect on the relationship between number of illnesses and depression.[43] As others have suggested, positive social support may reduce intrusive thoughts that can affect quality-of-life measures, mental health outcomes, and possibly illness intrusiveness.[34] While most studies of social support of GBM with prostate cancer have been qualitative, our results support these qualitative results by suggesting that social support can be especially important for unpartnered men.[9, 44] To our knowledge, ours is the first study to document the buffering effect of positive social support with regard to illness intrusiveness in GBM with cancer.

Our data are limited by the small sample size, cross-sectional nature of the data, and, potentially, measurement issues. Given that we studied a relatively small group of GBM with prostate cancer and that only 28 men were unpartnered, our statistical analyses are underpowered to demonstrate significance. Men were within four years of their diagnoses, the average in both groups being around two years, and assessed once. The direction of the findings is unknown. For example, increased illness intrusiveness might lead over time to a weakening of positive support, as shown in earlier research.[41] Moreover, these relationships may differ for men at various points of the cancer survivorship trajectory and could be stronger during the treatment phase, when support needs tend to be highest.[48] Another concern is the assessment of positive social support, which was a general measure of support. It is possible that a questionnaire that assessed these aspects of social support with regard to specific cancer-related experiences or needs might have shown a stronger relationship to illness intrusiveness. Finally, there are a number of issues that were not measured in our study that might have provided more insight into what influences illness intrusiveness in GBM with prostate cancer. Despite limited research on illness intrusiveness in cancer, one study found that more stressful life events were associated with lifestyle disruptions in cancer.[16] In view of our current knowledge of stressful experiences for GBM with prostate cancer, future research could examine specific stressors, such as navigating doctor-patient communication and negotiating intimate and sexual relationships, to see how illness intrusiveness is specifically affected by these variables.

These findings, in the context of the growing literature on GBM with prostate cancer, have a number of clinical implications for healthcare providers. A qualitative study found that gay men with prostate cancer reported unique social-support needs compared to those reported in the literature for heterosexual men, such as access to prostate cancer support groups specifically for GBM.[49] In addition, instrumental support was reported as low across the recovery phase. Single men reported instrumental support coming from friends, family, and paid caregivers, which differs from the care experienced by heterosexual men, who often have wives and children to assist with caregiving. Healthcare providers need to offer information on local and online prostate cancer support groups that are aimed at meeting the needs of GBM. With regard to unpartnered men, healthcare providers also need to assess the availability of instrumental and emotional support, not just in the immediate postsurgical period but also during the treatment and recovery phase. Although the subject has not directly been examined in these analyses, several studies have documented the fact that gay men tend to be less satisfied than heterosexual men with their relationships with healthcare providers.[1, 4, 5, 46, 47] Healthcare providers are urged to actively seek education and training to provide culturally competent care to this vulnerable group of men, which may help to offset illness intrusiveness of prostate cancer.

REFERENCES

1. Hart TL, Coon DW, Kowalkowski MA, et al. Changes in sexual roles and quality of life for gay men after prostate cancer: Challenges for sexual health providers. *Journal of Sexual Medicine.* 2014; 11 (9): 2308–2317.

2. Wassersug RJ, Lyons A, Duncan D, et al. Diagnostic and outcome differences between heterosexual and nonheterosexual men treated for prostate cancer. *Urology.* 2013; 83 (3): 565–571.

3. Allensworth-Davies D, Talcott JA, Heeren T, et al. The health effects of masculine self-esteem following treatment for localized prostate cancer among gay men. *LGBT Health.* 2016; 3 (1): 49–56.

4. Ussher JM, Perz J, Kellett A, et al. Health-related quality of life, psychological

distress, and sexual changes following prostate cancer: A comparison of gay and bisexual men with heterosexual men. *Journal of Sexual Medicine.* 2016; 13 (3): 425–434.

5. Ussher JM, Perz J, Rose D, et al. Threat of sexual disqualification: The consequences of erectile dysfunction and other sexual changes for gay and bisexual men with prostate cancer. *Archives of Sexual Behavior.* 2017; 46 (7): 2043–2057.

6. Scholz U, Knoll N, Roigas J, Gralla O. Effects of provision and receipt of social support on adjustment to laparoscopic radical prostatectomy. *Anxiety Stress & Coping.* 2008; 21 (3): 227–241.

7. Huntley AL, King AJ, Moore TH, et al. Methodological exemplar of integrating quantitative and qualitative evidence—supportive care for men with prostate cancer: What are the most important components? *Journal of Advanced Nursing.* 2017; 73 (1): 5–20.

8. Thomas C, Wootten A, Robinson P. The experiences of gay and bisexual men diagnosed with prostate cancer: Results from an online focus group. *European Journal of Cancer Care.* 2013; 22 (4): 522–529.

9. Hoyt MA, Frost DM, Cohn E, et al. Gay men's experience with prostate cancer: Implications for future research. *Journal of Health Psychology.* 2017; doi: 10.1177/1359105317711491.

10. Devins GM. Illness intrusiveness and the psychosocial impact of lifestyle disruptions in chronic life-threatening disease. *Advances in Renal Replacement Therapy.* 1994; 1 (3): 251–263.

11. Devins GM, Mandin H, Hons RB, et al. Illness intrusiveness and quality of life in end-stage renal disease: Comparison and stability across treatment modalities. *Health Psychology.* 1990; 9 (2): 117–142.

12. Devins GM, Edworthy SM, Guthrie NG, Martin L. Illness intrusiveness in rheumatoid arthritis: Differential impact on depressive symptoms over the adult lifespan. *Journal of Rheumatology.* 1992; 19 (5): 709–715.

13. Antony MM, Roth D, Swinson RP, et al. Illness intrusiveness in individuals with panic disorder, obsessive-compulsive disorder, or social phobia. *Journal of Nervous and Mental Disease.* 1998; 186 (5): 311–315.

14. Bloom JR, Stewart SL, Johnston M, Banks P. Intrusiveness of illness and quality of life in young women with breast cancer. *Psycho-Oncology.* 1998; 7 (2): 89–100.

15. Schimmer AD, Elliott ME, Abbey SE, et al. Illness intrusiveness among survivors of autologous blood and marrow transplantation. *Cancer.* 2001; 92 (12): 3147–3154.

16. Devins GM. Psychologically meaningful activity, illness intrusiveness, and quality of life in rheumatic diseases. *Arthritis and Rheumatism.* 2006; 55 (2): 172–174.

17. Bettazzoni M, Zipursky RB, Friedland J, Devins GM. Illness intrusiveness and subjective well-being in schizophrenia. *Journal of Nervous and Mental Disease.* 2008; 196 (11): 798–805.

18. Edelstein K, Coate L, Massey C, et al. Illness intrusiveness and subjective well-being in patients with glioblastoma. *Journal of Neurooncology.* 2016; 126 (1): 127–135.

19. Devins GM, Bezjak A, Mah K, et al. Context moderates illness-induced lifestyle disruptions across life domains: A test of the Illness Intrusiveness Theoretical Framework in six common cancers. *Psycho-Oncology.* 2006; 15 (3): 221–233.

20. Ullrich PM, Carson MR, Lutgendorf SK, Williams RD. Cancer fear and mood disturbance after radical prostatectomy: Consequences of biochemical evidence of recurrence. *Journal of Urology.* 2003; 169 (4): 1449–1452.

21. McCarthy BW. Treatment of erectile dysfunction with single men. *In* Rosen RC, Leiblum SC, eds. *Erectile disorders: Assessment and treatment.* New York: Guilford Press; 1992: 313–340.

22. Kowalkowski MA, Hart SL, Du XL, et al. Cancer perceptions: Implications from the 2007 Health Information National Trends Survey. *Journal of Cancer Survivorship.* 2012; 6 (3): 287–295.

23. Goh AC, Kowalkowski MA, Bailey DE Jr., et al. Perception of cancer and inconsistency in medical information are associated with decisional conflict: A pilot study of men with prostate cancer who undergo active surveillance. *BJU International.* 2012; 110 (2, pt. 2): E50–56.

24. Vij A, Kowalkowski MA, Hart T, et al. Symptom management strategies for men with early-stage prostate cancer: Results from the Prostate Cancer Patient Education Program (PC PEP). *Journal of Cancer Education.* 2013; 28 (4): 755–761.

25. Hosain GM, Latini DM, Kauth M, et al. Sexual dysfunction among male veterans returning from Iraq and Afghanistan: Prevalence and correlates. *Journal of Sexual Medicine.* 2013; 10 (2): 516–523.

26. Kowalkowski MA, Chandrashekar A, Amiel GE, et al. Examining sexual dysfunction in non-muscle-invasive bladder cancer: Results of cross-sectional mixed-methods research. *Sexual Medicine.* 2014; 2 (3): 141–151.

27. Kowalkowski MA, Goltz HH, Petersen NJ, et al. Educational opportunities in bladder cancer: Increasing cystoscopic adherence and the availability of smoking-cessation programs. *Journal of Cancer Education.* 2014; 29 (4): 739–745.

28. Devins GM, Dion R, Pelletier LG, et al. Structure of lifestyle disruptions in chronic disease: A confirmatory factor analysis of the Illness Intrusiveness Ratings Scale. *Medical Care.* 2001; 39 (10): 1097–1104.

29. Barrera M, Sandler IN, Ramsay TB. Preliminary development of a scale of social support: Studies on college students. *American Journal of Community Psychology.* 1981; 9 (4): 435–447.

30. Lubben JE. Assessing social networks among elderly populations. *Family & Community Health.* 1988; 11 (3): 42–52.

31. Krause N, Markides KS. Measuring social support among older adults. *International Journal of Aging & Human Development.* 1990; 30 (1): 37–53.

32. Krause N. Negative interaction and satisfaction with social support among older adults. *Journals of Gerontology: Series B: Psychological Sciences & Social Sciences.* 1995; 50B (2): P59–P73.

33. Paterson C, Robertson A, Nabi G. Exploring prostate cancer survivors' self-management behaviours and examining the mechanism effect that links coping and social support to health-related quality of life, anxiety and depression: A prospective longitudinal study. *European Journal of Oncological Nursing.* 2015; 19 (2): 120–128.

34. Roberts KJ, Lepore SJ, Helgeson V. Social-cognitive correlates of adjustment to prostate cancer. *Psycho-Oncology.* 2006; 15 (3): 183–192.

35. Matheson L, Watson EK, Nayoan J, et al. A qualitative metasynthesis exploring the impact of prostate cancer and its management on younger, unpartnered and gay men. *European Journal of Cancer Care.* 2017; doi: 10.1111/ecc.12676.

36. Mehnert A, Lehmann C, Graefen M, et al. Depression, anxiety, post-traumatic stress disorder and health-related quality of life and its association with social support in ambulatory prostate cancer patients. *European Journal of Cancer Care.* 2010; 19 (6): 736–745.

37. Gore JL, Krupski T, Kwan L, et al. Partnership status influences quality of life in low-income, uninsured men with prostate cancer. *Cancer.* 2005; 104 (1): 191–198.

38. Bergman J, Gore JL, Saigal CS, et al. Partnership and outcomes in men with prostate cancer. *Cancer.* 2009; 115 (20): 4688–4694.

39. Benedict C, Dahn JR, Antoni MH, et al. Positive and negative mood in men with advanced prostate cancer undergoing androgen deprivation therapy: Considering the role of social support and stress. *Psycho-Oncology.* 2015; 24 (8): 932–939.

40. Zhou ES, Penedo FJ, Lewis JE, et al. Perceived stress mediates the effects of social support on health-related quality of life among men treated for localized prostate cancer. *Journal of Psychosomatic Research.* 2010; 69 (6): 587–590.

41. Sohl SJ, Levine B, Case LD, et al. Trajectories of illness intrusiveness domains following a diagnosis of breast cancer. *Health Psychology.* 2014; 33 (3): 232–241.

42. Cohen S, Wills TA. Stress, social support, and the buffering hypothesis. *Psychological Bulletin.* 1985; 98 (2): 310–357.

43. Ahn S, Kim S, Zhang H. Changes in depressive symptoms among older adults with multiple chronic conditions: Role of positive and negative social support. *International Journal of Environmental Research and Public Health.* 2016; 14 (1).

44. Rosser BR, Hunt SL, Capistrant B, et al. Understanding prostate cancer in gay, bisexual, and other men who have sex with men and transgender women: A review of the literature. *In* Ussher JM, Perz J, Rosser BRS, eds. *Gay and bisexual men living with prostate cancer: From diagnosis to recovery.* New York: Harrington Park Press, 2018.

45. Lepore SJ, Revenson TA. Social constraints on disclosure and adjustment to cancer. *Social and Personality Psychology Compass.* 2007; 1: 313–333.

46. Ussher JM, Rose D, Perz J. Mastery, isolation, or acceptance: Gay and bisexual men's construction of aging in the context of sexual embodiment after prostate cancer. *Journal of Sex Research*. 2017; 54 (6): 802–812; doi: 10.1080/00224499. 2016.1211600.

47. Rose D, Ussher JM, Perz J. Let's talk about gay sex: Gay and bisexual men's sexual communication with healthcare professionals after prostate cancer. *European Journal of Cancer Care*. 2017; 26 (1).

48. Dale W, Bilir P, Han M, Meltzer D. The role of anxiety in prostate carcinoma: A structured review of the literature. *Cancer*. 2005; 104 (3): 467–478.

49. Capistrant BD, Torres B, Merengwa E, et al. Caregiving and social support for gay and bisexual men with prostate cancer. *Psycho-Oncology*. 2016; 25 (11): 1329–1336.

CHAPTER 13

The Effects of Radiation Therapy for Prostate Cancer on Gay and Bisexual Men's Experiences of Mental Health, Sexual Functioning and Behavior, Sexual Identity, and Relationships

William West, B. R. Simon Rosser, Benjamin D. Capistrant, Beatriz Torres, Badrinath R. Konety, Darryl Mitteldorf, Michael W. Ross, and Kristine M. Talley

CHAPTER SUMMARY

As part of a larger study of prostate cancer in gay, bisexual and other men who have sex with men (GBM) in North America, we conducted individual semistructured telephone interviews with 6 GBM who received radiation treatment and 19 who underwent radical prostatectomy. GBM who underwent radiation treatment reported multiple sexual challenges similar to those published for men who underwent radical prostatectomy. Two key differences were identified. GBM who received radiation reported additional bowel and urinary urgency challenges that were not reported by GBM who had radical prostatectomies, which had implications for receptive anal sex. Conversely, GBM who received radiation were less likely to report severe erectile dysfunction, anatomical changes, and total ejaculate loss than GBM with radical prostatectomies. Clinical implications include the importance of addressing these differences in sexual outcomes when discussing treatment options with GBM, possibly as part of a broader discussion of role-in-sex and how to minimize the negative effects of treatment.

KEY TERMS

gay and bisexual men, prostate cancer, qualitative study, radiation treatment

Ussher, Jane M., Perz, Janette, Rosser, B. R. Simon, eds., *Gay & Bisexual Men Living with Prostate Cancer*
dx.doi.org/10.17312/harringtonparkpress/2018.06.gbmlpc.013
© 2018 Harrington Park Press

INTRODUCTION

In research focusing on long-term outcomes of prostate cancer treatment for heterosexual men, the prevalence and incidence of erectile dysfunction and urinary incontinence appear similar after surgical and radiation treatments.[1] However, there are significant differences across treatment types in evaluations of short-term outcomes.[2] Radical prostatectomy results in an immediate decline in sexual function that often improves over time.[2] Erectile dysfunction in radiation patients generally appears several months to a year after treatment. After radiation, once dysfunction appears, recovery is more difficult.[2] Radiation treatment also has an effect on ejaculate. Over time, the amount of ejaculate decreases until there is none.[2] The effect of radiation on penile length has not been adequately studied. Because the rectum is also radiated, an additional concern is both acute and chronic effects in some patients, such as fecal incontinence, pain, bleeding, and susceptibility to perforation.[2] For gay, bisexual, and other men who have sex with men (GBM), long-term rectal pain leading to inability to engage in receptive anal sex is a potential concern, but studies of this topic are lacking. These sexual changes can result in changes in mental health, sexual behavior, and relationships (see chapters 1–6).[3–6] There is a need for further research that focuses on the subjective experiences of those undergoing radiation treatment.

In this chapter we discuss themes that emerged in interviews with GBM who were treated with radiation and those who had prostatectomies. The themes fall into two distinct but interrelated categories: (1) physical (sexual) changes and (2) psychological or emotional changes. Analysis of these two categories leads to a modified theory that can be tested to determine if changes in clinicians' approaches can ameliorate some of the negative outcomes experienced by patients.

This analysis was conducted as part of a broader research study into the effects of prostate cancer treatment on GBM.[7–10] To document the effects of different treatments on sexual and urinary functioning, we published two papers on the effects of radical prostatectomy surgery on GBM.[9, 10] The first paper focused on the sexual functioning effects of radical prostatectomy treatment in 19 GBM and identified three main changes: anatomical (e.g., changes to the shape and size of the penis), behavioral (including erectile dysfunction), and across the sexual response cycle.[9] In the second paper on mental health, sexual identity, and relationship sequelae, five themes emerged: (1) shock at the diagnosis, (2) reactive depression, (3) sex-specific situational anxiety,

(4) grief, and (5) an enduring loss of sexual confidence.[10] In this chapter, which is the first to focus specifically on the effects of radiation treatment for GBM, we draw on the key findings from these previous two papers to situate the experience of the six GBM with prostate cancer in our sample who underwent radiation treatment.

STUDY DESCRIPTION

This research used a qualitative design of one-to-one, semistructured, in-depth telephone interviews. The methods and measures are detailed elsewhere.[9] Briefly, participants were recruited through Malecare, the United States' leading men's cancer support group (both online and in-person groups) and advocacy organization. Of particular note for this analysis, Malecare offers specific online support groups for GBM with prostate cancer as well as for GBM with erectile problems. Each participant was asked to discuss his experience with prostate cancer, detailing when he was diagnosed, his risk factors, the treatment(s) undertaken, his health status since treatment, whether sexual rehabilitation was offered and what type(s), and his experience in rehabilitation. The data analysis was informed by principles of thematic analysis[11] and grounded theory approaches.[12] One investigator (Torres) undertook the primary coding of all data. The results presented here reflect the primary author's use of a constant comparative method from grounded theory, investigating the differences and similarities between the experiences of GBM treated with radiation and of those who had radical prostatectomies, whose experiences are reported elsewhere.[9, 10]

RESULTS

Three groups of changes emerged from the 6 GBM treated with radiation (RAD) compared with the 19 GBM treated surgically (SUR): reactions to anatomical changes, behavioral changes, and sexual response changes (table 13.1).

The distinct anatomical changes for participants treated with radiation focused on urinary and bowel function, particularly increased urgency. This contrasts with the prostatectomy group, in which nearly every participant mentioned changes in penis size and other changes such as curvature and color. The radiation group did not mention these changes unless prompted by a question. For example: "Yeah. Since you're bringing that up, I didn't mention it, but it [shrinkage] happened.

I don't think it's an inch, probably more like a half inch" (RAD01). Neither group reported being warned of these anatomical changes. Both groups mentioned changes in ejaculate. For the prostatectomy group, it was the immediate lack of ejaculate after surgery, whereas for the radiation group, it was changes in consistency or a more gradual decline (see table 13.1).

The emotional reaction to anatomical changes for the radiation group was focused on urinary function and rectal changes, whereas the prostatectomy group vocalized repeatedly changes to the penis and ejaculate loss. Emotional intensity was gauged not just by tone but also by intensifiers and aporia. Descriptions of changes in urinary function focused on both urgency and experiences of burning upon urination: "Now, I have a little bit of burning with urination. That's probably about the only side effect from the radiation. For a while, I was getting up frequently at night and urgency and stuff like, also urinary pains" (RAD04). Similarly, men who had experienced radiation reported pain or pressure and bleeding with bowel movements: "There's a colorful expression, the phantom turd, . . . in radiation you get sunburned in your colon, rectum. The nerves of the rectum, they interpret the sunburn from the radiation as pressure" (RAD03).

The anatomical changes that were similar between men treated with radiation and with prostatectomy included changes to penis anatomy (size, shape, and color), loss of ejaculate, and erectile dysfunction. Notably, though all GBM who had a radical prostatectomy reported changes to their penises, participants treated with radiation did not mention changes to their penises unless prompted by the interviewer. Like men who underwent a radical prostatectomy, men treated with radiation referred to changes to ejaculate. However, they described a change in consistency or loss of volume rather than the loss of ejaculate reported by participants following radical prostatectomy.

Erectile dysfunction (ED) was a common theme for both groups. Almost all reported experiences ranging from temporary minor challenges to chronic, permanent ED. Erectile strength was a stated concern, but here respondents questioned what was due to surgery and what was due to normal aging. ED was a more persistent concern among the prostatectomy group because the effect was immediate after surgery. Most GBM in both groups reported being warned of ED before treatment, but some added that clinicians' understanding of the difference in erectile strength needed for anal versus vaginal insertion left

TABLE 13.1

Sexual Changes: Comparison of GBM Who Underwent Radiation Treatment with Those Who Underwent Radical Prostatectomy for Prostate Cancer

	Radiation Treatment Group (*N* = 6 GBM)	Radical Prostatectomy Group (*N* = 19 GBM)
Anatomical changes	Approximately a year and a half out, I had a bout with radiation proctitis [i.e., inflammation of the lining of the rectum], and that lasted about two days. (RAD03)	It's like I had a penis transplant. That was the hardest thing . . . the cancer was easy! (SUR06)
	You've got to get up right now. Burning; the [urinary] burning was there . . . the jalapeño sunrise. (RAD03)	The biggest surprise for me was how my penis was unrecognizable. It did not look the same. They don't tell you that . . . it scared the daylights out of me. (SUR04)
	Primarily, I had occasions of very little warning when I needed to have a bowel movement or even when I had to urinate, the warning would be nothing like what I had been used to before treatment with the radiation. In the next two or three years, probably as many as half a dozen instances where I was just running for the bathroom or where I ended up dirtying my clothes before I got to the bathroom but gradually, these problems seemed to subside. (RAD01)	
Changes in ejaculate	After the radiation, I was still capable of producing semen, but it changed its color from a milky white to a translucent white and seemed like there was less of it. The ejaculate is lessened. There's not as much as there used to be. (RAD01)	Part of that change is loss. I can't tell you how much I miss cum. I miss it. I use a coconut shampoo because it feels and looks like cum. I love to touch that stuff. (SUR19)
	[Radiation treatment] took away the ejaculation and it has made it less and less enjoyable. (RAD03)	

TABLE 13.1

Sexual Changes: Comparison of GBM Who Underwent Radiation Treatment with Those Who Underwent Radical Prostatectomy for Prostate Cancer

	Radiation Treatment Group (*N* = 6 GBM)	Radical Prostatectomy Group (*N* = 19 GBM)
Behavioral changes	People that are into the top and bottom anal stuff, it does change their landscape considerably. (RADO2)	I was a top. I am a top, I guess. I have been very sexually active my entire life, and it was very important to me. Losing it was just devastating. (SURO5)
	The only thing [i.e., change in anal sex] is the larger the penis, it is more painful whereas before it didn't matter the size (RADO6)	There is pain if I use toys [to stimulate self, anally]. It's like someone is cutting me inside. (SUR15)
Sexual response changes	Sexual desire phase: The libido is pretty much gone. Part of it though is psychological, I think, because I've lost the ability to ejaculate. That's gone. (RADO3)	Sexual desire phase: My libido is much less than it was before [the surgery]. It comes and goes much more. (SUR13)
	That is so fundamental to how I perceive myself as a man, as a sexual being. (RADO5)	Plateau: Watching porn is helpful . . . to get you excited. It's difficult to prolong sexual excitement and to keep it going. If I lose the erection, it's hard to get it back. (SURO2)

much to be desired: "They referred to the standard of an erection capable of vaginal penetration, that was the standard that was used, and I just didn't get into it with them" (SURo3).

Rectal changes were repeatedly noted in the radiation group but were not noted by the surgery group. Urgency, often intense, was a common theme. Pressure and sometimes bleeding were also noted: "Radiation proctitis is [experienced when] the blood vessels in your rectum come to the surface or express themselves onto the surface very boldly and, when anything passes through, it just scrapes them wide open and there'd be blood everywhere" (RADo5).

Both groups adjusted their sexual behavior to accommodate changes brought on by their respective treatments. One consequence among the behavioral changes for men treated with radiation was more reports of changing role-in-sex from anally receptive to insertive because of the more profound rectal anatomical changes; the surgery group reported the opposite. Across groups, some men reported being unsure if, or when, they could resume receptive anal sex. Both groups also reported changes across the sexual response cycle. In both groups, the one phase that surprised the most was loss of libido or sexual desire, as reported in earlier research.[9, 10]

The second major thematic category was emotional reactions to diagnosis, treatment, and the consequences of treatment (table 13.2).

Many participants in both groups reported feeling shocked or terrified (or both) by their diagnosis. This was true whether the man reported an extensive family history or no history of prostate cancer. This reaction is not surprising. In studies based on heterosexual men treated for prostate cancer, their levels of emotional health—as measured by the SF-36-item subscale on emotional well-being—worsen immediately after diagnosis,[13] possibly returning to prediagnosis levels at longer-term follow-up.[14] Not all prostate cancer survivors' mental health appears equally affected by treatment, however. In previous research, heterosexual men treated with radical prostatectomies were reported to have scored significantly better on this measure over time than men who underwent pelvic radiation or watchful waiting.[13] Because there have been no quantitative studies in GBM prostate cancer survivors comparing radiation to prostatectomy treatment in terms of emotional well-being, we do not know if these results generalize to GBM. As table 13.2 summarizes, comments from participants in our study displayed almost equal distress at and following diagnosis, as well as similar challenges in sex-specific anxiety and loss of sexual confidence. Participants treated with radiation also reported a variety of emotions during the treatment period. Further research is needed to examine this issue in a larger sample of GBM, using mixed methods.

In terms of depression, GBM treated with prostatectomy described a reactive depression shortly after surgery, which focused on loss of and mourning for their sexual behavior or earlier sexual self: "I wasn't suicidal—I was just very depressed" (SUR09). GBM who underwent radiation also reported depression, but it was contextualized in response to culturally tone-deaf clinicians. For example, one participant reported becoming uncomfortable with his urologist, and ultimately changing to radiation treatment, after the specialist repeatedly ignored the patient's disclosure of his sexual orientation as gay (see chapter 8): "He

TABLE 13.2

Emotional Reactions: Comparison of GBM Who Underwent Radiation Treatment with Those Who Underwent Radical Prostatectomy for Prostate Cancer

	Radiation Treatment Group (*N* = 6 GBM)	Radical Prostatectomy Group (*N* = 19 GBM)
Emotional reaction to diagnosis	[Diagnosis was] very troubling. The information that I'd had about it was that it was, it could be fatal. I caught mine early. I guess to answer the question directly, I was very distressed. (RAD02) Initially it was very frightening and kind of dispiriting. . . . I was kind of numb, I didn't even really understand what he was saying. (RAD05)	Initially shocking, because I was only 52, and I thought I was in extremely good health, and then terrifying because I just assumed I was going to die soon. . . . It was just absolute and utter disbelief mostly because I thought I was so fit and I thought I was so healthy. (SUR04) I wasn't suicidal—I was just very depressed. (SUR09)
Emotional reaction going through treatment	The process itself wasn't so devastating. It was just all the research that I had to do to determine what treatment I was going to take. Once I made a decision as to what I was going to do, it was fine. I had no problems. It was all the research that I did [that] led up to my final decision. (RAD06) I went in with a prostate PSA reading of about 4 or 5, 4.5, and after my sixth month it had dropped to .7. I was very thrilled. (RAD02) With [stereotactic body radiation therapy] . . . I was sort of knocked out but I think that was really self-induced stress. My friend, he drove me to and fro for the five visits. I slept on the way home but honestly it was just because I was so worked up. (RAD05)	(Not applicable; participants were unconscious during surgery)

(continued)

TABLE 13.2 *(continued)*

Emotional Reactions: Comparison of GBM Who Underwent Radiation Treatment with Those Who Underwent Radical Prostatectomy for Prostate Cancer

	Radiation Treatment Group (*N* = 6 GBM)	Radical Prostatectomy Group (*N* = 19 GBM)
Sex-specific situational anxiety	I do think that's one thing that [is different for gay men] because, for gay guys, sex is more involved. Maybe it's true. Maybe straight guys are just as disturbed by that. The thing that bothers me the most I think is all those things that you think of as part of being a male. Some of that stuff is going to be a little bit tougher now. (RAD04)	Now, all the spontaneity is gone, which is a shame. (SUR12) It's stressful to meet some guy and really want to be with him and want to please him, and to recognize that I may not be able to. What that's done, in a funny kind of way, is I feel like I'm trapped in hookup hell. (SUR01)
Change in sexual confidence	I've adapted. I'm not so self-conscious about it anymore. You get this scenario going in your head that you're old, you've had cancer, and that's the end of . . . but that has not proven to be the case now. I guess October will be two years for me, or November will be two years for me. If any-thing, the sex is as enjoyable. (RAD02)	I feel less than the average gay person. (SUR17) [It's] impacted me in that it has contributed to my lack of confidence in myself as a sex-ual being. (SUR19)

[the surgeon] said, 'I can get you in next week if you'd like.' I am gay. He said, 'Bring the wife in, and we can discuss it.' I'd already told him several times I was gay. He was very uncomfortable with that" (RAD01). A second participant reported depression secondary to learning that the treatment had not been entirely successful: "[I had] doubts about [my] radiologist's competence. Maybe these doubts appeared only a couple of years later when I realized that my cancer and my PSA had risen again and it was determined that I had to have further treatment on the prostate" (RAD02).

Grief was commonly reported in both groups and almost univer-sally linked to loss of gay male identity and sexual potency: "I do think that's one thing that [is different for gay men] because, for gay guys, sex is more involved. Maybe it's true. Maybe straight guys are just as disturbed by that. The thing that bothers me the most I think is all those things that you think of as part of being a male. Some of that stuff is going to be a little bit tougher now" (RAD04). Sex-specific situational anxiety expressed itself generally in similar ways for both groups, as reported previously (see chapters 2, 6, and 10): "It's stressful to meet some guy and really want to be with him and want to please him, and to recognize that I may not be able to. What that's done, in a funny kind of way, is I feel like I'm trapped in hookup hell" (RAD01).

Compounding this problem for the radiation group were urinary control issues and diarrhea. Both these symptoms were seen as major impediments to initiating sexual encounters after treatment. The final theme was an enduring loss of sexual confidence, one expressed with regularity by both groups (see table 13.2).

DISCUSSION

The key finding of this analysis is that treatment with radiation has profound effects on GBM prostate cancer survivors. We compared the sexual effects experienced by GBM who underwent radiation to those experienced by GBM who had radical prostatectomies.[9, 10] In terms of sexual challenges, several similarities and differences were noted. Key similarities include GBM reporting penile shrinkage, erectile difficulties, less ejaculate, changes in their subjective sense of orgasm, and loss of sexual confidence and sense of being a man (i.e., decreased sexual self-esteem), as reported in previous research (see chapters 1–7 and 11).[15–17] GBM in both groups spoke of challenges in addressing these functioning concerns, including challenges in rehabilitation (e.g., a vacuum device leading to bleeding) and changes in role-in-sex (generally from being the insertive partner to being the receptive partner in anal sex) (see chapters 6, 10, and 11).

However, key differences also emerged. Though none of the men who received radical prostatectomies mentioned urinary urgency or bowel problems, several men who underwent radiation reported complications both in bowel and urinary urgency not involving sex and bowel radiation effects sufficient to change the experience of receptive anal sex. On a positive side for radiation, while GBM in both treatment groups reported a loss of ejaculate that they found disturbing, some men who received radiation still reported an ability to ejaculate and only limited changes (e.g., change in ejaculate color), whereas men with radical prostatectomies reported total absence of ejaculate. Climacturia was reported by several men in both treatment groups. In terms of enduring loss of sexual confidence, GBM treated with prostatectomy were more likely to describe their loss of sexual confidence as "devastating." Some described themselves as "severely damaged" as men because of their lack of sexual functioning (see chapter 2). This perception could reflect the fact that the erectile functioning and ejaculate challenges following prostatectomy are more sudden and severe, which allows less time for psychosexual adjustment to occur.

There are several directions for future research. First, we encourage other researchers to examine GBM's experiences by type of treatment so that the differences by treatment can be validated. Second, we caution that radiation treatment is itself a very wide category and that different types of radiation treatments may have subtle differences in outcome that warrant more exploration. Third, given that a key difference found between the radiation group and the prostatectomy group was in irradiation of the bowel, clinicians counseling GBM on whether to choose radiation or surgery for prostate cancer treatment should explicitly discuss the effects on anal sex. Given our results, men who identify as "tops" or prefer the insertive role in anal sex may experience greater distress associated with erectile challenges following surgery. Conversely, men who identify as "bottoms" or prefer the receptive role in anal sex may experience greater challenges following radiation treatment. Other considerations aside, testing protocols that specify treatment effects by mode in sex could help GBM make informed treatment choices, improve outcomes, and advance shared decision-making practice in prostate cancer treatment (see chapter 20).

A final key difference between the radiation and surgery groups was noted. At least in the United States, all participants reported being referred first to a urologist. Those who chose radiation consistently sought a second (and sometimes numerous other) opinion, whereas some who underwent surgery did not.

A prevailing theme that unites both groups of GBM was the sense of surprise. Even when warned of post-treatment effects such as erectile dysfunction, GBM who underwent either radiation or surgery were surprised and, in some cases, shocked by the extent of the effects. Some GBM claimed they had no warning. One patient asserted that changes to his penis were so extreme he felt like he had had a penis transplant and that this outcome was worse than the cancer itself. When another complained about penis shrinkage to his specialist, his provider discounted his complaint, stating there had been none. What is clear from these interviews is that patients often did not fully realize the effects of various treatments (see chapter 2). And, if some dysfunction was discussed, the discussion failed to predict the degree of actual distress likely to be experienced (see chapters 6, 7, and 8). Patients also reported that they often were given little to no power in decision making. Some participants described their providers as little more than "used car salesman" hawking either surgery or radiation, depending on their specialty. Shared decision making, as described in chapter 20, is designed to overcome what was lacking in these patient-provider interactions.[18, 19]

Given the degree of confusion and distress exhibited in patient responses, it could be beneficial to treat clinically localized prostate cancer as a preference-sensitive condition. The clinician portraying professional equipoise should practice shared decision making with the patient.[20] *Equipoise* can refer to exploring all options with the patient without advocating for any particular option. Shared decision making means exploring these options in light of the patient's values and the possible treatment effects.[18] Pros and cons of each approach should be explored in terms of gay sexuality, and existing data and evidence should be discussed. This practice would go a long way to ameliorating what at least one patient directly commented on: "The crazy thing about this disease is nobody agrees on anything. You talk to a radiologist and 'You got to do radiation.' The urologist said, 'You need to do surgery.' I talked to [proton company] and had them check me out, and [they said] proton therapy was the way to go" (RAD04).

CONCLUSION

GBM with prostate cancer treated with radiation report significant sexual changes. The key finding from this research is that, though the effects of radiation are similar in many ways to those of radical prostatectomy, there are important differences. Specifically, the effects on bowel functioning and possibly urinary functioning are significant following radiation treatment, although these may be offset by less severe changes in ejaculate and erectile functioning than those experienced following radical prostatectomy. In shared decision making between GBM patients and their providers, the implications of differences in treatment on insertive and receptive anal functioning should be raised as part of the discussion on which treatment option(s) will have the least effects on a particular man's sexual functioning and, ultimately, quality of life.

ACKNOWLEDGMENTS

This study was conducted with funding from the National Cancer Institute (Grant award no. 1 R21 CA182041).

REFERENCES

1. Litwin MS, Hays RD, Fink A, et al. Quality-of-life outcomes in men treated for localized prostate cancer. *Journal of the American Medical Assocation (JAMA)*. 1995; 273 (2): 129–135.

2. Tal R. Prostate cancer and sexual dysfunction in gay men. *In* Perlman G, ed. *What every gay man needs to know about prostate cancer*. New York: Magnus Books; 2013: 47–75.

3. Hart S, Coon D, Kowalkowski M, Latini D. Gay men with prostate cancer report significantly worse HRQOL than heterosexual men. *Journal of Urology*. 2011; 185 (4, Suppl.): e68–e69.

4. Hartman ME, Irvine J, Currie KL, et al. Exploring gay couples' experience with sexual dysfunction after radical prostatectomy: A qualitative study. *Journal of Sex & Marital Therapy* 2014; 40 (3): 233–253.

5. Ussher JM, Perz J, Kellett A, et al. Health-related quality of life, psychological distress, and sexual changes following prostate cancer: A comparison of gay and bisexual men with heterosexual men. *Journal of Sexual Medicine*. 2016; 13 (3): 425–434.

6. Wassersug RJ, Lyons A, Duncan D, et al. Diagnostic and outcome differences between heterosexual and nonheterosexual men treated for prostate cancer. *Urology*. 2013; 82 (3): 565–571.

7. Capistrant BD, Moon JR, Berkman LF, Glymour MM. Current and long-term spousal caregiving and onset of cardiovascular disease. *Journal of Epidemiology and Community Health*. 2012; 66 (10): 951–956.

8. Capistrant BD, Torres B, Merengwa E, et al. Caregiving and social support for gay and bisexual men with prostate cancer. *Psycho-Oncology*. 2016; 25 (11): 1329–1336.

9. Rosser BRS, Capistrant BD, Torres B, et al. The effects of radical prostatectomy on gay and bisexual men's sexual functioning and behavior: Qualitative results from the *Restore* study. *Journal of Sex and Relationship Therapy*. 2016; 31 (4): 432–445.

10. Rosser BRS, Capistrant BD, Torres B, et al. The effects of radical prostatectomy on gay and bisexual men's mental health, sexual identity, and relationships: Qualitative results form the *Restore* study. *Journal of Sex & Relationship Therapy*. 2016; 31 (4): 446–461.

11. Braun V, Clarke V. Using thematic analysis in psychology. *Qualitative Research in Psychology.* 2006; 3 (2): 77–101.

12. Corbin JM, Strauss AL. *Basics of qualitative research: Techniques and procedures for developing grounded theory.* 3rd ed. Los Angeles: Sage; 2008.

13. Litwin MS, Lubeck DP, Spitalny GM, et al. Mental health in men treated for early stage prostate carcinoma. *Cancer.* 2002; 95 (1): 54–60.

14. Korfage IJ, de Koning HJ, Roobol M, et al. Prostate cancer diagnosis: The impact on patients' mental health. *European Journal of Cancer.* 2006; 42 (2): 165–170.

15. Ussher JM, Perz J, Rose D, et al. Threat of sexual disqualification: The consequences of erectile dysfunction and other sexual changes for gay and bisexual men with prostate cancer. *Archives of Sexual Behavior.* 2017; 46 (7): 2043–2057.

16. Dowsett GW, Lyons A, Duncan D, Wassersug RJ. Flexibility in men's sexual practices in response to iatrogenic erectile dysfunction after prostate cancer treatment. *Sexual Medicine.* 2014; 2 (3): 115–120.

17. Hart TL, Coon DW, Kowalkowski MA, et al. Changes in sexual roles and quality of life for gay men after prostate cancer: Challenges for sexual health providers. *Journal of Sexual Medicine.* 2014; 11 (9): 2308–2317.

18. Centers for Medicare & Medicaid Services. Beneficiary engagement and incentives: Shared decision making (SDM) model. 2017; https://innovation.cms.gov/initiatives/Beneficiary-Engagement-SDM/. Accessed May 30, 2017.

19. Charles C, Gafni A, Whelan T. Shared decision-making in the medical encounter: What does it mean? (Or it takes at least two to tango). *Social Science & Medicine.* 1997; 44 (5): 681–692.

20. Elwyn G, Coulter A, Laitner S, et al. Implementing shared decision making in the NHS. *British Medical Journal.* 2010; 341: c5146.

CHAPTER 14

Toward a More Comprehensive Model of Prostate Cancer Care Inclusive of Gay and Bisexual Men and Transgender Women

Donald Allensworth-Davies, Thomas O. Blank, Brian de Vries, and Emilia Lombardi

CHAPTER SUMMARY

Despite the recent growth in cancer care research specific to sexual-minority populations, comprehensive care models of prostate cancer inclusive of gay and bisexual men (GBM) and transgender women (TGW) are lacking. The prostate cancer care process is described as occurring in four phases: (1) screening, (2) diagnosis, (3) treatment, and (4) post-treatment and survivorship. Research in the past ten years has shown that while the biology of prostate cancer is similar regardless of sexual orientation or gender identity, the psychosocial needs of gay, bisexual, and transgender persons are quite different from those of their straight peers. In this chapter we describe a comprehensive care model for GBM, TGW, and others with diverse sexual and gender identities at risk for prostate cancer; the model includes these four phases and was informed by a national survey of gay prostate cancer survivors that we conducted.[1] It is our hope that this model of prostate cancer care can be used as a foundation for both clinicians and GBM and TGW patients in understanding and addressing some of the unique needs at each stage of the prostate cancer care process.

KEY TERMS

bisexual, cancer treatment, gay, prostate cancer, transgender

INTRODUCTION

One important step as part of the continued evolution in prostate cancer psychosocial research in sexual-minority populations is to begin developing and testing conceptual frameworks and developing models

Ussher, Jane M., Perz, Janette, Rosser, B. R. Simon, eds., *Gay & Bisexual Men Living with Prostate Cancer*
dx.doi.org/10.17312/harringtonparkpress/2018.06.gbmlpc.014
© 2018 Harrington Park Press

for understanding and differentiating between psychosocial *predictors* and psychosocial *outcomes*, especially within the context of prostate cancer care and quality of life (QoL). In this chapter we propose a model of the prostate cancer care experience of gay and bisexual men (GBM) and transgender women (TGW) to help inform prostate cancer care and the design of future prostate cancer research (figure 14.1).

Although difficult to illustrate visually, the longitudinal nature of this model is important because QoL is a complex construct that includes both physical and mental health, and it is far from static. For example, in 2010–2011 we administered a national QoL survey to 111 gay prostate cancer survivors to assess post-treatment prostate cancer QoL outcomes.[1] The QoL reported by the men that we surveyed was quite different from their QoL at the time of diagnosis, and for nearly all, it remained forever changed.[2] Only by measuring QoL throughout screening, diagnosis, treatment, and post-treatment/survivorship can we fully understand QoL changes as well as the implications for health and use of health services. We discuss the context of this model and the different stages below.

PSYCHOSOCIAL EFFECTS OF PROSTATE CANCER CARE IN GBM AND TGW POPULATIONS

SCREENING AND DIAGNOSIS

A number of prediagnosis considerations specific to sexual-minority populations may influence their ability or willingness to pursue prostate cancer screening.[3-5] These considerations may include an unwillingness to seek healthcare services because of a lack of health insurance, fear of discrimination from providers, lack of perceived severity of medical conditions or symptoms, and past dissatisfaction with services.[6] GBM and TGW may also be engaging in behaviors that place their health at risk (and some of which may also increase their cancer risk), such as alcohol, drug, or tobacco use and risky sexual behavior, which may cause feelings of resistance toward interacting with the healthcare system. They may also have actively competing conditions, such as psychiatric morbidity, HIV/AIDS, and chronic diseases that are unrelated to prostate cancer but that may delay prostate cancer screening. Some may seek screening if they have a family history of prostate cancer, or if they know that they are in a group with increased risk, such as African Americans.[7, 8] Still others may not undergo screening until

FIGURE 14.1 Conceptual model of prostate cancer care for gay/bisexual men and transgender women

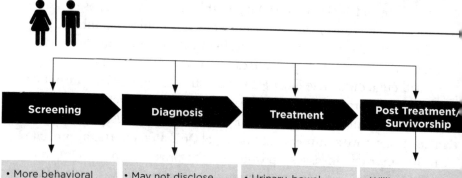

Screening	Diagnosis	Treatment	Post Treatment/ Survivorship
• More behavioral risk factors (e.g., alcohol, drug, or tobacco use)	• May not disclose sexual orientation or gender identity owing to fear of discrimination/receiving substandard quality of care	• Urinary, bowel, and sexual function concerns may overlap	• Willingness to disclose sexual orientation or gend identity and comfor with provider(s) ma affect compliance with follow-up care
• More psychiatric comorbidity		• Sex more broadly conceptualized and may include:	
• More likely to be HIV+	• May perceive providers or care environment as insensitive and/or inhospitable	o anal sex	• Because sex is conceptualized differently, may be more adaptable to changes in function
• Even if partnered, may be in a sexually nonmonogamous relationship		o oral sex	
		o masturbation	
	• Patient requires help in treatment decision making, emotional support, and postsurgical planning. May not have a partner or family member to assist in these roles	o kissing/massage	
		o role-play/toys	• If partnered, type of support available and effect on relationship may be different from those for straight men (e.g monogamous relationship may becom nonmonogamous)
• May have a partner who has already been diagnosed with /treated for prostate cancer		• Sexual function in some form still central to identity among gay/bisexual men, including erectile function and ejaculate	
• Lower baseline self-esteem owing to stigma as a sexual minority			
• May not be "out"	• Willingness to disclose sexual orientation and comfort with provider(s) may affect engagement in treatment decision making	• Non-masculine identity would provide different concerns regarding side effects and treatment	• If not partnered, may have few or no sources of practical, emotional support
• May have internalized homophobia/transphobia			
• May not present or identify as male			• Few outside suppor resources available to gay or transgender prostate cancer survivors (e.g., support groups)

they present with symptoms or have the prostate-specific antigen (PSA) test conducted by their primary care provider in a regularly scheduled physical. However, there are also factors that could encourage patients to actively seek screening, such as being out to and regularly seeing their primary care provider or having a partner who has already been diagnosed with and treated for prostate cancer.

Screening recommendations for TGW, compared to GBM, at this time are uncertain, however, because prostate cancer is believed to be a rarer occurrence in this population despite the prostate's not being routinely removed as part of sex reassignment surgery.[9] Most of the reported cases of prostate cancer in TGW were in individuals who started hormone therapy later in their lives or who had received hormone therapy for several years.[9-11] Assuming that this rare occurrence of prostate cancer is representative of the population, then prostate cancer screening could be limited to TGW who began hormone therapy later in life or those who have a family history of prostate cancer.[9] Yet, given that TGW are also often unwilling to seek healthcare owing to fears of discrimination and stigma,[12] or may not be able to access care because of a lack of insurance and ability to pay,[12] the true prevalence of prostate cancer in this population can only be estimated. From a screening perspective, McNamara and Ng offer the most practical recommendation for patients and providers — "Screen what you have"[3] (i.e., all persons with a prostate should undergo prostate cancer screening). TGW, like GBM, should be counseled about the risks and benefits of prostate cancer screening, while taking their individual surgical history and hormonal status into account.[3]

TGW, and others who do not adopt a male identity but have a prostate, will have different sexual orientations and screening needs from those who identify as men, regardless of sexual orientation. The results of prostate cancer treatment also attack aspects that relate to masculine social roles (e.g., a functional penis, libido), but those who do not value such activity will not be as affected and may have different concerns (e.g., ability to maintain estrogen treatment as part of transgender care or the diagnosis's influence on their ability to attain gender-reassignment surgery). Clinicians need to be open to people who have different perspectives and needs from those of straight cisgender men with prostate cancer.

TREATMENT

Treatment options. Treatment options for localized prostate cancer encompass a wide array of approaches, including watchful waiting or active surveillance, surgery, radiation therapy, hormone therapy, or some combination of these.[13] Surgery may be used in a variety of ways—for example, to remove and evaluate the lymph nodes to determine whether the prostate cancer has spread (pelvic lymphadenectomy) or to remove the prostate, surrounding tissue, and seminal vesicles if the prostate cancer is localized (radical prostatectomy).[13] Radiation therapy uses high-energy X-rays or other types of radiation to kill cancer cells or prevent them from growing. Which treatment option is best depends on the stage of the disease, likelihood of spread, and aggressiveness of the cancer. Other important factors are the patient's age, general health, whether the cancer has been newly diagnosed or has recurred, and feelings about potential treatments and their possible side effects.[13]

Treatment decision making. A growing literature has emerged over the past several years on the importance of the decision-making process in selecting a prostate cancer treatment as well as the roles of providers and patients in this process (see chapters 4, 9, and 10). For some patients to feel that they have made an informed treatment decision, a complex process may unfold both internally and with the treating provider. Others may not wish to be involved in making a treatment decision and prefer to be told by their provider which treatment is best for them. The decision-making process also assumes that the patient understands the information that is being presented, that the treating provider has adequate time to present all the available options, and that the provider describes the side effects of each option and can help the patient choose a treatment that is in keeping with the patient's values and desired functional outcomes after treatment.[14-16]

Creating a hospitable environment for GBM and TGW patients can help facilitate open communication during the treatment process as well as increased patient satisfaction with treatment (see chapters 8 and 10).[17] At the treatment stage, it is important for the provider to recognize that how comfortable GBM and TGW patients feel in disclosing their sexual orientation is one factor that may help determine the extent to which they are willing to participate in the treatment decision-making process. However, the assumption here is that the patient also desires to be part of the process; some GBM and TGW patients (and others) prefer that the physician choose the best option. For GBM and TGW, active involvement in their prostate cancer treatment decision making may be difficult if not impossible if they are not comfortable revealing their sexual orientation or gender identity to their healthcare providers. Fearing discrimination, stigma, receipt of substandard care, or denial of access to care, many choose not to reveal their sexual orientation.[6] However, disclosing one's sexual orientation and gender identity to a healthcare provider can be crucial in selecting a prostate cancer treatment that is tailored and responsive to each patient's unique needs, especially given that all treatments may adversely affect sexual function and possibly other aspects of QoL, such as incontinence (see chapter 8). In addition, failure to establish rapport and communication between physicians and patients has been found to be associated with decreased levels of adherence to physician recommendations and treatment plans, as well as decreased rates of patient satisfaction.[18] In the context of prostate cancer, this failure of rapport could greatly increase the risk of medical complications following treatment as well as cancer recurrence if GBM and TGW patients fail to comply with post-treatment follow-up.

In describing treatment options for GBM and TGW, it may also be useful to consider that many GBM and TGW patients conceptualize sex as a range of activities that can include anal sex, oral sex, masturbation, kissing, massage, role-play, or sexual toys (see chapters 10 and 11). For this reason, urinary, bowel, and sexual function concerns may overlap in a way that they do not for straight men.[1, 4, 19] Sexual function, including erectile function and ejaculate, is also central to GBM's identity; at the same time, they may be more flexible in how their sexual identity is defined (see chapters 2, 5, and 6).[17] TGW and others who do not adopt a male identity will have a very different perspective, as TGW may not value erectile function and ejaculate, but may be more concerned with how the treatment will affect their lives as TGW (e.g., maintaining estrogen therapy).[9, 10, 20] All these considerations can influence how well patients and their partners adapt to changes following treatment.

Effects of prostate cancer treatment. An additional area of concern is that of health worry. Waiting for an ultrasound or biopsy result generates initial worry and anxiety that increase once a prostate cancer diagnosis is confirmed, as Rosser and colleagues outline in chapter 1. The resulting worry and anxiety in turn can lead to generalized anxiety disorder, panic symptoms, or insomnia (or a combination of these).[18, 19] Emerging evidence on adult LGBT mental health also suggests that as a sexual minority, GBT patients have a higher degree of tension, worry, and stress, both more generally and in the healthcare environment, because of perceived stigma or discrimination, internalized homophobia or transphobia, or distrust of healthcare providers at the time of prostate cancer screening than their heterosexual peers[6, 21] (see chapter 8). This worry and stress could subsequently increase as a result of the diagnosis and treatment process.

For many men, treatment of prostate cancer has profound effects on masculine identity and self-esteem.[1] Men who are taught by our culture to portray themselves as strong and unemotional suddenly find themselves in a position of vulnerability. Previous research suggests that the combination of poor sexual functioning and adherence to traditional norms of masculinity may also result in poor social, role, and mental health functioning following treatment for prostate cancer.[21] Yet despite these associations of masculine identity and self-esteem with QoL following prostate cancer treatment, the question remains whether these associations remain true for GBM.

POST-TREATMENT AND SURVIVORSHIP

In this stage, the effects of the previous stages of the care process on QoL begin to manifest themselves. If the patient has had open communication with the providers throughout the process, then we would expect self-esteem either to remain unchanged or to improve, feelings of stigma and discrimination to be less, treatment regret to be low, and trust in healthcare providers and compliance with follow-up care recommendations to be high. Prompting patients, including unpartnered patients, to identify a person or persons whom they can rely on to help during the recovery process and to consider what additional support they may need after treatment may also be useful at this time.[4] Patients may adapt to changes in urinary, bowel, or sexual function by redefining sexual identity or gender identities and sexual behaviors, and, if partnered, possibly by renegotiating the terms of their sexual relationship as well, as chapters 10 and 11 describe. Monogamous relationships may become open relationships or vice versa in order to continue to meet the needs of both partners.[18] The provider may again wish to discuss with the patient possible resources for information and additional support, especially if the patient is not partnered.

Decisional regret. Higher levels of decisional regret following treatment for prostate cancer have been found to be associated with a variety of factors, including age; urinary, bowel, or sexual side effects experienced as a result of treatment; increases in Gleason or PSA scores; and decreases in role and social functioning.[22-25] Patients with treatment regret (i.e., feelings of having made the wrong treatment decision and wishing to undo that decision) may also be at greater risk for depression, anxiety, or poor general mental functioning. With a group of predominantly nonwhite, low-income, and uninsured men, Hu and colleagues reported that fear of cancer recurrence was also a significant determinant of treatment regret.[26] For GBM and TGW patients, treatment regret may also be influenced by whether they have revealed their sexual orientation and gender identity to their treating provider and felt comfortable discussing their treatment concerns and if that might have led to another decision or option.[27]

Social support. An aspect of well-being that has broad implications across all phases is social support. As a correlate of social well-being, it is an important coping strategy that has received extensive attention in the context of QoL for cancer patients and has been found to play a critical role in physical and psychological well-being.[4, 18] Social support and the use of other coping strategies have been shown to buffer the negative side effects of the cancer experience, both psychologically and physiologically.[28] Among prostate cancer survivors, Mehnert and colleagues also reported that lack of positive support and detrimental social interactions (such as overprotective behavior, dismissive or conflictual behavioral patterns, or pessimism) were predictors of psychological comorbidity and mental health problems.[29] Partner support is also of concern because patients depend on their partners for emotional and practical support. Research suggests that though straight men tend to rely on spouses and biological family members for support, GBM and TGW may rely more on self, partner, and chosen family.[4]

One form of support that is relevant for some men following prostate cancer treatment is support groups. Support groups can function as an important mechanism in the exchange of prostate cancer education and information as well as create an environment in which personal emotions can be shared with others who have been through a similar experience. Support groups in general are often positively evaluated by their participants and have also been found to exert a positive influence on psychosocial well-being.[4] While increasing in number, there are still few GBM- and TGW-specific prostate cancer support groups. Many GBM may not feel comfortable attending support groups of predominantly heterosexual men because of fears of stigma and discrimination or concern that they would be limited in their ability to openly share their experiences and emotions with other members of the group and thereby obtain the support they need.[4] Unfortunately, the rarity of prostate cancer among TGW and other diverse gender groups means that there is little opportunity for either support groups or individual peer support for these individuals.

IMPLICATIONS FOR CLINICAL CARE

As this chapter notes, GBT individuals represent a hidden sexual minority in prostate cancer care, and this assessment is especially true of older GBM and TGW who may have come of age in an era when being GBT was still classified as a mental disorder and who may have been ostracized by their families.[6, 30] Many LGBT persons choose not to disclose their sexual orientation to healthcare providers because they do not feel comfortable doing so or they fear receiving substandard care as a result.[6] However, the experiences associated with learning to live as a sexual minority in a predominantly straight cisgender society (e.g., knowing when it is safe to disclose oneself as being GBM or TGW) may also act as sources of emotional strength during crises, such as prostate cancer diagnosis, that GBT experience later in their lives.[31]

Given the serious implications of a prostate cancer diagnosis and the radical changes in urinary, bowel, and sexual function that often accompany prostate cancer treatment, feelings of fear, sadness, and embarrassment are not uncommon.[1, 32, 33] Studies suggest that maintaining a positive attitude and good communication with one's provider are important determinants in prostate cancer QoL and treatment satisfaction.[17, 27, 34–38] In addition, healthcare providers may give verbal and nonverbal cues to the patient that their practice environment is not LGBT friendly or, because of a lack of knowledge about partners, friends, or other nontraditional supports, may not be able to access the GBM's support networks to help him in making arrangements for post-treatment recovery.[38]

In terms of social support from friends, families, and support groups, though there are very few GBM- or TGW-specific prostate cancer support groups in this country, some of these patients have been able to identify social support for themselves both during and after the treatment process. Partners, friends, and coworkers are often sources of both emotional support and assistance with tasks such as transportation and grocery shopping while patients are undergoing prostate cancer treatment and recovery.[4] This mechanism is not surprising because GBM and TGW who are open about their sexual orientation or gender identity may be estranged from their families of origin.

In conclusion, the value in studying sexual-minority and transgender populations in prostate cancer care lies in identifying not only how GBM and TGW patients are different from straight cisgender men but also how they are similar. What can straight men learn from GBM and TGW patients in reshaping their sexual activities and identities following prostate cancer treatment? What can GBM and TGW patients learn from straight men about preserving their post-treatment self-esteem and minimizing their treatment regret? To the extent that prostate cancer care for GBM and TGW can not only ensure that the perspectives and experiences of these patients are represented but also help inform QoL for *all* patients with prostate cancer, the closer we will be able to come to a truly integrative model of prostate cancer care that is inclusive of, without being divided by, sexual orientation and gender identity.

ACKNOWLEDGMENTS

The initial development of the model described in this chapter was based on research supported by a grant from the National Cancer Institute (principal investigators, D. Allensworth-Davies and J. Clark, no. 1R03CA136114-01A1). The content of this chapter is solely the responsibility of the authors and does not necessarily represent the official views of the National Cancer Institute or the National Institutes of Health. The authors would also like to thank the gay prostate cancer survivors who agreed to participate in this study.

REFERENCES

1. Allensworth-Davies D, Talcott JA, Heeren T, et al. The health effects of masculine self-esteem following treatment for localized prostate cancer among gay men. *LGBT Health*. 2016; 3 (1): 49–56.

2. Allensworth-Davies D. *Assessing localized prostate cancer post-treatment quality of life outcomes among gay men*. Boston: Boston University School of Public Health; 2012.

3. McNamara M, Ng H. Best practices in LGBT care: A guide for primary care physicians. *Cleveland Clinic Journal of Medicine*. 2016; 83 (7): 531–541.

4. Capistrant BD, Torres B, Merengwa E, et al. Caregiving and social support for

gay and bisexual men with prostate cancer. *Psycho-Oncology.* 2016; 25 (11): 1329–1336.

5. Thomas C, Wootten A, Robinson P. The experiences of gay and bisexual men diagnosed with prostate cancer: Results from an online focus group. *European Journal of Cancer Care.* 2013; 22: 522–529.

6. Institute of Medicine. *The health of lesbian, gay, bisexual and transgender people: Building a foundation for a better understanding.* Washington, D.C.: National Academies Press; 2011.

7. Howlader N, Noone A, Krapcho M, et al. *SEER cancer statistics review (CSR), 1975–2014.* Bethesda: National Cancer Institute; 2017.

8. Blocker DE, Romocki LS, Thomas KB, et al. Knowledge, beliefs and barriers associated with prostate cancer prevention and screening behaviors among African-American men. *Journal of the National Medical Association.* 2006; 98 (8): 1286–1295.

9. Trum HW, Hoebeke P, Gooren LJ. Sex reassignment of transsexual people from a gynecologist's and urologist's perspective. *Acta Obstetricia et Gynecologica Scandinavica.* 2015; 94 (6): 563–567.

10. Miksad RA, Bubley G, Church P, et al. Prostate cancer in a transgender woman 41 years after initiation of feminization. *Journal of the American Medical Assocation (JAMA).* 2006; 296 (19): 2312–2317.

11. Turo R, Jallad S, Cross WR, Prescott S. Metastatic prostate cancer in transsexual diagnosed after three decades of estrogen therapy. *Canadian Urological Association Journal.* 2013; 7 (7–8): 544–546.

12. Lombardi E. Public health and trans-people: Barriers to care and strategies to improve treatment. *In* Meyer IH, Northridge ME, eds. *The Health of Sexual Minorities.* Boston: Springer; 2007: 638–652.

13. National Cancer Institute. Prostate Cancer Treatment. 2016; www.cancer.gov/cancertopics/pdq/treatment/prostate/Patient.

14. Birnie K, Robinson J. Helping patients with localized prostate cancer reach treatment decisions. *Canadian Family Physician.* 2010; 56 (2): 137–141.

15. Mishel MH, Germino BB, Lin L, et al. Managing uncertainty about treatment decision making in early stage prostate cancer: A randomized clinical trial. *Patient Education and Counseling.* 2009; 77 (3): 349–359.

16. Zeliadt S, Ramsey S, Penson D, et al. Why do men choose one treatment over another? A review of patient decision making for localized prostate cancer. *Cancer.* 2006; 106 (9): 1865–1874.

17. Hart TL, Coon DW, Kowalkowski MA, et al. Changes in sexual roles and quality of life for gay men after prostate cancer: Challenges for sexual health providers. *Journal of Sexual Medicine.* 2014; 11 (9): 2308–2317.

18. Blosnich JR. Sexual orientation differences in satisfaction with healthcare: Findings from the Behavioral Risk Factor Surveillance System, 2014. *LGBT Health.* 2017; 4 (3): 227–231.

19. Ussher JM, Perz J, Rose D, et al. Threat of sexual disqualification: The consequences of erectile dysfunction and other sexual changes for gay and bisexual men with prostate cancer. *Archives of Sexual Behavior.* 2017; 46 (7): 2043–2057.

20. Sharif A, Malhotra NR, Acosta AM, et al. The development of prostate adenocarcinoma in a transgender male to female patient: Could estrogen therapy have played a role? *Prostate.* 2017; 77 (8): 824–828.

21. Conron KJ, Mimiaga MJ, Landers SJ. A population-based study of sexual orientation identity and gender differences in adult health. *American Journal of Public Health.* 2010; 100 (10): 1953–1960.

22. Lin Y-H. Treatment decision regret and related factors following radical prostatectomy. *Cancer Nursing.* 2011; 34 (5): 417–422.

23. Davison BJ, So AI, Goldenberg SL. Quality of life, sexual function and decisional regret at 1 year after surgical treatment for localized prostate cancer. *BJU International.* 2007; 100 (4): 780–785.

24. Diefenbach MA, Mohamed NE. Regret of treatment decision and its association with disease-specific quality of life following prostate cancer treatment. *Cancer Investigation.* 2007; 25 (6): 449–457.

25. Diefenbach M, Mohamed NE, Horwitz E, Pollack A. Longitudinal associations among quality of life and its predictors in patients treated for prostate cancer: The moderating role of age. *Psychology, Health & Medicine.* 2008; 13 (2): 146–161.

26. Hu JC, Kwan L, Krupski TL, et al. Determinants of treatment regret in low-income, uninsured men with prostate cancer. *Urology.* 2008; 72 (6): 1274–1279.

27. Rose D, Ussher JM, Perz J. Let's talk about gay sex: Gay and bisexual men's sexual communication with healthcare professionals after prostate cancer. *European Journal of Cancer Care.* 2017; 26 (1).

28. Roesch SC, Adams L, Hines A, et al. Coping with prostate cancer: A meta-analytic review. *Journal of Behavioral Medicine.* 2005; 28 (3): 281–293.

29. Mehnert A, Lehmann C, Graefen M, et al. Depression, anxiety, post-traumatic stress disorder and health-related quality of life and its association with social support in ambulatory prostate cancer patients. *European Journal of Cancer Care.* 2010; 19 (6): 736–745.

30. Blank T, Asencio M, Descartes L, Griggs J. Aging, health, and GLBTQ family and community life. *Journal of GLBT Family Studies.* 2009; 5: 9–34.

31. Fredriksen-Goldsen KI, Kim HJ, Bryan AE, et al. The cascading effects of marginalization and pathways of resilience in attaining good health among LGBT older adults. *Gerontologist.* 2017; 57 (suppl. 1): S72–S83.

32. Rosser BRS, Capistrant BD, Torres B, et al. The effects of radical prostatectomy on gay and bisexual men's sexual functioning and behavior: Qualitative results from the *Restore* study. *Journal of Sex and Relationship Therapy.* 2016; 31 (4): 432–445.

33. Hartman ME, Irvine J, Currie KL, et al. Exploring gay couples' experience with sexual dysfunction after radical prostatectomy: A qualitative study. *Journal of Sex and Marital Therapy.* 2014; 40 (3): 233–253.

34. Torbit LA, Albiani JJ, Crangle CJ, et al. Fear of recurrence: The importance of self-efficacy and satisfaction with care in gay men with prostate cancer. *Psycho-Oncology*. 2015; 24 (6): 691–698.

35. Lee TK, Breau RH, Eapen L. Pilot study on quality of life and sexual function in men-who-have-sex-with-men treated for prostate cancer. *Journal of Sexual Medicine*. 2013; 10 (8): 2094–2100.

36. Lee TK, Handy AB, Kwan W, et al. Impact of prostate cancer treatment on the sexual quality of life for men-who-have-sex-with-men. *Journal of Sexual Medicine*. 2015; 12 (12): 2378–2386.

37. Ussher JM, Perz J, Kellett A, et al. Health-related quality of life, psychological distress, and sexual changes following prostate cancer: A comparison of gay and bisexual men with heterosexual men. *Journal of Sexual Medicine*. 2016; 13 (3): 425–434.

38. Bonvicini KA, Perlin MJ. The same but different: Clinician-patient communication with gay and lesbian patients. *Patient Education and Counseling*. 2003; 51 (2): 115–122.

CHAPTER 15

Malecare

Twenty Years of Innovation and Service to Gay and Bisexual Men and Transgender Women with Prostate Cancer

Darryl Mitteldorf

CHAPTER SUMMARY

This chapter tells the story of the world's leading gay, bisexual, and transgender (GBT) prostate cancer psychosocial support group network, Malecare. Challenged to develop the world's first prostate cancer support group for gay men, a small group of social workers and psychologists developed a set of unique modalities to help GBT people with the psychosocial and sexual stressors associated with prostate cancer diagnosis and treatment. A new nonprofit organization called Malecare was formed to create novel programs, using those new interventions to help underserved men diagnosed with cancer. During the last two decades, Malecare has become a source of medical innovation, healthcare change, and psychosocial understanding for all men diagnosed with cancer throughout the world.

KEY TERMS

bisexual cancer, bisexual health, gay cancer, gay health, LGBT cancer, LGBT health, prostate cancer, psychosocial, support groups, transgender cancer, transgender health

BEGINNINGS

I am a social worker. During the mid-1990s, I was working in European refugee resettlement camps. It was rewarding, sleep-depriving, and honorable work to help torture survivors from lesser-developed countries find their footing in prosperous and safer societies. One day I got

Ussher, Jane M., Perz, Janette, Rosser, B. R. Simon, eds., *Gay & Bisexual Men Living with Prostate Cancer*
dx.doi.org/10.17312/harringtonparkpress/2018.06.gbmlpc.015
© 2018 Harrington Park Press

a letter from my dad saying that he had prostate cancer. Not knowing what that meant and not being able to get him to talk about it on the phone, I dropped everything and returned home. I soon learned that he wasn't going to die anytime soon, but that he did have an advanced stage of his disease and would need extensive help with treatment navigation.

My dad was brilliant at doing things for others, crap at helping himself. I thought he needed other men his own age to talk to about his health. I thought a cancer group might be a good opportunity for him to have some conversation and an outlet for venting. I wanted him to see that he, as well as other men, could continue to live enjoyable and worthy lives with their cancer. Unfortunately, he and I shared a common complaint—we both hate commuting, and the nearest prostate cancer support group was nearly an hour away.

I thought: I'm a social worker, I can start a group. I joined with a national prostate cancer patient organization and started a prostate cancer support group at a local hospital. So in November 1997 my dad and about 30 other men sat in a hospital auditorium while I introduced a urologist to talk about prostate cancer. Then I offered to meet with the men in a smaller group setting after the lecture. Few took me up on the offer. My dad grew weary and stopped attending after the second meeting.

My dad's presentation of self seemed familiar to me because it was similar to that of the refugees I had been helping in the resettlement camps. Like a refugee, he was dealing with a type of adjustment disorder and the stressors that are unique to adults with sudden life changes. For him, and other men, this once-a-month so-called support group that I led was useless. More frequent and reliably scheduled group meetings that engage and provide psychosocial support would be better, in a style similar to what we used in the resettlement camps. Unfortunately, in 1997 there were no cancer survivor support group models that matched what I was looking for. So I developed one.

THE SUPPORT GROUP

We were based in a hospital in lower Manhattan in New York City, so there were many men happy to find a support group that they could easily attend after work. Men, many of whom attended with their wives, would stay for the lecture but leave before we could develop a more open-to-everyone kind of conversation. Also, I noticed that there were several men who seemed much more uncomfortable than others. I wanted to understand why. During the last of our lecture-style meetings,

I gathered four of them and asked. One was notably quite vocal about not feeling comfortable being out in the group. Another said that the only reason he was sticking around to talk with me was because I had brought up anal insertive sex as being different from vaginal insertive sex.

These four men and I sat around talking about prostate cancer from a gay man's perspective. They talked about all sorts of things that were totally outside the heterosexual experience of prostate cancer. Specifically, the men had concerns about sexual identity and integrity relative to androgen deprivation treatment, which is similar to the punishment foisted on gay men in England during the 1940s, 1950s, and 1960s. They mentioned discomfort even in talking about cancer with gay friends when everyone in the New York gay community was focused on HIV/AIDS activism. They worried about the entirety of their sexual identities being disrupted as a consequence of prostate cancer treatment and the unique psychosocial challenges that disruption presents. And they recounted the extraordinary challenges generated by heterosexual presumption by the medical community. Most prevalent of all was their experience of a total lack of recognition of men who have sex with men as a unique psychosocial cohort that was experiencing prostate cancer. Then and there, I understood that what was needed was a group meeting just for men who enjoy sex with men. As we discussed what a support group for gay men with prostate cancer might look like, I remember saying a phrase I think I may have been the first to utter, "gay psychooncology," and seeing a brightness restored to all four men's faces.

By then it was 1998. I sent a letter to the national organization that we were affiliated with, asking if its members knew of any other gay men's groups and requesting that they list our meeting, specifically, as a gay men's group. We didn't expect the reaction we received. There was no discussion; they just kicked us out. Our New York City group was removed from the organization's support group directory, and we no longer received copies of its newsletter. Despite numerous phone calls to the organization's home office and to the president of its board of directors, I never received an explanation.

MALECARE BEGINS

Because I was determined to continue the gay men's prostate cancer support group, I thought it would be essential to have a formal and legal foundation for my work. I started a nonprofit organization called Malecare. I placed flyers in community centers, gay bars, and elsewhere, and I had success in attracting new men to the group. Around late 1999, several social workers and psychologists joined me as volunteers in helping run Malecare. We were all convinced we were onto something unique and thoroughly helpful.

The monthly lecture-and-breakout-group model in use by many cancer support groups other than Malecare quickly proved inadequate for helping gay men diagnosed with prostate cancer. In my view, monthly lectures offered by prostate support groups then and now often offer only a modicum of support and are more like marketing events, not only for doctors and hospitals seeking new patients, but also for pharmaceutical companies that view support groups as vehicles for promoting their products.

A man in need of psychosocial support needs meetings that occur more frequently than once a month. Imagine missing one meeting and having to wait at least another full month until the next. Cancer doesn't afford that much time for waiting. Also, lectures are not support groups. Lectures generally consist of an individual speaker delivering an informative talk for the majority of the scheduled time. The audience sits facing the speaker, rather than each other. Audience members usually get to ask a question and not much else. Lectures rarely afford men the opportunity to share their stories at length or to interact with each other in any depth. A helpful support group is five to fifteen men, sitting around a table, being led in conversation about their cancer by a social worker or psychologist, for 90 minutes. That was the first of several innovative modalities that Malecare would bring to the prostate cancer patient community in the United States.

BECOMING A NATIONAL ORGANIZATION

Around 2001 many people were saying that they read about Malecare on the Internet. Dozens of clinicians around the United States asked if they could copy or affiliate with our work. Many more social workers and psychologists volunteered to build and maintain Malecare. As our groups became more refined, we developed simple protocols that could easily be taught via Skype or phone calls to clinicians outside New York City. For example, one Malecare innovation was to have first-time attendees speak first, starting them off with the request "In 90 seconds or less, tell us why you are here." Obviously, everyone takes more than 90 seconds to share his story and hear comments from the other group members. We found that getting the new guy (or guys) to speak first relieved both individual and group anxiety and more efficiently integrated the new guy into the body of the existing group.

Using this very-simple-to-teach system, Malecare has created a network of in-person, patient-centered psychosocial support groups in the United States and an online support group network that is accessible throughout the world. Our quality maintenance and patient-safety assurance have allowed hospitals and community health centers to be accepting and inviting of our groups. Also, our unique group modality differentiates Malecare as an organization of substance, leadership, and innovation, which gives our local hosts the benefits of association with a well-regarded national brand.

COLLABORATION

On a very cold Saturday afternoon in 2012, I was sitting in a daylong prostate cancer conference in New York City. Several doctors spoke to an audience of 50 or so patients. The conference closed with a talk by David Sandoe, a wonderful man from Australia, who spoke about how he had surgery and, despite impotence, was having a wonderful relationship with his wife. "No worries, mate. . . . When you lose your ejaculate after surgery, there's no more mess." So I guessed that this guy and his wife didn't care about ejaculate. David sat down at a table to enjoy a cup of coffee and I went over to join him, introducing myself as a support group leader, just like himself. Did he understand that it might be difficult for the gay men in the audience to relate to what he was saying? I asked this with constrained arrogance. "Oh, you know, I think you are right," he responded, "but I didn't know that there were any gay men in the audience. I guess it is not quite right for me to have assumed that."

David was a patient member of the Prostate Cancer Foundation of Australia (PCFA). We then began a long conversation, perhaps two hours long, about gay and bisexual men (GBM) and prostate cancer survivorship. From that conversation, Malecare's first major international collaboration was born. Starting in 2013, the PCFA, in partnership with Malecare in the United States, established six gay men's support groups. They also developed booklets covering diagnosis, treatment, side effects, and well-being specifically for GBM.[1] This collaboration has become a model that lent itself to collaborations with similar organizations in the United States, Canada, and the United Kingdom, along with emerging prostate cancer organizations from Iceland to South Africa. Because of these collaborations, Malecare saw the value of creating an alliance of prostate cancer organizations from around the world, to share cross-border treatment opportunities and strategies for inclusion of all men in access to care. The Global Prostate Cancer Alliance was founded by Malecare as a free and open system of communication among like-minded, nonprofit patient-helping organizations.

TRANSGENDER WOMEN

Some time in 2000 I was working part-time as a social worker with a community-based mental health organization. One of my clients was an older transgender woman who had difficulty sleeping because of frequent urination. She had resisted suggestions to see a urologist about prostate cancer, mostly, in her reasoning, because she was not a man and did not see any reason to get tested for "men's things." That she still had a "men's thing," meaning a prostate, crystallized a toxic dynamic faced by many older transgender women (TGW): a struggle to reconcile the realities of anatomy with the truth of their identity and gender.

We worked for half a year together as her symptoms, including lower back pain, got worse and worse. A few months of consultations and tests brought her to a diagnosis and the beginning of treatment for metastatic prostate cancer. Her initial treatment required 40 days of radiation spread over eight weeks. She complied with the treatment but had one nonnegotiable demand: that her treatment be scheduled as the very first appointment of the day, so that she could minimize waiting room contact with men diagnosed with prostate cancer. She was able to seek treatment as long as she could see herself as a woman diagnosed with prostate cancer rather than as a woman diagnosed with a man's cancer. This requirement created an interesting issue for prostate cancer support group attendance. To her, attending a gay men's group was just as toxic as attending a straight man's group.

So Malecare developed what we believe is the first support group for transgender women. Unfortunately, in the year 2000 we could attract only two women to attend the group. An online group failed to develop a critical mass, too. We started to wonder if a broader approach might be more sustainable and equally helpful—a psychosocial support group to which all LGBT cancer survivors would be welcome.

MALECARE AND THE NATIONAL LGBT CANCER PROJECT

We asked our patient community and ourselves what psychosocial commonalities might exist for all lesbian, gay, bisexual, and transgender cancer survivors. After three years of effort, we developed a deep understanding of which stressors and psychosocial challenges could be helped in a well-managed LGBT cancer survivor support group. One of the challenges involved community identity. In 2004 women could readily find lesbian-focused cancer support, and GBM could find quality gay and bisexual support in Malecare. But many men and women felt themselves a part of something larger. We found that the phrases "LGBT cancer survivor" and "LGBT psycho-oncology" resonated deeply and helped restore the dignity of LGBT-identifying cancer survivors. Social workers, psychologists, and oncologists with whom we spoke thought that our ideas about LGBT cancer survivors as a unique cohort were innovative and potentially helpful.

So in 2005 Malecare founded the National LGBT Cancer Project, the world's first nonprofit organization focused on LGBT cancer survivorship. We created online support groups, using the brand Out With Cancer. We helped several community cancer centers across the United States form in-person Out With Cancer groups, using our training for their staff. The National LGBT Cancer Project has been replicated around the world, and we could not be more proud. People will copy good things, and, with rare exception, that is good for everyone.

WORKING WITH PHARMACEUTICAL COMPANIES

Malecare honors pharmaceutical companies that create treatments that save our lives. We believe it is our responsibility to advocate for these same companies' marketing their treatments in equitable and affordable ways, with a no-compromise goal of universal access to healthcare. Several times a year pharmaceutical companies, biologic and genetic test developers, and medical device manufacturers ask heads of patient-focused nonprofits, like Malecare, to review potential marketing materials for consumers.

Almost all the materials I reviewed seemed to target white, middle-class men and their age-appropriate wives. A telling moment for me was the time I handed a pharmaceutical company's marketing person one of Malecare's brochures, which shows a gay couple with their son. The marketing person complimented Malecare on our novel approach, showing a set of "brothers" engaged in prostate cancer awareness. Upon hearing that the image was that of a partnered couple and their son, that same marketing person said, "Is that possible?" Though we were speaking in a major American city around 2003 or 2004, she didn't understand that gay men could raise children.

A marketing person for a major company was clueless about a major segment of her market—which, from Malecare's perspective, meant that a major pharmaceutical company did not have a concern about gay men who use their products, even after two decades of HIV/AIDS awareness. That company simply was not doing market research on our community. Did they not care? Certainly they expected to sell their product to gay men. But pharmaceutical marketing people seem to assume that gay men would be responsive to heterosexually positioned materials because they were so used to seeing such materials.

Malecare identified three issues regarding our mission to make pharmaceutical companies more responsive to our community:

1. To alter the way prostate cancer treatments are marketed so that gay men are included both in imagery and in texts

2. To acknowledge unique stressors for gay men in support materials

3. To improve identification and accrual of gay and bisexual men in clinical trials

We gave ourselves five years, from 2005 to 2010, to achieve tangible results.

As of May 2017, our efforts have had good outcomes with some companies, and disappointing or null results with others. For the latter group of companies, gay and bisexual men continue to be irrelevant. All those companies' prostate cancer marketing materials are purely heterocentric, and they do absolutely no outreach to the GBM community or even offer support to our work, as they do to all other prostate cancer organizations. We suggest that patients test out all prostate cancer websites with a simple search for the term *gay*.

RESEARCH

Early on, we saw the need to innovate and lead a marketing effort for more research regarding GBM and TGW with prostate cancer. We did not have a clue what disparities, if any, might exist, but we knew it was important to find out. And our support group attendees wanted to know, too. Many men entered our groups, happy for the comradeship and ease of conversation, but confused about whether there was something about being gay that might make prostate cancer a truly different experience.

Because we were being asked to help accrue patients for clinical trials, it was an easy proposition to demand that the trials include demographic questions about gender, sexual identity, and type of relationship a participant was involved in. Remarkably, we were refused at every turn. Not one clinical trial manager empathized with our requests. In fact, almost all were quite adamant that the differentiation would prove irrelevant. Most toxic was the fact that many of the researchers voiced homophobic concerns that the mere inclusion of a question regarding sexual identity would dissuade further participation in their research study. Researchers thought they were in safe territory in ignoring Malecare, as long as we focused only on gay men.

So, to fight back, some time around 2003 I changed our mission goal to say that Malecare is working to become the world's leading non-profit organization for men's cancer survivorship. We needed authority and muscle power. The authority would come from our own self-funded research, and the muscle would come from size.

We were determined to become large in numbers of group attendees. To do that, we began to develop additional support groups that would be inclusive of men of all sexual identities. Malecare was and still is one of the very few organizations to conduct weekly 90-minute, sit-around-a-table-and-share group meetings. We found a niche ready to fill. And fill it we did, very quickly building our census to nearly three times the size of the next-largest competing nonprofit. We were also the first large nonprofit organization to identify men with advanced-stage prostate cancer as a cohort with unique psychosocial and treatment issues. Our advanced-stage support groups increased our size by an additional third.

Starting around 2008, Malecare had a massive database of patients, all eager to share their thoughts and experiences with the hope of improving treatment outcomes. Researchers were knocking at our door several times a month. But, getting GBM and TGW investigative criteria inserted into survey and clinical research remained a huge challenge. Researchers who agreed to work with Malecare under our terms saw their subject accrual completed in short order. Researchers also said that they found valuable insights from Malecare's group leadership and our deep understanding of the psychosocial issues of our group attendees.

We thought we were making progress, but between 2009 and 2012 an interesting problem emerged. As Malecare patients saw the papers that were produced from those early studies, they stopped participating in research. From focus groups of our group attendees we learned that our men were angry that Malecare was not mentioned as a partner in almost all the papers. They felt that if Malecare was not mentioned, then they as individual patients were not credited or acknowledged. It was a surprise to me and our staff that these men were participating not only to improve treatments, but also to build awareness of support groups in and of themselves. And they were right to feel that way.

These men wanted other men to find the same helpful value in Malecare groups that they had found, and they simply were not going to participate in anything that would not further that goal. Our staff and I decided that Malecare would participate only in research in which we felt we could provide significant input into all aspects of the particular investigation. We sought to have one or more of our staff as co-investigators and to ensure that our contributions would constitute more than subject accrual assistance. Malecare is a ready and able community partner to all researchers who respect our organization collegially, and we can now demonstrate through numerous published papers and high-level grant awards that our inclusion benefits everyone.

INNOVATION AND THE FUTURE

Malecare is now positioned as one of the world's leading prostate cancer patient organizations. During the last 20 years, we've learned that partnerships and collaborations are the fastest and most equitable and sustainable method of spreading our work around the world. From our Global Prostate Cancer Alliance we've learned that engagement of international prostate cancer coalition stakeholders and organizations from many disciplines, from consumer to doctor, advocate to minister of health, nurse to researcher, helps facilitate program implementation. Malecare works with nonprofit organizations that are already working within local communities. We offer training and support materials to these organizations and help with marketing and promotion. We stay connected with these local nonprofits in keeping with our theme of "treating locally, connecting globally." In this way prostate cancer patients from communities of all sizes and locations share information and support, across borders and without fear.

Our strong suit is collaborating in innovative programming and promoting new thinking about prostate cancer. In 2011 we began a research program called Start a Cure, which has led to several peer-reviewed papers, abstracts, posters, one patent, and one patent pending.*

Our online support group network is one of the largest in the world. And our technical innovations, such as Cancergraph (a clinical trial, accrual, mobile app system, and patient side-effect recording device), help thousands.

Twenty years ago, Malecare played a key role in initiating the field of gay psycho-oncology and LGBT psycho-oncology, which are now respected fields of research in which brilliant investigators develop new modalities to help patients. For the next 20 years, Malecare will continue to find ways to increase access to healthcare and to advocate for prostate cancer treatments that are effective, affordable, and morbidity-free. The spine of our mission remains the same as when we started: to reduce fear and ease adjustment to the diagnosis and to restore dignity and happiness to all men diagnosed with prostate cancer and, with our research program and CancerGraph, to survivors of all cancer types.

REFERENCE

1. Prostate Cancer Foundation of Australia. Prostate cancer pack: Information for gay and bisexual men. 2014; www.prostate.org.au/awareness/for-recently-diagnosed-men-and-their-families/gay-and-bisexual-men/download-information/.

* U.S. Patent no. 9,168,002, October 27, 2015: A device and method for real-time simultaneous measurement of radiation at specific parts of the body. Understanding cumulative radiation exposure in people undergoing ionizing radiation for diagnostics and medical treatment is essential in reducing secondary tumors from primary radiation therapy. U.S. Provisional Patent Application no. 62/370,092, September 7, 2016: Mobile health-monitoring Cancergraph, a symptom and side-effect recording and reporting mobile app, patent pending.

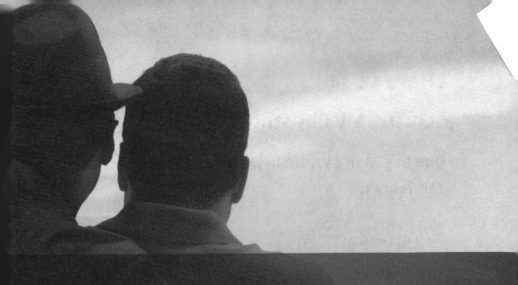

SECTION THREE

PERSONAL EXPERIENCES

CHAPTER 16

"Losing My Chestnut"

One Gay Man's Wrangle with Prostate Cancer — Ten Years On

Gary W. Dowsett

CHAPTER SUMMARY

This chapter documents my personal encounter with a prostate cancer diagnosis and initial treatment ten years ago. Such personal accounts can offer insight into health issues and concerns otherwise unrecognized in healthcare, along with the particular kinds of science and research that underpin them. Such accounts have been used extensively in health research and politics, particularly when affected communities have a stake and a need to right some wrong. I wrote this article with that aim in mind. It was written in 2008 at the request of the editor of the journal *Reproductive Health Matters,* Marge Berer, to contribute to a set of testimonials on cancer experiences for an issue of the journal focused on reproductive cancers.[1] For this version, I have updated aspects to reflect changes in the prostate cancer field and added a short afterword, "Ten Years On."

KEY TERMS

cancer treatment, gay men, prostate cancer, sexual dysfunction, sexuality

Ussher, Jane M., Perz, Janette, Rosser, B. R. Simon, eds., *Gay & Bisexual Men Living with Prostate Cancer*
dx.doi.org/10.17312/harringtonparkpress/2018.06.gbmlpc.016
© 2018 Harrington Park Press

INTRODUCTION

I am a sexuality activist, researcher, and theorist with 40 years of experience working, thinking, writing, and debating in sexuality and gender politics, and nearly 35 years of working in HIV/AIDS. I can talk about sex underwater! For me, like everyone else, the first time—losing my cherry—was an important moment marking a new phase of my life, and I have talked with amusement about that moment with friends and in my work. I want to tell another tale here, one about losing my chestnut this time.

Cancer. That was the word I dreaded but had been anticipating as a diagnosis for nearly a decade. Prostate cancer is the most common cancer in men after lung cancer and, it seems, growing in prevalence to equal breast cancer in many resource-rich and developed countries. Indeed, there are approximately 12,000 new diagnoses in Australia each year (almost a quarter of a million in the United States). It comes at you in scales, scores, and stages, with actuarial tables on ages, survival rates over time—it is definitely "men's business" and is handled in a matter-of-fact, man-to-man way. There is not much room for emotion in the urologist's office. Diagrams of your "chestnut" (it looks a bit like one in the drawings) with its little wings (seminal vesicles) make it look like a logo for international airmail, but it is held to earth by a kite string–like urethra. You can live without it, but how well you live is the next question after how long.

In 2007 I was diagnosed with prostate cancer. I also received the recommended action—in my case, a radical prostatectomy, complete removal of my chestnut—and a sketch of the prospects for a future life. Then, with a manly shake of hands, I found myself on the street heading somewhere, home, work, a bar, with a cloud dulling my senses and numbing my heart. At least for a while. A decade before, I had had an infection in the prostate. How did I know? Some blood in my semen. How did I see that? As a gay man with a reasonably active sex life, I knew about safe sex. "Cum on me, not in me" was a key slogan used in gay men's HIV prevention for years. Need I say more? My general practitioner (GP—i.e., internist, family physician) ordered a prostate-specific antigen (PSA) test—the major diagnostic tool for assessing prostatic problems—and did the usual direct (or digital) rectal examination (DRE). The DRE revealed a somewhat enlarged prostate, but for my age (heading toward my late forties then) this was not entirely unusual. But the surface of the prostate he felt was smooth—no bumps—a good sign, as bumps indicate a possibly cancerous growth starting to press against the outside capsule that contains the prostate. The PSA test result came back a "six," considered a bit high for my age and possibly indicating some problem, but not necessarily cancer. Elevated PSA scores occur with a range of prostatic conditions, including the enlarging that comes with aging.

Off to the urologist—the men (mainly) who "own" prostates. A further PSA test, another DRE, and a urine-flow test led to a decision to undertake a biopsy. This so-called simple day procedure under a general anesthetic left me peeing blood for a month. The blood should not have taken that long to clear. As with every new procedure and the associated tests, I looked for the good news. There was no sign of cancer. An infection of the prostate was diagnosed and a quite long course of antibiotics prescribed. Duly healed. But I kept watch, asking for a PSA test and DRE annually from my GP, and neither showed any changes for nearly eight years. There were a few more moments with blood in semen, but my GP (at a gay men's health practice) concluded that these were not of concern because of the steady PSA scores, which remained at six for all that time.

Then, at the end of 2006, as part of my annual check-up, the PSA test returned a score of eight. It is such jumps in scores that are more worrying than slow elevation, and it was off to the urologist again—a new one, younger, in a specialist urology clinic attached to one of the better private hospitals in Melbourne, Australia, where I live. Another DRE (no bumps) and a PSA test (it had dropped to seven) were good signs, it seemed. It could have been another infection that fed the PSA blip, given the steady sixes over the years, but with the elapsed time since the last biopsy, the urologist advised that I have another one, as a PSA score of seven was high for my age (55). I put it off for a while because of overseas travel for work, and I finally underwent the procedure in April 2007, fully expecting (hoping for) anything other than cancer.

It was cancer. The word I dreaded.

The options were canvassed, and a radical prostatectomy was recommended because of my scores and age—young for this, although diagnoses are increasingly made at younger ages as PSA testing becomes frequently used as a screening test (even if not officially recommended as such), and more men become aware of prostate problems through public health education and are seeking advice earlier. The prognosis for full recovery and survival after a prostatectomy is getting better. There was then an 85% chance of remaining cancer-free at ten years; it is now 98%. However, this simple figure hides a multitude of ifs and buts that one finds out about later. I sought a second opinion. Same diagnosis, same recommendation, same prognosis; no choice really if I wanted to live at least longer than if I did nothing. Now, being a kind of nerdy, intellectual type with all the resources that a university academic has at his disposal, I hit the Internet and the databases for everything I could find. Well, there is a lot of medical science out there, many big outfits at work, and there are considerable differences of opinion on the increasing use of prostatectomy and at younger ages, and quite a deal of health education advice, chatty little booklets and websites. I learned I faced a range of odds, depending on how big the cancer was, its stage (there are four of them with various subtypes and descriptors, indicating whether it is contained or has metastasized; the biopsy cannot reveal everything), and what the eventual Gleason score was. I was told my Gleason score of seven (intermediate level concern) comprised 80% three and 20% four in the postsurgery pathology tests, but the seven itself on biopsy was a concern. Today a score of seven, like mine (three plus four), would be considered a possible candidate for active surveillance rather than immediate treatment; a seven of four plus three score would most likely warrant treatment. This is now; that was then.

Also, there was a range of probable side effects to consider. A prostatectomy is no simple fix. The surgery could have left me with a urinary continence problem that might dog me for the rest of my life and with unpredictable sexual dysfunction. There is unavoidable temporary and permanent nerve damage to this nerve-dense part of the abdomen. The second opinion also revealed that I would never ejaculate again no matter what else did or did not occur, and that was a real blow, for it signaled symbolically more than anything else that sexual pleasure would never be the same again. It was also a fact notably absent from much of the health literature on prostate cancer, which is surprisingly coy when it comes to the sexual side effects of treatment. The reproductive health side effects for men young enough and with an interest in having children are also rarely mentioned, as prostate cancer is assumed largely to be an older man's disease. Sexual and reproductive health in this game is equated mostly with erectile function.

It is all a bit heterosexist too. All the brochures I was given by helpful nurse counselors never mentioned gay men with prostate cancer. One from the Queensland Cancer Council buried toward the back a small photo of two men, but the word "gay" was not mentioned anywhere. When questioned by a colleague about this, the reply was that the Council never mentions the sex of the partner in the text, so it is gender nonspecific. Any gay man can tell you how specific that actually is by the way sexual relations and activities are rendered in the text itself; just using "partner" does not render any text nonheterosexist. No mention is made of gay men who might also be HIV-positive, or where a gay male couple might both have the disease. And, of course, there is no mention of gay sex. There was one reference at the back of the booklet, which at that time was the only book on gay men and prostate cancer in the world.[2] I ordered it immediately. It was quite useful, if not very rigorous or helpful on the latest developments. Its testimonials from men recovering from various treatments were cautionary and did not invite great optimism for a future life, fully recovered. But my growing recognition was that there is no full recovery from this even if the cancer was successfully removed.

I had a month to wait until a vacancy came up on my surgeon's list. It was to happen at the private hospital where his clinic was based. My private health insurance would add to the funding available from Australia's national health system, Medicare; but I would face not insignificant out-of-pocket copayment costs, a result of the messy hybrid national health system we have in this country. During that month, I organized my work, letting my staff know and making contingency plans for research projects.

Family, friends, and colleagues rallied round wonderfully. My natal family all live in other states, but offered support and were always on the end of a phone if I needed them. My "sewing circle" of gay friends rostered themselves for support, transport, company, visits. Who says there is not gay family! Being (then) single and unpartnered, this sharing of the burden of care and support in so many ways was both a surprise (was I actually deserving of this?) and hard to take for someone who has always been fiercely independent and self-reliant. I also sought the services of a counselor before and for three months after the surgery, as I had realized that the (inevitable) mental health side effects were not deemed something warranting postoperative medical care.

The surgery went according to plan. I was offered only an "open" prostatectomy. Even though laparoscopic and robotic techniques were used at the time, they were not widely available, and many of the current advances in radiation therapy were only on the horizon. In fact, the whole thing was like a fully scripted play: four days in hospital, ten further days at home with a catheter to manage, its withdrawal, then continence management, recovery over time, and back to work in two months or thereabouts. It all sounded fairly straightforward. Very fearful about the surgery and the outcome, I headed off to hospital at 6:30 A.M. Undressing in my hospital room, and after a quick good-bye to a friend who accompanied me that far, I was taken down to the theater, then a quick word with the anesthetist, a needle in the arm, and "bingo," I woke up three or four hours later with no diseased chestnut.

What I did have was pain. I was flat on my back with a self-managed morphine drip in one arm (I had had hopes that this bit might be a bigger buzz than it was), a tube draining my abdomen, all heading left of the bed, the catheter heading right. My legs were encased in gorgeous white pressure stockings ("they will come in useful for long distance flying afterwards," said the nurse—I was incredulous!). I was basically pinned there like that for two days, woken *every* hour for blood pressure and pulse tests, gratefully receiving backwashes from the night nurse, and definitely not at all hungry but very thirsty. I was sweating all the time and it was the middle of our winter outside. Finally, the pain relief was authorized by the surgeon and things slowly progressed along their preordained path.

This was nursing by numbers: the timing and procedures organized around shifts and the daily processes of hospital life. Day three saw me sitting in a chair for a while. Then, it was out with the drain—look the other way and think of England. The portable catheter bag was fitted. Walking up and down the corridor regularly was recommended and duly practiced. Showering with the bloody catheter and its bloody bag was choreographed and duly practiced; and before I knew it, it was time to go home. Surely not. I barely had even begun to recover, had had no sleep for days, and was still in some pain. But this is modern medicine; it is all done by the book.

Going home was a blessed moment. No one checked to see if I had anyone at home to support me . . . umm. I had, but they did not even ask. Two dear friends, a retired gay couple, actually came to nurse me for a month after the surgery—that was a remarkable gift. They were relieved occasionally by my gay family in shifts. Being at home became an obsession with process as well, managing the catheter (an endless chore), showering and dressing, eating, undressing, resting, walking, talking about process—all pursued with stoic determination to do as much as I could myself, even with my friends there caring for me. One's world becomes so small, framed by the confines of one's dwelling and focused on the minutiae of domesticity.

I read Nelson Mandela's autobiography to remind myself that things were not as bad as I sometimes thought—he had had prostate surgery too. We had a daily reading from *Pollyanna* (so gay!) over morning tea. Eating became the central driver of a timetabled day—no wonder older people find themselves eating dinner at 5 P.M. Sleeping was the worst part. I had to sleep on my back for ten days until the catheter was removed. I sweated bucketsful every night. No one told me to expect that. My bedding was soaked every few hours, and it was not from a leaking catheter. I lost almost 10% of my body weight within a fortnight of the surgery. My ribs were individually observable and palpable, and my butt—never callipygian at its best—disappeared. An angry red scar running from navel to pubis testified to what I had gone and was going through.

An unexpected call from the surgeon, reporting that the pathology test on the prostate revealed there was no evidence of cancer cells in the seminal vesicles or positive surgical margins, was greeted with an instant flood of tears. I had not realized that my stoicism floated on a volatile emotional sea—something I was going to have to come to grips with as time wore on and a part of living through this experience that was never mentioned in the educational material, by the nurse counselors, or ever spoken of by the medics. This is a man's disease and you take it like a man.

For those so minded, not only was my Gleason score a seven, as explained earlier, but also my cancer stage could be described on the tumor-nodes-metastasis (TNM) system as "T1c"—the cancer cannot be felt during a rectal exam, but is discovered in biopsy after an elevated serum PSA level; "N0"—prostate cancer has not spread to lymph nodes; and "M0"—there is no evidence of distant spread or metastases from prostate cancer. These results, with the PSA score of seven before surgery, my age, and a skilled surgeon, had put me on the best footing I could be on to start this next stage of my life.

The day the catheter was removed marked another milestone: seconds before its removal, the nurse reverse-filled my bladder with saline, whipped out the catheter, and, issuing a stern "hold it," had me walk a few paces to the toilet before releasing. I did all that and she calmly said,

"Good, you won't be incontinent." Big news comes in laconic remarks. She handed me a complimentary pack of Depend "guards for men" and sent me on my way with blessed relief. This, however, soon gave way to the logistics of battling incontinence over the following weeks, with unreliable if improving bladder control, endless pelvic floor (Kegel) exercises, nerve-racking uncertainty during my first visits to a restaurant and to a concert, and learning to live without the extra control a prostate contributes to the bladder. I had to reread my body; its sensations were unreliable (possibly because of the nerve damage during surgery) and its messaging just was not working as I understood it—when I thought I was peeing I wasn't; when I thought I was dry, I suddenly wet myself. I was at times furious and quite desperate about it. At other times, I just laughed like a child. Clearly, the nerve damage was not all permanent; things improved fast, the odd accident notwithstanding, and Depend and I soon parted company, although for years I traveled with one in my briefcase. Not sure why, really.

As for sexual dysfunction—what am I prepared to share with you, dear reader? Sexual dysfunction is almost entirely configured as erectile dysfunction in prostate cancer: Can you get an erection, how firm is it, will it stay up, for how long? Sexuality as I understand it—comprising the whole shopping list from interest to arousal, to pleasure and pleasuring, to intimacy and orgasm, to discourse and meaning-making—does not feature in the world of prostate cancer. My surgeon, a youngish bloke and pretty good at his job, promised we would start discussing sex at the six-week mark. When I reminded him of that, he instantly reached for the prescription pad and wrote a script for Viagra. Whoa, I thought; that was not what I was talking about. I had read in the brochures about erectile dysfunction and I knew that recovery of function was a very variable business. I had been posting and discussing this issue already in a "gay men and prostate cancer" Yahoo group, and there was a lively exchange going on about recovery of function and sexual pleasures, including new ones, and quite a deal of humor (and loss) in these postings. It was never going to be smooth sailing, that I knew; but I thought we would be talking about sexuality, not just about getting a "woody." I know about "woodies"; they are my personal and professional stock in trade. Living though cancer makes the professional personal.

Anyway, at this stage, I had already had the odd orgasm (some quite odd, given the nerve damage, and at first without any hint of an erection), and was coming to grips with orgasming without ejaculation—I will forever miss that. My surgeon declared I was certainly "ahead of the pack"—the story of my life! While the average age for prostate cancer surgery is now 59, the disease is more often thought of as an older man's issue. Being a bit younger than the average at the time, I certainly hoped I'd have a better than average recovery. It is also a tribute to my surgeon's skill that I had even this level of function at that stage, and it would be churlish not to acknowledge that. But a presurgery conversation about the always improving nerve-sparing techniques designed to save sexual function had not been encouraging. He suggested that for a young (for this disease), sexually active man like me, they take great care to do the least damage possible to the nerve bundles surrounding the prostate, but added: were I a 70-plus sexually non-active man . . . he drew a square with his index fingers in mid-air then chucked it over his shoulder. My heart sank for those 70-plus men who may no longer be sexually active with partners, but for whom the guilty pleasure of erections and masturbation was a silent secret now, lost forever to assumptions about age and pleasure. This was another moment when you realize how poorly men and our sexuality are thought about in medicine and health.

Back to my sex life . . . for I was/am determined to have one. All the pamphlets assume that the issue is about getting an erection for penetrative purposes, and that there is a willing little woman waiting there, legs apart, happy to let you practice for however long it takes to make it function again. No discussion of pleasure, intimacy, loss, desire, reciprocity, relationality or, indeed, alternatives to intercourse. I reminded my surgeon that I was a gay man, with fairly versatile sexual interests, and wondered also when it might be safe or wise to recommence anal intercourse (from both angles). Well, after a long technical digression on the distance between the prostate (or where it once was) and the anus—something I am actually very familiar with—I had received no answer. Journeys home from medical consultations are sometimes longer than the car ride. I went back to the Yahoo group for some good advice. Where I will get to on regaining sexual function is a tad unknowable, it seems, and somewhat unpredictable. As the nerves continue to heal slowly, it is really a case of practice, patience, and persistence. But I have been assured again that I am well "ahead of the pack."

There are other moments but not enough space here to tell them all. An ill-advised attendance at the Australian National Prostate Cancer Conference a few months after returning to work left me angry at the neglect of gay men, our partners, and concerns entirely from the research agenda and the programmatic response. The positioning of men as prostate cancer "patients" and "consumers" [sic] is light years behind HIV/AIDS, where people living with HIV are worked with, not just on. The social science and public health prostate cancer research agenda is nowhere as well developed as it is for breast cancer. The understanding of men's sexuality that underpins the field is also at best rudimentary; it is as if 40 years of feminist and queer theory and activism have somehow passed urology by unnoticed.

To all intents and purposes, my life went back to normal over the following two or three years—well, that is how it appeared to the doctor, my colleagues, and even myself in those hours when my mind was on what I was doing. Not so. There is before and after. There were moments of dark uncertainty and quiet despair for quite a long time. There was a private part of me that no one reached. Sometimes, I doubted a future; other times, I saw only a truncated one—would the cancer recur, when? There was (and is) the mirror to remind me of a body forever changed inside and out. There has been an endless "coming-out" process (right here, right now, again) as a cancer "survivor"—I have been coming out as a gay man all my life, but this is different. Pursuing a sexual life was complicated—one guy just gawked and said: "Oh, my God, what did they take out?" Just call me "Alien"! There was (and is still) anger and loss to deal with. Am I stronger for the experience, have I matured through the hardship, have I become a better person, do I deal with life one day at a time, and reevaluate what really counts in life, counting my blessings as a result? Maybe, but fuck that! I just want my chestnut back!

AFTERWORD: TEN YEARS ON

It has now been ten years almost to the day as I updated the text above and now write this afterword. I am grateful to the editors for the opportunity to say more about my experience of living with prostate cancer as a gay man.

Perhaps the most important thing to say is that I am still here ten years on!

Survival rates for men living with prostate cancer are improving very fast. I won't say if you are going to have cancer that this is the one to have, because the very existence of such high five-year and ten-year survival rates in the medical literature indicates that some men do not live as long as I have. Recurrence and fear of recurrence are constant companions for many who have experienced cancer, and these produce an underlying level of daily stress that never recedes. It is stimulated by annual PSA tests, keeping an askance watch on cancer cell movements. Other regular reminders are friends informing me they too have been diagnosed — probably eight over the last ten years — and seeking advice on what to do next. I have even been asked to talk with the occasional unknown friend of a friend or relative who has learned that he has prostate cancer. This is partly because I now work in the field myself and am considered to have some expertise and experience.

Am I a prostate cancer "survivor"? I really dislike the term. I regard myself as a man "living with prostate cancer," though the medics might regard me as "cured." Even if I am lucky enough never to experience cancer recurrence, I live in some fear of that possibility. Daily, I live with the consequences of treatment, particularly whenever I see my scarred naked body. When I have sex, not ejaculating is a constant reminder. It is part of my academic research work. Other men like me become support group leaders, lobby for funding in research, become ambassadors and peer educators to raise prostate cancer awareness. For me, this is being a man living with prostate cancer.

Ten years on my prostate health is fine, as far as I know. My PSA has remained very low. One brief scary increase in my PSA score, but not anywhere near high enough to warrant any intervention, soon receded. No one knows why. There is something liminal (i.e., being permanently on a threshold of something) about living with prostate cancer; I am always "looking over my shoulder," just in case. My general health now at age 65 is a bit less than optimal: some arthritis, high-ish cholesterol, and I'm less fit than I should be (whatever that means) and certainly not as energetic as I once was. I plan to retire soon, in part to ensure I have a retirement of a reasonable length . . . just in case.

Almost immediately after my treatment, I began to research prostate cancer in gay men. A pilot study allowed me to start investigating whether other gay men had similar experiences of being inadequately handled by the prostate cancer field. I confirmed that my experience was certainly not unique. There was at that time the small beginnings of a now-growing body of work that revealed how poorly gay men living with prostate cancer are understood, diagnosed, treated, and supported. That small beginning led to a number of research grants and collaborations. Suffice it to say, there is now an appreciable subfield in prostate cancer research on gay and bisexual men, and I am very pleased to have made my own small contribution to it.

That work has been part of my way of living with prostate cancer. I am certainly not the first academic to make his life his work; but for me more was a stake. After 35 years of working in HIV/AIDS research and being a gay activist for even longer, I could not abide the ignorance and neglect of gay men's needs in the prostate cancer field. I could not believe the fundamental ignorance of human sexuality that underpinned the medical and psychosocial literature on prostate cancer for gay men, but really for all men. It felt like a sexual dark age had somehow escaped the enlightenment of 40 years of second-wave feminism and gay liberation (including LGBT politics and queer theory), and all we have learned globally about human sexuality in 35 years from HIV/AIDS. Things are changing in this regard in the prostate cancer field, slowly and inexorably. I want to be sure that it will be better for those who follow me. That is another way I live with prostate cancer.

Just over five years ago, in what still seems a miraculous blessing to me after fifteen years of unpartnered life, I met my current partner. That change has made an enormous difference to my life. Beyond the shared joys of love, there are mutual pleasures and companionship in daily life, travel, food and wine, entertaining friends, cultural and artistic events, hobbies, and so on. We are both academics, and many of the uncertainties and exigencies of university life in Australia today are also a shared "pleasure." So is our sexual life together. This is actually quite different from what I hinted at above. Then, I pursued and negotiated casual sexual encounters as a context for rebuilding a sexual life after my treatment. I was quite lucky in meeting a number of very understanding partners during that time. In my now very active and partnered sex life, what can I tell you, dear reader? Well, that's kind of private. I will say that nothing works like it did before prostate cancer; it is a constant task to work at it in the here and now, and sexual success has to be constantly redefined and reimagined. There are great pleasures to be enjoyed, and moments of disappointment. My partner is a wonderful, understanding, and very sexy man. I never gave up on pursuing a satisfying sex life, and I've been richly rewarded for those efforts.

Today, I am still a gay man living with prostate cancer as I daily engage with it, interrogate it, seek to change it, and live with its uncertainties, its ever-present consequences, and its discursive terrors. Do I miss my chestnut? Absolutely. Have I learned to live without it? Yes, it hasn't been easy, but the answer is still yes. Do I want it back? Of course! I hope they 3D-print one soon . . . as long as it works!

ACKNOWLEDGMENT
This chapter is reproduced with the kind permission of *Reproductive Health Matters*, the journal in which it was originally published.

REFERENCES
1. Dowsett GW. "Losing my chestnut": One gay man's wrangle with prostate cancer. *Reproductive Health Matters*. 2008; 16 (32): 145–150.
2. Perlman G, Drescher J, eds. *A gay man's guide to prostate cancer*. Binghamton, N.Y.: Haworth Medical Press; 2005.

CHAPTER 17

What about Me?

Ross Henderson

CHAPTER SUMMARY

This is my personal account of having been diagnosed with prostate cancer (PC) at the age of 46. As a young man I was unaware of the physical, emotional, and psychological effects that accompany such a diagnosis as well as the ramifications of radical prostatectomy. This chapter follows my journey, through the highs and lows of the experience, with particular focus on my involvement in the formation of the gay and bisexual men's PC support group Shine a Light. I also aim to share information with those people receiving a PC diagnosis in the hopes of making their journey with the disease a little easier and more comfortable.

KEY TERMS

cancer diagnosis, case study, gay man, prostate cancer, recovery, sexuality, treatment

When I turned 45, I felt I had reached a significant milestone in my life called middle age. I was well in myself, single, and free, with a good job, a great family, and marvelous friends. I had come out as gay when I was 37—late in life, for a whole variety of reasons—and was now enjoying my newfound freedom as a sexual man. I was finally integrated in a holistic sense.

At 46 years of age, I decided to have the checkup that I had been postponing for the last twelve months. My general practitioner (GP) is a gay man in his sixties, with a great sense of humor; he is skilled and knowledgeable, very caring, careful, and wise, and he always took time to understand me. I love him; he is a marvelous man and a brilliant doctor. Cholesterol, STIs, HIV status, blood pressure, blood sugars were all tested. My GP had also been testing me since I was about 40 for

Ussher, Jane M., Perz, Janette, Rosser, B. R. Simon, eds., *Gay & Bisexual Men Living with Prostate Cancer*
dx.doi.org/10.17312/harringtonparkpress/2018.06.gbmlpc.017
© 2018 Harrington Park Press

prostate cancer. The more common age for testing is 50 (unless there is a history of the disease in the family). The dreaded DRE (digital rectal examination), while unpleasant, takes only a minute, and what's a minute of discomfort when it can prevent a serious illness? It was all just a matter of course. I would be out of there as soon as possible and on my way to the gym, good health, and well-being. I didn't realize then that this day would change my life forever, especially hearing my doctor's slightly concerned voice informing me about my enlarged prostate.

"Probably nothing to worry about," he said, "but worth obtaining a PSA reading." It could have been any one of a number of things, but because of my young age, prostate cancer was considered highly unlikely. A PSA test? Upon inquiry, I was told it was a test that measures the level of prostate-specific antigen (PSA) in the blood, and it can help diagnose prostate disease. I felt embarrassed that I didn't even know what it was.

Arriving home, I started thinking about the PSA result. It was probably nothing to worry about, and my understanding was that prostate cancer affects mostly men in their sixties, seventies, and upwards. There was no history of prostate cancer in my family, although my biological father died at the age of 23, and both my grandfathers had died in their early fifties, so I guess we didn't really know all the facts from either side of the family. When I arrived home, I rang my good friend Chris. He'd researched an enlarged prostate on Google and learned that it could be attributed to many things other than cancer. What a relief! I could stop worrying.

Still, I was distracted all week, both at home and at work. I spoke to my dear friend Mirna at work one afternoon; she is also a counselor. I told her of my test and my alarm at what the results might indicate. It wasn't until many months later that she told me that I had appeared different that day and that, despite her reassurances, it seemed that somewhere deep inside of me I had already guessed that I had cancer. She had heard it in my voice. I already knew.

I had to go back to my GP a week later to obtain the results of my blood tests. My GP ushered me into his office, gave me all the blood results (which were all excellent), leaving the PSA until the very end. It was 5.9. He mentioned again that, while there was probably nothing to worry about, it would be advisable to see a urologist and seek his professional opinion. He knew I was anxious—he could see it, hear it in my voice.

I immediately made an appointment with a highly recommended urologist for a few days later. He was a serious man; it went with the territory. He performed another DRE. More unpleasantness. His voice showed some concern; there was a rough patch on the surface of the prostate. A high-ish PSA, an enlarged prostate, and a rough surface—three things not in my favor. I felt sick. The doctor suggested another PSA test, as well as a biopsy, which was scheduled for early in December. This was to be day surgery. The doctor said that it was a simple procedure, no pain, but there would be some interference to the prostate and this would cause my semen to become bloodied and that I would ejaculate what looked like dark brown diesel oil. The day of my biopsy came and went smoothly.

It was Sunday night, December 6, 2009. I drank a couple of glasses of red wine, mindlessly watched television, and contemplated the next day, when I would probably receive my biopsy results. The phone suddenly rang. It was about 8:30 P.M. It was my urologist.

His voice was clear and serious. There had been thirty cores taken, and only one core had been positive for cancer—a very small tumor right in the center of the prostate. "Will I die?" I asked, matter-of-factly. "No," the answer came back quickly and firmly. "We have caught it early, it's very small, and it's right in the middle, not towards the outer shell of the prostate—which is good news." I couldn't think properly. He relayed some of the facts and statistics to me. I found it hard to concentrate, maybe because of my anxiety or the wine or a combination of both. He wanted to see me at the end of the week to discus things further.

The few days after receiving the news, I felt surprisingly good. The cancer was treatable and beatable. They could cut it out of my prostate and I would return to good health. Nothing will have changed—just a small hiccup in the bigger scheme of things.

My doctor's appointment was late at night. My dear stepdad came with me. I had been told that it is always useful to take someone with you as an extra pair of ears and an attitude of greater objectivity. He was the perfect person to accompany me. He is very methodical, sensible, and smart, and he listens attentively. Together we had prepared a series of questions that we needed to ask—what my treatment options were being the first.

The hospital floor was in darkness except for one small light at the end of the corridor. It looked so gloomy and ominous. The doctor welcomed us in. My stepfather and I sat down and listened to the barrage of options that lay before me and all the associated facts and data that come with a diagnosis of prostate cancer—radiotherapy, brachytherapy, surgery, prostatectomy, the Da Vinci robot, PSA scores, Gleason scores, American results, Australian results, figures, data, impotence, incontinence. Facts, facts, and more facts. The good news was that he felt he could get rid of the cancer (the number-one concern!), but the bad news was that there were side effects with each of the various approaches.

After surgery, for example, there would be no semen or ejaculate present, the seminal vesicles would be removed along with the prostate, and there could be a 50% chance of impotence and a small chance of incontinence. I was told I would still be able to have an orgasm, though. *Huh? That didn't make sense!* There was so much my head was trying to comprehend. Where was the social worker to deal with the emotional fallout of this conversation? I felt scared, bewildered, overwhelmed, and faint. *Was this really happening?* I stared into space and saw the doctor's lips moving, although no sound emerged. I think he decided that we had spoken for long enough and that he didn't want to overload me with any more information (*too late for that!*), so he welcomed me back to discuss and review the options at a later date. Think things over. The good thing, according to the doctor, was that we had plenty of time; we didn't have to rush.

Just before we left, I asked the doctor for a private word. My stepfather vacated the room and went and sat in the waiting room outside. Tears welled up in my eyes. "Doctor, I am 46, a single, gay man who hasn't yet found his life partner. This news is devastating to me. What happens to these men who have poor outcomes after treatment and end up both incontinent and impotent?" He looked at me and said the scariest word in the world to me: "Depression." "What happens to their sex life?" The doctor referred to the fact that sex can become less spontaneous and might need to be more planned. One can take medication (Viagra or Cialis, of course), a self-administered injection, an implant that costs approximately $11,000 in Australia; and the incontinence (while unlikely for my age) could be managed using incontinence pads.

Really, these are my options? I felt so old. "Can I speak to a social worker, or is there a support group I can attend?" The doctor advised me that there was no social worker, that the support group was mainly composed of much older men in their sixties and up, and that I might feel a sense of alienation within the group given my younger age. He certainly wasn't recommending it. "Will I still feel an attraction toward men without having my prostate?" I asked. "It will be like admiring a picture," came the reply. *A picture! It sounds like I will be admiring the fucking Mona Lisa.*

I wanted to ask so many more questions, intimate ones about my sex life, and yet I felt awkward doing so. I looked at the photo of him and his wife and children, beautifully framed and so proudly placed on his desk. *What about anal sex? Penetrative sex? Receptive sex? How will the absence of semen affect my orgasm? How can you reach orgasm with a flaccid penis? Will I still be a sexual man? Will I feel attractive to other men?* These were all such personal questions interconnected with my identity, and I needed answers to reduce my anxiety, and yet I just couldn't bring myself to ask them. I felt embarrassed revealing myself to this man and caught up in a heterosexist world, just as I always had.

I left the hospital and said good-bye to my stepdad. I had arranged to meet my friend Chris afterward to discuss my results. I was totally wired. Chris and I walked and talked around the block, across the street, around the park, back around the block—me leading the way, Chris following me wherever I decided to go, both conversationally and geographically. What did all this news mean for my identity, my masculinity, my ego, my sexuality, my love life, my lust life, my relationships, my future? Why couldn't I handle this more maturely, confidently, like other men? Why couldn't I take it in my stride, methodically, like my stepfather would have, instead of feeling so hysterical about it? I was so ashamed of myself. Why was I creating such a big deal out of this? The doctor could save my life and rid the cancer from my body before it spread. Surely this was the most important point: to be cancer-free. What about impotence, though? And the idea of being incontinent simply made me feel so much older than my 46 years.

My mother had not been well and had been in the hospital having complicated back surgery. I had been in the exact same hospital at the same time having my biopsy, just two floors below. The family and I had not told her of my cancer diagnosis, as we did not want her to worry and wanted her to recover fully from her operation first. She would find out soon enough, although it was not a conversation I was looking forward to; I knew it would really upset her. The day came a week later, and I asked my stepdad to explain the diagnosis to her and what it meant. I knew I would cry when I saw her after she had digested the news. I have really seen my mother cry only twice: first, when I told her I was gay, and again now, when I told her that I had cancer.

Telling my friends that I had cancer was the next thing to manage. It was like coming out all over again. I felt so ashamed. I admitted to them in my kitchen one morning how I felt the cancer was my fault, my doing. I had lived a fairly reckless life in my twenties and thirties, smoking a lot of pot, drinking copiously most weekends, eating lots of red meat and not enough fish, not exercising, smoking cigarettes for eighteen years, and having many sexual partners (though I practiced safe sex). I felt remorse that I had not led a healthier life when I had had the opportunity to do so.

Why have I been so stupid? What have I done to deserve this? Is this some kind of bad karma? Had all my worries about being gay finally resulted in a buildup of tension and anxiety and stress resulting in prostate cancer? It's all been my doing!

I had been told by the doctors to review the literature on prostate cancer, watch some DVDs on the topic, read information and pamphlets, talk to survivors, ask questions and seek answers, practice meditation, and get some exercise. The literature unavoidably concentrated on heterosexual couples in their later years, discussing their situation. Even when the text referred to one's "partner" rather than one's "wife," it was laden with heterosexual images. I felt so alienated from the support resources and material. *Where are my resources? Why aren't I included? What about me?*

I started to see my old counselor again, a psychologist who was to become a major part of my life over the next six months. She had run my coming-out group when I was 33—when I had just started to come out to myself and accept who I was. She is an amazing woman, highly skilled, compassionate, trustworthy, good-humored, and totally committed to her clients and her profession. She is one of the nicest people I have ever met. The day that I went to see her, I announced in a lethargic voice that I had been diagnosed with prostate cancer. I explained my feelings of anxiety about my future, and my feelings of depression returning—the depression that she had worked on tirelessly with me years before. She heard me and empathized with me—which was so important—and she helped me connect with another young, gay survivor of prostate cancer to talk with him about his experience and how he had managed, despite the results of his surgery not being that successful. I needed this connection desperately; I needed to ask all my personal questions of someone who was young and gay and had traveled similar terrain. I needed hope and reassurance that I would be okay. I felt that he would understand; he did, and I felt remarkably better after my conversation with him. This connection seemed such an essential part of my mental and emotional coping.

I received a second opinion from another specialist in the field that reinforced the recommendation that the most suitable option for me, given my age, tumor size, and Gleason score of 7, was the radical prostatectomy using the Da Vinci robot and nerve-sparing techniques. Prostate cancer normally strikes men in their sixties and up. Most men will die *with* prostate cancer and not *of* it. In younger men it can be a faster-growing cancer. My expected life span was longer, and radiotherapy carried long-term side effects of erectile difficulties and the possibility of the cancer's returning in areas located next to the damaged area, such as the bladder and the bowel. I desperately wanted to talk to other young men and to hear stories with positive outcomes. Everything so far seemed so pessimistic. I wished there had been a cancer support group for young, gay men. Unfortunately, I was told there was no such thing available.

My stepbrother and his husband live in Wellington, New Zealand. I love them and have a special relationship with them. They demonstrated their support for me by linking me up with a friend of theirs who was the same age as I and gay, and who'd had external beam radiation a few years before. I rang him and talked endlessly to him over the phone, asking all those personal questions I needed answers to, seeking his recommendations, hearing his choices and their subsequent results. There is one sure thing when discussing prostate cancer that you can't avoid: you connect immediately with the heart of someone's being, the essence of being a man, his sexuality, and who he is.

My urologist also kindly sent me a letter recommending that I speak to another man who was younger than I (in his thirties) and had recovered amazingly well from his surgery. Within one week of his surgery his erectile functioning and continence had returned. This was highly irregular, as I had heard that it can take up to three years for functioning to resume, and in most cases it will never return to its full potency—if potency returns at all. This was what I needed to hear: a positive story from a younger man. Over the next few months I was to hear a range of stories from friends and relatives. So many people had stories linked to a friend or relative. There were some wonderful stories and some awful ones. I heard of the difficulty many men had in making treatment choices. This was certainly an unusual aspect of this particular type of cancer. Few cancers offer treatment options.

It was six months before I made up my mind to choose the surgery option, an agonizing six months of obsession and high levels of anxiety.

I had been unsuccessfully trying to adopt the watchful waiting option. The tumor was minute, I reminded myself. I was so scared of losing my potency and continence that I would have done anything that prevented the treatment, despite the incessant nagging from my family to have the surgery. Everyone talked about the Big C, but I was worried about the Big I and its effects on my mental health. My psychologist was simply amazing through this period, seeing me weekly and sometimes even daily. She helped me place things in perspective, talked about more positive possibilities, challenged my negative, catastrophic thinking, and helped me relax and stay calm, reframing things and helping me create meaning out of what I was going through. She drew attention to my strengths and resources, and she acknowledged my many support systems.

It was now February and I was back working, albeit not being fully present and engaged in what I was doing; a couple of times I had panic attacks in the middle of my classes. It was a bumpy six months of tossing around the options, indecision, talking to people, doctors, sexual health rehabilitation specialists, and patients. The final clincher for me, though, was when the urologist said that if I were his brother, he would be advising that I act now and not leave it any longer. This turned out to be magical encouragement as, unbeknown to me, the cancer had started to spread within the prostate.

Jacki is one of my closest friends and has supported me so totally throughout this incredible journey. Given my current circumstances, that I was about to lose my prostate and hence my semen and capacity to ejaculate, she asked me whether I had thought of sperm donation before my operation. It suddenly dawned on me that this would be the last possible opportunity for me to become a father. (I have since learned that sperm can be drained from the testes as a viable alternative to ejaculation.) The prospect of probably never becoming a parent was something I believed I had dealt with many years before, upon coming out as a gay man. Now that whole idea resurfaced, and I found myself deliberating over the possibility yet again. *Do I want to become a father? A sperm donor?* I pondered this for another month, the time ticking by and the operation now due in only five days. I had decided that there would be no harm in freezing my sperm. I made my appointment the following day to go to the clinic, giving myself the possibility of parenthood or sperm donation at some later date. I was told that the cutoff date for donation was fifty years of age. I had just scraped in.

I made my way to the clinic, completed the paperwork, and saw the young men in the waiting room. I was taken to my private room and given a plastic bottle, and my attention turned toward the numerous *Penthouse* magazines on the small table in the middle of the room. *Great!* There was a TV for viewing the pornography. *This is surreal.* I was so very anxious—anxious about the impending operation, anxious about "performing" with this very tight deadline, anxious about the whole idea of becoming a parent. Needless to say, my anxiety won over my ability to perform the required task, and yet again a huge feeling of shame and failure overtook me. I was angry with myself for my procrastination over the previous month, making me feel so powerless in the face of the impending deadline. I left hurriedly in a daze of confusion and said good-bye to my final chance to become what I had always been groomed for—a father. I was devastated.

The surgery lasted about three hours, and there were two surgeons and an anesthetist present. I woke up in my room afterward, and the doctor came in to see me. He said that the operation had gone very well. They had removed the prostate gland and seminal vesicles, and he thought that he had managed to successfully spare the nerves that surrounded the prostate, a difficult and tricky procedure. I relaxed into my pillow with a huge feeling of relief. How great to hear such news! The cancerous prostate was gone. I guess the next thing was to wait until my body started to heal itself; my erections would, I hoped, return and my incontinence would disappear.

My recovery at home went tremendously well, especially when I heard the final pathology result: that the cancer looked as if it had been contained within the shell of the prostate. There would be no need for radiation treatment. I experienced three weeks of incontinence and only one major bed-wetting mishap. I was so relieved to have the catheter out, literally in a one-second pullout motion by the nurse. It was also about three weeks into my recovery when I awoke in the early hours of the morning to find and feel an outstanding erection. I smiled and jumped out of bed and looked at myself naked in the mirror. I was both overwhelmed and excited. I was potent and after only three weeks! I had prepared myself for a three-year wait—if it happened at all. I was so relieved! It's almost embarrassing to have wished so much for my erectile return, but it was a big thing for me, especially being single and reliant on a more casual sex life, where performance is considered paramount.

JOINING A GAY AND BISEXUAL MEN'S PROSTATE CANCER SUPPORT GROUP

One year after the surgery, I spoke to a social worker in Melbourne who worked for the Cancer Council there. She advised me of a pilot group that was starting up in Sydney to explore the needs of gay and bisexual men who have a prostate cancer diagnosis. Coincidentally, I had also seen an ad in the gay press for this group looking for men to come forward with their stories. I rang and spoke to the organizer and social worker straight away and put my name down to attend the pilot group, which would run for three consecutive Tuesdays. This was to be an invaluable part of my healing, creating meaning out of what had been a difficult time in my life; as a counselor, I knew that creating meaning for clients out of their experience is an important part of their therapeutic recovery.

The three workshops were run professionally by Greg, a highly experienced social worker in the area of men's health. Greg is also gay and had dealt with his own type of cancer, leukemia. He collated data about our experiences through three stages: diagnosis, treatment, and aftercare. The three weeks went by very quickly and I met a wonderful group of fifteen gay- and bisexual-identifying men, all with interesting stories to tell. I was the second-youngest in the group and found some solace talking to the other young men in the group. Except for two or three, the participants were single—which I personally found an interesting statistic—and there was a range of different personalities and cultures in the room. I felt that I was contributing to something quite special during this period, and I eagerly and vocally added my thoughts and shared my experiences. We looked at how things could be improved from a gay man's perspective—we had been the "forgotten group." Now I felt included. I was finding my voice in trying to shape things differently for future gay and bisexual men going through the challenges accompanying a prostate cancer diagnosis.

The Shine a Light group in Sydney was born in 2011 and has been running the first Saturday of every month for seven years at the ACON (AIDS Council of New South Wales) offices in Surry Hills. The group is an open group for men affected by prostate cancer—who identify as gay or bisexual—and their partners. I have often been asked why we need a separate group for gay and bisexual men, and my answer is to provide a safe place for these men to discuss their concerns and their sexual lives free from any heterosexist norms, judgments, and prejudices, which many gay and bisexual men have encountered at some point in their lives. It is a nonjudgmental space for discussing our thoughts, sharing our emotions, relating how we have coped or possibly haven't. Our group is open to people who have had any one of the many possible treatment options and who are dealing with the various effects on mind, body, and soul. We have a range of speakers, such as dieticians, surgeons, urologists, sexual rehabilitation specialists, and educators in alternative sexual practices. We attend to the needs of different people in the room as best as we can. We laugh and we cry. The main goal is to connect with one another and share stories, highs and lows, ups and downs, with like-minded people. It is a chance to share knowledge and support one another. It is a social opportunity that gives added meaning to those on this journey, helping them through a frightening time in their lives. It is about making friends.

I am 54 now, and another milestone has been reached and a new chapter in my life has begun. Life seems amazingly good. I have balance restored. I have meaning in my life; I have become an ambassador to the Prostate Cancer Foundation of Australia. I have made some marvelous friends from the Shine a Light group. I attend training days to improve the functioning of our support group. I have had a role to play in the development and distribution of new resources for gay and bisexual men. I feel included in the support material and resources available to gay and bisexual men and feel I have contributed my voice to the well-being of these men, who are in various stages of dealing with their prostate cancer diagnoses. I remain a lecturer and have a counseling practice. I provide support to many men, both gay and straight, of all ages and cultural backgrounds, and hear about their experiences, the good and the not-so-good. I feel relieved and grateful for my good health. My last PSA test result was 0.03, essentially undetectable.

I want to finish by saying thank you to my surgeon, who did such a brilliant job on all three fronts of removing the cancer and restoring me to full continence and near 100% potency levels, and to all my wonderful family and friends who have helped and supported me on my journey and who have played an integral part in my recovery and in my life.

CHAPTER 18

An Invader in the Pleasure Dome

Perry Brass

CHAPTER SUMMARY

This account is the first in a series on a gay man facing prostate cancer originally published in *Gay City News*, edited by Paul Schindler. It covers the process of diagnosis and decision making about treatment from the perspective of Perry Brass, a gay activist and writer. This article discusses his emotional reactions to diagnosis, interactions with health professionals associated with diagnosis and treatment decision making, and the final decision made about treatment.

KEY TERMS

choice of radical prostatectomy, emotional reactions to cancer diagnosis, gay men, personal account of cancer, preventing erectile dysfunction, prostate cancer, prostate drugs, treatment decision making, value of PSA

This past March, I received a call from Dr. Art Rastinehad, the young urologist who had just performed the latest prostate biopsy on me — the fifth done on me over the last decade — informing me I have prostate cancer. Though for years I had faced the possibility of this diagnosis, no one ever is *really* prepared for it.

For a moment, I stopped breathing. It instantly brought back to me my father's horrible, painful death from colon-rectal cancer when I was 11, and the fear that my life, with all its routines and pleasures, was really going to change. How was I going to handle that?

At 68, I learned I was going to be a cancer patient. The thought terrified me.

I could barely speak when I hung up. I managed to tell my husband, Hugh Young, then Ricardo Limon, my closest friend. After that, I could barely talk about it for days. I just held it inside me, or tried as best I could to deny it.

Ussher, Jane M., Perz, Janette, Rosser, B. R. Simon, eds., *Gay & Bisexual Men Living with Prostate Cancer*
dx.doi.org/10.17312/harringtonparkpress/2018.06.gbmlpc.018
© 2018 Harrington Park Press

In truth, I'd been expecting this diagnosis (while at the same time hoping against it), owing to my chronically high PSA level. PSA, or prostate-specific antigen, is determined by a blood test that tracks a protein in your blood released by infections in the prostate. These infections can range from more treatable forms of prostatitis to cancer itself. A "perfect" PSA is 0, meaning no infection at all. After 0, a number spread is given to the readings. For a decade mine had ranged from a 6 to an 8—without any indications of prostatitis. So I didn't have a prostate infection per se, but I did have this high PSA. I was also taking finasteride, a drug normally prescribed for an enlarged prostate—the problem that causes men to have to pee over and over in the middle of the night—and finasteride itself halves your PSA. In other words, my 6 was actually a PSA of 12, my 7 a 14, my 8 a 16.

Any PSA over a 4 makes urologists take notice, and my first biopsy, done in Brooklyn, was performed with almost no anesthesia other than a local in the form of a cream. I was literally bent over a table, and told by the urologist that I'd experience only a "slight pinch." I screamed loud enough to be heard in Manhattan; *it was like having a rattlesnake shot up my ass seven times.* The reality is a small needle sent up your rectum to get to your prostate. Like a harpoon, it retrieves minute samples of prostate material to be analyzed by a pathologist. A few weeks later, it came back negative. What a relief! I was off the hook.

Still, my PSA never got lower than the safety of 4, and that in itself bothered the next several urologists I saw. One of the indicators of cancer is a bouncing PSA; its veering from one number to another too fast suggests there is an infection, possibly cancer, working through you. For years mine had been doing just that, rarely settling on one number. I had three other biopsies over the years—by then I insisted I be knocked out by anesthesia for each.

And each came back negative, puzzling both me and my doctors. "You are," Dr. Rastinehad explained to me in March, "a Gleason 7. Or 3 + 4."

In treating prostate cancer, your Gleason number, derived by a pathologist from your biopsy, is important; it describes where the cancer is located and in what density. A "3 + 4" meant that my cancer was located in two areas and was aggressive, but not as aggressive as a "4 + 3." Gleason 6 means that your cancer is manageable. There are men with that number who do nothing: they are in "active surveillance" and may submit to a biopsy every few years, get their PSA tests taken often, and hope for the best. At 7, you are already in the territory of risk that your cancer can spread—metastasize to your bones and pelvis—thereby progressing to a Gleason 8, or, worse, a 9, which is called stage 4 prostate cancer.

So getting this diagnosis when I did was *fortunate;* I even describe it as a "stroke of luck," in that I finally found out where my cancer had been hiding. Rastinehad told me exactly where the cancer was and why it had not been found in earlier biopsies. Exactly how this happened is also part of my story.

Last October, Mark Horn, a longtime friend, revealed that he'd had prostate cancer—PC for short—for eight years. His Gleason score was a 6, qualifying him for active surveillance. I told him about my struggles with repeated biopsies, which in themselves can be risky procedures, doing possible harm to the prostate and, at a minimum, usually result-ing in bleeding in your urine, feces, and semen for a week or so after-ward. Mark strongly suggested that before my next biopsy I get an MRI (magnetic resonance imaging) of my prostate. The MRI would show areas of the prostate that are questionable owing to their a lighter den-sity, an indicator of infection or cancer. Using this MRI, it's easier for a urologist to focus exactly where to aim the biopsy needles.

I went to my urologist, Dr. Craig Nobert, who felt that I was due for another biopsy, and I asked him for an MRI. He responded, "I can get you one, but they're not very conclusive."

Mark had told me to insist, and I did. Very generously, Nobert referred me to his colleague Rastinehad, a younger urologist at Mt. Sinai who has been working with the use of MRIs and prostate biopsies for several years. I immediately felt a great deal of confidence being in Rastinehad's hands, even though this use of MRIs and biopsies is still considered experimental by some insurers.

I completed the MRI, and in March went to Beth Israel Hospital to have Rastinehad do the biopsy, not under a general anesthesia but rather using an effective local. To target the biopsy needle with even greater specificity, he used an ultrasound at the same time—a proce-dure that required me to have my legs raised in stirrups, something I'd never experienced before. Half-dozing through the procedure, I felt occa-sional slight but unsettling pinches. I received more anesthesia when I asked for it, but when my legs were removed from the stirrups they were very wobbly.

For the next nine days, while the samples were analyzed by a pathol-ogist, I really didn't want to think about the whole business, deciding I *would* be negative again; it just *had* to be. Then Rastinehad called with the results and told me that the problem all along had been that the cancer was located extremely close to my urethra; any urologist not using an MRI and an ultrasound would never get that close for fear of permanently damaging that urine duct. The truth was that I might have been positive for years, the cancer simply being missed by all my previous biopsies. My luck was in having used an MRI; without it, I could have gone undiagnosed until I became symptomatic enough to have bone pains and bleeding and had landed squarely in stage 4 prostate cancer.

Predicting the progression of prostate cancer—how fast it is growing, and where it will end up—is difficult. Its location and other factors, including genetics (very important), age, and lifestyle, all play a part. Smokers and men who are heavy, for example, are in more danger. Some contributing factors regarding diet have not been fully confirmed, but there are doctors who suggest that men with a raised PSA level eliminate all red meat, a source of testosterone, from their diet. Yet one friend my age, a lifelong vegetarian, came down with PC five years before I did—and his case raises other questions. He's been in a long-time domestic relationship with two other men; all three of them were diagnosed with PC within the space of three years. Can PC be, in any way, transmitted sexually, or can chances of developing it be accelerated by sex? There has been some evidence that prostate massage can be good for you, and even anal sex, if done carefully, can be helpful to your prostate. But there have been no scientific studies done on this topic or other ways in which sexual life experiences (including contracting STDs) affect prostate cancer.

Being a gay, older man facing prostate cancer, I was not alone: I have about a dozen friends who've fought this disease, and there is a somewhat loose network of support for us—gay men confronting a battle with a cancer that can kill. Each year, approximately 33,000 men die of prostate cancer; it is hard to tell how many are gay, but gay prostate cancer has become an issue in a community that is both aging and accepting its aging.

Youth, however, is no barrier to the disease. In recent years, the average age of prostate cancer patients has declined; men as young as 40 are now being diagnosed with it. Why? It could have to do with prescription drug use, intake of testosterone additives, fat-laden diets, stress, and other factors, including genetics. For example, African American men today are experiencing higher than average rates of prostate cancer, and because more of them are uninsured, they are dying from the disease at a higher rate than men from any other ethnic background. Among young men diagnosed, one outcome is more rapid progression of the disease, making it all the more important that younger men start getting digital examinations—a doctor performing a finger probe of the prostate through the rectum—earlier than most physicians are willing to offer them, and also have their PSA levels checked.

PSAs in themselves are controversial. Some studies have shown that they are inconclusive and lead to biopsies that don't need to be done or to faulty diagnoses. I've yet to meet a urologist who discounts them, however; all those I've seen say they are an extremely effective tool for flagging cancer that is coming.

After my diagnosis, when I returned to my original urologist, Craig Nobert, he quickly read my mind. "Most men, when they hear that word 'cancer,' the whole conversation stops," he said. "It shouldn't." Nobert took me through all the options, with their pluses, minuses, and possible complications. Initially, I intended to go with radiation beam therapy and the "seeds"—small radioactive particles surgically implanted in the prostate to target the cancer. This option was certainly less threatening to me than having my prostate surgically removed. Hormone therapy—aimed at reducing my testosterone level to zero to starve the cancer of male hormones, the element that it grows on, and carried out in tandem with chemotherapy and radiation—was also a disturbing prospect. Several of my friends had gone that route and been basically pushed into a menopausal state of hot flashes, breast enlargement, mood swings, depression, and skin outbreaks. I dreaded that.

Nobert suggested a second opinion—which is standard for patients facing the sort of life choice I was confronting. In the end, I got four, after first returning to Art Rastinehad, basically for moral support. He told me I was in great physical shape and should consider a radical prostatectomy. It's major surgery but, still in my 60s, I was strong enough to stand it. The payoff is that it would simply cut the *source* of the cancer out of me.

Then I went to a wonderful radiologist at Mt. Sinai West, Dr. Andrew Evans, who told me that with a Gleason score of 7, radiation and the seeds provided a good prognosis, with basically no pain and little recovery time. He also, however, underscored a warning Nobert had earlier given me: once you do radiation, if the cancer *has* spread and you *need* to do a radical prostatectomy afterward, the burn damage from the radiation makes it difficult to salvage those very important nerves in the prostate that lead to sexual response; as a result, getting an erection can be difficult.

If that wasn't strong enough medicine, he added, "It's like taking apart a grilled cheese sandwich *after* it's been grilled."

Going outside the Mt. Sinai system for another perspective, I saw Dr. Jim Hu, an excellent urological surgeon with a great reputation at Weill Cornell Medical Center who had performed a large number of prostatectomies. By this point, any denial I had was crumbling. I was a cancer patient; I had to face it. Still, I was falling apart every time I went into a PC discussion in a medical setting. I would start crying without any warning, barely able to contain myself. Though I let a few more people know about my diagnosis, I was still mostly keeping it to myself. My husband, Hugh, suggested psychotherapy, but I found that even the energy to do that was missing: I needed to get my treatment resolved, and each "second opinion" only hammered that in.

I spoke again to Mark Horn, who by this time had completed another biopsy, in which his Gleason had jumped to 7. "I'm going to do a robotic radical prostatectomy," he told me. "And I want to do it as fast as I can. I've had a great run on active surveillance, but I can't take a chance with this. Also, I'm in good shape, and I want to do this while I'm still young enough to get through this operation without problems."

The conversation with Mark suddenly crystallized everything for me. I did not want to undergo radiation if the result would be that dreaded "grilled cheese" effect—I would not risk having major erectile dysfunction for the rest of my life. And hormones scared the crap out of me, as did any form of chemotherapy—certainly at this point. Mark also told me that he was getting one of the best prostate cancer surgeons in the country to do it: Dr. Ash Tewari, the head of urology at Mt. Sinai, the man who basically oversees Art Rastinehad's and Craig Nobert's work. I asked Mark if he thought there was any chance I'd get Tewari to do my operation, and he warned he was very solidly booked.

I quickly called Tewari's office and made an appointment for a week later. Very anxious, I arrived to find a warm and supportive doctor who asked me, "What can I do for you?" I answered, "You can do this operation on me, like you're doing for my friend Mark Horn."

He smiled. "Mark's my friend, too. I'll be glad to do it."

ACKNOWLEDGMENT

This chapter was originally published in *Gay City News*, edited by Paul Schindler; http://gaycitynews.nyc/invader-pleasure-dome/. It is the first in a three-part series. For the second and third installments, see http://gaycitynews.nyc/stepping-prostate-cancer-surgery/ and http://gaycitynews.nyc/recovery-life-prostate-cancer/. Also a one-year-later follow-up was published: http://gaycitynews.nyc/invader-pleasure-dome-one-year-later/.

CHAPTER 19

Looking Back

Engaging Prostate Cancer as a Gay Man at the Turn of the Twenty-first Century

Gerald Perlman

CHAPTER SUMMARY

This chapter reflects my experience with prostate cancer as a gay man seeking help in the painfully heterosexist environment of 2000. The narrative looks back at my feelings, my reactions, my concerns, and my revelations and awakenings as I struggled with my own confusing search for help, compassion, and understanding in an environment that was quite unfriendly to gay men. I write of my wrestling with issues of helplessness, identity, anger, sex, shame, and loss, and how I went from being a participant in a support group for gay men to facilitator of that group of courageous men, all of whom found themselves in a similar situation.

KEY TERMS

gay men, heterosexism, HIV/AIDS, impotence, incontinence, prostate cancer, radiation, sex, side effects, support groups

LOOKING BACK: DIAGNOSIS AND CONFUSION

I was diagnosed with and treated for prostate cancer late in the year 2000. During the ensuing years, my PSA readings have been in the undetectable range. And this has been a relief and a blessing. In fact, I hardly think about prostate cancer anymore unless I see an article in a magazine or newspaper, or I am asked to write a chapter such as this one. And aside from some late radiation effects that influence my ability to get as full an erection as I had when I was in my late fifties and early sixties, I have come away from the process relatively unscathed.

Ussher, Jane M., Perz, Janette, Rosser, B. R. Simon, eds., *Gay & Bisexual Men Living with Prostate Cancer*
dx.doi.org/10.17312/harringtonparkpress/2018.06.gbmlpc.019
© 2018 Harrington Park Press

Of course, aging plays a factor here as well. But, fortunately, we live in the age of Viagra and Cialis, and that has helped correct some of the negative by-products of aging as well as of the prostate cancer treatment.

It was August, a time when, like many others in my profession, I take a vacation from my psychotherapy practice. It is a time I try to catch up with many of the things I had put off during the year. Visiting a urologist was one of the things I needed to cross off my list. I had been routinely screening my PSA since I was 50. That is the recommended age at which white men should begin monitoring their PSA levels; the recommended age is earlier for men who have a family history of prostate cancer. For black men, it should begin at age 40.[1] My PSA always hovered around 4.1, which is just over the 0 – 4 range considered normal. My openly gay physician thought nothing of it, so neither did I. But I was having trouble with urination. I would urinate often and with a weak stream. It disturbed my sleep. I passed it off to age or BPH (benign prostatic hypertrophy), a noncancerous enlargement of the prostate that can cause urinary problems, usually in older men.

Because of my urinary problems, my physician suggested I consult a urologist. He recommended a man who practiced in Greenwich Village in New York City and was said to be "gay-friendly." Were there no gay urologists in New York City? My physician was unaware of any, and I searched in vain. Today I am aware of many proudly "out" gay urologists. But in the year 2000, they weren't advertising.

Several weeks later, I consulted the "gay-friendly" urologist, who could find nothing definitive from the digital rectal exam (DRE) he gave me: an unpleasant, over-lathering of lubricating lotion, followed by his sticking his finger up my anus to probe my prostate gland (which should be about the size of a chestnut or walnut and feel like the tip of one's nose). At the end of that procedure, I was given a load of tissues and told to wipe myself up.

My PSA by then had risen to 5.2. This was considered an aggressive bump up. He suggested I get a biopsy, which I did. It was a much more painful experience than I had expected. About 6 – 12 thin needles are inserted through the rectum (which is the most common procedure), or through the urethra, or through the perineum (the area between the anus and the scrotum) into the prostate to extract tissue samples of the gland. My advice, although you may get some pushback from the urologist, is to insist on an anesthetic. And expect to have blood in your urine for up to several weeks.

Two weeks after the biopsy, there I was, apprehensive, seated across from this "gay-friendly" urologist. He didn't seem friendly to me, gay or otherwise. His face was dour. This didn't bode well. He said, "I have some bad news for you." Then, from across the desk that separated us, he slid a piece of paper that read "Diagnostic Report" in bold red letters. In what seemed like even bolder red letters I read, "Prostatic Adenocarcinoma; Gleason Score 6 (Grades 3 + 3) and 15% of submitted tissue is involved in Specimen 3." Everything else was in black ink and seemed normal.

I was traumatized. My brain froze. My body stiffened. I couldn't, nor did I want to, move. The urologist was babbling about the numbers and the pictures and who knows what else. I couldn't attend to him because my mind and body had gone numb. I had dissociated. Then, after what seemed like an eternity, he handed me several outdated pamphlets, which pissed me off. My anger awakened me. Really, outdated pamphlets!

I could sense his discomfort, his sense of helplessness, and his desire to get me out of his office. He suggested I make an appointment with his office-mate, who was a surgeon. I didn't want to do that. I wanted to run, to wake up from a nightmare in a place where cancer didn't exist. And I knew that once I left his office, it would hit hard: that at the age of 58, out of the blue, I had just been diagnosed with prostate cancer.

I walked the city for about an hour, experiencing anxiety, helplessness, and confusion. Where do I go from here? What are my options? In those days, watchful waiting was not recommended, particularly if you were under the age of 60.

For many days, I did nothing. I was afraid and in denial. Then I read about New York City's Mayor Rudolph Giuliani's struggle with prostate cancer.[2] He opted for brachytherapy (radioactive seed implantation) in conjunction with hormone treatment. And I had heard that Joe Torre, the New York Yankees' manager, had chosen radical prostatectomy, the so-called gold standard for prostate cancer treatment at that time. What else was there? I knew about cryotherapy, proton beam therapy, hormone therapy, alternative diet therapies, and so on. Some of these procedures had dreadful side effects or sounded too untested. Cyber-knife treatment was not available then. And robotic nerve-sparing surgery was in its infancy.

I read everything I could get my hands on. There was nothing definitive or reassuring. No clear path. And the books had titles like *The Prostate: A Guide for Men and the Women Who Love Them;*[1] *Men, Women,* and *Prostate Cancer: A Medical and Psychological Guide for Women and the Men They Love;*[3] *The Lovin' Ain't Over: The Couple's Guide to Better Sex after Prostate Cancer.*[4] It wasn't about Michael and Bruce, you can be sure. There was nothing relating to gay men. And while the books were generally informative, they left me feeling excluded as a gay man, once again.

Of course, today things are a little better; there have been several books and articles written in the last decade aimed at gay men with prostate cancer. The first, which I coedited, *A Gay Man's Guide to Prostate Cancer*, came out in 2005.[5] A sequel was published under the title *What Every Gay Man Needs to Know about Prostate Cancer: The Essential Guide to Diagnosis, Treatment, and Recovery.*[6] More recently, Gilad E. Amiel and colleagues wrote a chapter about gay men and prostate cancer in *Cancer and the LGBT Community.*[7] As a self-proclaimed "sexuality activist, researcher, and theorist," Gary W. Dowsett has given us a look into his personal journey with prostate cancer in an article entitled, "Losing My Chestnut: One Gay Man's Wrangle with Prostate Cancer" (see chapter 16 of this book).[8] And of course, now there is this book and a growing body of academic research.[9]

But at the turn of the twenty-first century, there were no gay guides, no books, no support groups. I was continuously coming up against heterosexist bias. It brought to mind the forms I had filled out at the first urologist's office. They had no gay sensibility. *Gay* seemed an inconceivable concept. A form put out by the pharmaceutical company Pfizer presents five questions regarding erectile functioning; these were scored on a scale from 1 to 5 (from generally difficult to not difficult). A score of 21 or less usually indicates erectile dysfunction. It was the second question that disturbed me the most as a gay man. It asked, "When you had erections with sexual stimulation, how often were erections hard enough for penetration?" Of course, they were assuming penetration of the vagina, not the anus. And what about a blow job? How hard must one be to get that? Or a hand job? And what about sex toys? The list can go on. Suffice it to say, I was put off and I told the nurse I was gay and didn't know how to answer this. To which she replied, "Try your best."

Making a decision like that can be the most difficult and loneliest of human responsibilities. For prostate cancer there is no magic wand, no guaranteed cure, and there are all those scary side effects. I had older straight male friends who put a priority on continence over potency. I am not sure if it is because I am a gay man or because I was a relatively young man at the time, but my priorities were quite different. Losing my erection was not going to happen. As if I had control over such a thing. But being sexually vital was so much a part of my sense of self. It related to my feeling loved, attractive, accepted, passionate, alive, and validated. I had been sexual as far back as I could remember. To be unable to have an erection, or worse, I thought, not be able to be sexually aroused and achieve an orgasm, seemed unimaginable at the time. More than seventeen years later, with sexual desire no longer in control of me, it is a relief to know that sex need not be conflated with love, validation, and so forth. There have been several major medical events in my life. And from each one I have learned something new about myself and others. My having prostate cancer helped me distinguish between sex and the many qualities I had attributed to it.

DISTRAUGHT AND SEEKING SUPPORT

I was a fan more of Joe Torre than of Rudolph Giuliani; nevertheless, after several months of deliberation, I decided to go the brachytherapy route, and I contacted Giuliani's physician. Having made the decision, I felt a weight lifted off my shoulders, for a while at least. My anxiety and depression returned soon enough, and I felt the need for a support group. I called the New York City Gay and Lesbian Center. No luck. I called every organization that might potentially have something to do with gay men and prostate cancer. I was batting zero. Finally, I came across Malecare, an organization founded by Darryl Mitteldorf, a straight male social worker who ran monthly groups for gay men with prostate cancer in addition to weekly groups for all men, regardless of sexual orientation, diagnosed with prostate cancer (see chapter 15). His was the first of such groups. There are now several Malecare satellites around the world. And there are other similar supports groups for gay men now that were not available at the turn of the century.

Cancer was my enemy, an alien that had invaded my body, my sexuality. I wanted it out. Some men can live more easily with the knowledge that there is a cancer growing within. They are more likely to take a position of watchful waiting, or active surveillance, as it is also called. In the year 2000 it was not considered a wise option. Now it is a respected alternative to the more invasive procedures available. If I were to be diagnosed today with my stage T1c cancer (a very low stage), I might have taken a wait-and-see attitude, which involves testing for PSA levels every few months and regular DREs. But seventeen years ago, I wasn't there. And as I noted, that option was frowned on by the medical community.

So I opted for the radiation treatment, which appeared to pose a lower risk of impotence than a radical prostatectomy. I also religiously did visualization exercises. It was like playing PacMan. I would visualize the alien cancer bodies being eaten up by the helper cells in my body. I don't know if it helped; but it couldn't hurt, so I did it. And by then, I had become a member of the gay men's prostate cancer support group and I wasn't alone anymore.

FROM DIAGNOSIS TO TREATMENT

Although I had been diagnosed in August, it wasn't until mid-December that I found myself lying on a gurney in a freezing cold hallway with the thinnest of blankets over me. I was shivering from cold and from fear. After what seemed like forever, I was wheeled into a room where I saw my primary surgeon, who would place the radioactive seeds in my prostate, and another doctor who had done the initial testing. He was there to guide my primary surgeon's placement of the needles via an ultrasound device. There were also a resident and an anesthesiologist in the closet of a room where I would be treated. I was given a local anesthetic. I could feel pressure, but no pain. Upon leaving, I was given a prescription for Flomax (a drug that relaxes the prostate gland and the bladder neck, allowing for an easier flow of urine). I was told that I could take aspirin or ibuprofen for any discomfort I might feel. An appointment to visit the surgeon was set up for a few weeks later.

The day after seeding I had no feeling in my penis. It was numb. I panicked. I called the surgeon. He had no idea why I would have no feeling in my penis. He suggested I call the anesthesiologist. The latter had never heard of such a thing. She told me she would do some research and get back to me. Oh, my God. My worst fears were being realized. The anxiety was overwhelming. She called back and said it was a one-in-a-million phenomenon. Most probably, a nerve had been temporarily injured when I was injected with the anesthetic. She was pretty sure it would return to normal in a day, but she couldn't be sure. I hung up the phone and cursed and cried. Fortunately, several hours later, sensation returned to my penis. I was euphoric. I called the doctors and let them know that all was well again. For the moment, at least. The next few days were sleepy and uncomfortable ones. I hadn't filled the Flomax prescription. I wasn't big on taking medicine at the time. Since my bout with prostate cancer, my attitude about taking medicine has changed significantly.

When I got to see the surgeon and the resident, I was asked about my well-being. I complained that I was having a difficult time urinating and it was very painful when I did; the pain was such that I dreaded having to urinate. I had to hold on to the walls and grit my teeth when I did. Sitting and urinating was somewhat less painful than standing. The surgeon explained that the prostate would eventually regress, but for now, it was swollen from the procedure and I was experiencing referred pain from the seed implantations. He told me I was healing and the difficult and painful urination would subside. He also asked if I was taking the Flomax, to which I replied, "No." "Well, you must take it," he said. "It will help the flow." So I did, and it did. Two pills a day for many months, plus prescription-dose ibuprofen (600 mg). I was told that this regimen would help until my prostate shrunk from the radiation, at which point I would no longer need the medication. Not true. Today I take a generic form of Flomax every other day. It turns out that my prostate pushes into my urethra. This was discovered by means of an ultrasound, which the second doctor administered after I refused to have another biopsy just because I had been complaining that my urinary flow was still weak.

One of the really scary things was that the first time I ejaculated and many times after that, my ejaculate was a Pepto-Bismol pink. Just as I had after the biopsy, I was spurting a combination of semen and blood. That subsided, and my ejaculations and erections were fine for many years. Incontinence was never an issue. And although the bleeding from my penis had ceased, blood was still coming out in terrifying clots from my anus. For thirteen months I suffered with this affliction. That it lasted so long was another one-in-a-million anomaly.

I dreaded going to the bathroom. I dreaded farting. I took to wearing sanitary napkins. It was frustrating and often embarrassing, and I was frightened and angry. Much reassurance and many home remedies from urologists didn't stop the bleeding. But then, thirteen months later, it did stop, and the problem never returned. One thing nobody had told me was that there would be "late radiation effects." It takes time for the effects of radiation to manifest themselves in the tissues surrounding the prostate gland. That happened about five years after the procedure. Until then, I had enjoyed full and sustained erections. After the late radiation effects appeared, I was still able to get aroused, I could get an erection, and I could ejaculate. But the erections weren't as they had been, and there was a decrease in the amount of ejaculate;

the only ejaculate came from my seminal vesicles (which are spared in seeding, as opposed to having no ejaculate after radical prostatectomy). I came in droplets. And when I take Flomax, I have a common side effect called retrograde ejaculation (i.e., nothing comes out; semen goes into the bladder instead of out through the urethra). This affected the quality of my orgasms. I took to scheduling my Flomax intake around the times I assumed I was going to have sex so it wouldn't interfere with my pleasure. For most gay men, the lack of ejaculate is a considerable loss. Some gay men have told me it makes having sex much less messy. I like the messiness, so for me it was a loss. But my husband, who is 11 years younger than I, has been wonderfully understanding and supportive. He has treasured my droplets and my 90% erections without my feeling that I was damaged goods. And I have moved into another psychic space. My performance anxiety is practically nonexistent. We have both come to accept what we then called "our new normal" before it was fashionable to do so. And, yes, Viagra helps. Curiously, over the years I have often had no need for it. The experience of getting an erection is an important one for most of us. I worked with a man who had a penile implant and he despaired that despite the fact he could get a full and lasting erection at will by pumping, he could not feel the thrill of getting hard. For some others with penile implants, this is not an issue.

THE GROUP AND THE ISSUES WE CONFRONTED

I had discovered the one group in the city, at the time, that focused on gay and bisexual men with prostate cancer. These days that group includes male-to-female transgender folks as well. With the help of the weekly mixed-sexual-orientation male-support group, the monthly gay and bi men's support group, and individual therapy, I began to process and integrate the profoundly stressful, sometimes terrifying and exhausting experience of diagnosis of, treatment for, and recovery from prostate cancer. More than eighteen months after my diagnosis, and feeling as though I had been living in an emotional Cuisinart, life began to settle down and return to some reasonable semblance of what I will loosely refer to as normalcy.

The founder of Malecare knew I was a clinical psychologist and certified group psychotherapist at the time. And since I was a gay man as well, he suggested that I take over his position as facilitator of the gay and bi men's group. It was a role I embraced gratefully for almost ten years. From that experience came the first comprehensive book for gay men with prostate cancer based on the scientific knowledge of the time and the actual experiences of the men in the group.[5]

A myriad of emotions and states of consciousness come flooding in, or are dissociated, upon one's hearing the word *cancer*. With the diagnosis and treatment of prostate cancer, because it is so intimately connected to a man's sexuality, reactions are often exacerbated. Sadly, it is fairly common knowledge that when men experience conflict or emotional turmoil in their lives, they, more than women, are likely to shut down and withdraw.[10] Men, in general, tend to bond through common activities and interests. It is therefore no surprise that much talk in male support groups is about information gathering, statistics swapping, and problem solving rather than emotions. I don't mean to minimize the importance of these activities. Irvin Yalom has highlighted the importance of information sharing as a basic curative factor in psychotherapy groups.[11] But for a man to express his feelings of despair, loneliness, anger, vulnerability, helplessness, shame, and loss is no easy task. Gay men are no less subject to these constraints than their heterosexual counterparts. The problem is exacerbated when gay men experience themselves as a marginalized subset of a larger group of men. A support group just for gay men with prostate cancer that is facilitated by a gay man with prostate cancer as well provides sufficient safety for the members to feel free enough to gossip, be flirtatious, be campy, and be as open as possible to sharing intimate aspects of their unique or similar experiences as gay men navigating the world of prostate cancer. That was certainly my experience as a participant in both a mixed-sexual-orientation group and a gay-men-only group.

We wrestled with many emotions. Our shared experiences bonded us. We learned from one another. We held one another emotionally. The men who had HIV/AIDS spoke movingly about being retraumatized as they struggled to come out for a third time: the pain, the fear, the shame. Whether we had HIV/AIDS or not, we all knew the shame of coming out and of having prostate cancer. If they had obvious side effects from their prostate cancer procedures, some men in the group worried about how and what, if anything, to tell a new partner or new hookup. Even men in long-standing relationships were concerned about their partner's reaction to incontinence, erectile dysfunction, burning sensations in their anus, and so forth.

At the doctor's office, most straight guys had their wives there as supporters, note takers, and information gathers. This is helpful because the men are usually so anxious they can't take in much of what is being said. But gay men, as they had initially struggled with being gay alone, were once again often alone in their struggle with prostate cancer. Even men who had partners left them home. They didn't want to upset their partner's work schedule, or they didn't want to "out" themselves to the doctor, or they needed to prove they could handle it themselves, the not-uncommon feeling among men of confusing isolation with independence. Even I, who have a longtime partner, now husband, went to the doctor's alone. I took the false bravado position of "It's no big deal and, honey, why don't you just go to work." I can't imagine many wives allowing their husbands to go without them. Men!

We all experienced anger. We were angry that we had the disease, angry at feeling like damaged goods again, angry at the lack of information pertinent to gay men, angry at the heterosexist assumptions in the medical field, angry at the withholding of information by many physicians, angry at the dismissive attitude many felt with straight doctors, even the so-called gay-friendly ones. We all felt angry at the lack of clear choices regarding treatment and pathways to health that could reassure us that the cancer wouldn't return. Younger men felt angry at having what they considered an old man's disease. We often felt lost.

Many of us felt the pain of loss regarding body integrity, sexual freedom, self-esteem, and control over one's life. We grieved over the loss of body parts and functions. Some men struggled with the changes in sexual feelings and sensations that often occur after some prostate cancer treatments. For example, some men experienced a loss of sensation in areas of the body that had once felt highly erotic; spontaneity may be lost, particularly if one needs pills, injections, insertions, or pumps to get and maintain an erection. Sometimes visual or fantasy stimulation may no longer work automatically to produce an erection. More tactile stimulation may be needed to get aroused. This was particularly true for men over 70 in the group. But, as they say, where there's a will there's a way, and I applaud the ingenuity of many of the men with whom I have worked. One fellow noted that he never left home without his cock ring. A man who ejaculated urine rather than semen became quite a star in the world of golden showers. For others, acquiring new areas of eroticism was a pleasant surprise. Not all gay men are genital-centric.

UNCERTAINTY AND RECOVERY

Hearing the words "You have prostate cancer" and coming to a decision about what to do about it is a very complicated and anxiety-ridden experience. Each man comes to a decision that seems right for him. And he lives with the results of that decision. It is different for each of us. I went through a great deal of anguish and pain as I engaged and wrestled with prostate cancer, but in the end, the journey has been transformative, both personally and professionally. It has given me the opportunity to lead groups and consult individually with other gay men who are struggling with prostate cancer. It has allowed me to edit two books and write several papers on the subject and to share some of my experience with the readers. On a personal level, it has forced me to reconsider the role of sex in my life. My attitude most often these days is "It is what it is." My ability to be open, to acknowledge my need of others, to be more authentic, and to feel far less toxic shame than I once did continues to evolve. The uncertainty of life never ceases to surprise me. John Lennon, among others, said that life is what happens while you're making other plans. Prostate cancer was certainly an unexpected event in my life. It has, however, pushed me to work on my capacity to accept life's uncertainty, and to struggle with surrendering to and accepting the reality of the unexpected in life. It isn't easy to accept the loss of youth, health, sexual certainty, body parts and functions, or the illusion of control. Prostate cancer and the vicissitudes of life have forced me to confront, marvel at, and grieve these aspects of my life. And in so doing, it has allowed me to be thrilled by a beautiful sunset, to smile at a baby, and to appreciate what is. Recovery is a continuous process.

REFERENCES

1. Walsh PC, Worthington JF. *The prostate: A guide for men and the women who love them.* Baltimore: Johns Hopkins University Press; 1995.
2. Giuliani R. *Leadership.* New York: Hyperion; 2002.
3. Wainrib BR. *Prostate cancer: A guide for women and the men they love.* New York: Dell; 1996.
4. Alterowitz R, Alterowitz B. *The lovin' ain't over: The couple's guide to better sex after prostate cancer.* Westbury, N.Y.: Health Education Literary Publisher; 1999.
5. Perlman G, Drescher J. *A gay man's guide to prostate cancer.* Binghamton, N.Y.: Haworth Medical Press; 2005.
6. Perlman G, ed. *What every gay man needs to know about prostate cancer.* New York: Magnus Books; 2013.

7. Amiel GE, Goltz HH, Wenker EP, et al. Gay men and prostate cancer: Opportunities to improve HRQOL and access to care. *In* Boehmer U, Elk R, eds. *Cancer and the LGBT community.* New York: Springer; 2015: 159–168.

8. Dowsett GW. "Losing my chestnut": One gay man's wrangle with prostate cancer. *Reproductive Health Matters.* 2008; 16 (32): 145–150.

9. Ussher J, Perz J, Rosser BRS. *Gay and bisexual men living with prostate cancer: From diagnosis to recovery.* New York: Harrington Park Press; 2018.

10. Markman HJ, Stanley SM, Blumberg SL. *Fighting for your marriage: Positive steps for preventing divorce and preserving a lasting love.* San Francisco: Jossey-Bass; 1991.

11. Yalom I. *The theory and practice of group psychotherapy.* 2nd ed. New York: Basic Books; 1975.

CHAPTER 20

A Shared Decision-Making Approach to Assessing Prostate Cancer Risk

A Gay Diary Case Study

B. R. Simon Rosser, William West, and Badrinath R. Konety

CHAPTER SUMMARY

In the United States, prostate cancer screening and diagnosis are advancing a shared decision-making approach whereby the patient and physician, and possibly other key persons such as a spouse, jointly investigate, test, diagnose, and develop a treatment plan tailored to the individual's specific needs. This first-person account uses a single-case, prospective-diary methodology to record the process from PSA testing to biopsy for a gay-identified man experiencing shared decision making in the age of the electronic medical record. The chapter documents the questions, reactions, and decisions that are foremost in the patient's mind as they occur. In addition, the involvement of the patient's husband in the process and the specialist's perspectives are summarized. The key finding is that shared decision making has several strengths, including facilitating patient buy-in and physician-patient communication. Identified weaknesses include the patient's taking at least partial blame when a medical procedure is performed incorrectly, as well as the process progressing at a speed determined in part by the patient. In the age of electronically delivered results, many of the key results and decisions were delivered remotely, facilitated by e-mail communication between patient and physician.

KEY TERMS

case study, gay and bisexual men, prostate cancer, shared decision making, treatment

Ussher, Jane M., Perz, Janette, Rosser, B. R. Simon, eds., *Gay & Bisexual Men Living with Prostate Cancer*
dx.doi.org/10.17312/harringtonparkpress/2018.06.gbmlpc.020
© 2018 Harrington Park Press

INTRODUCTION

Prostate-specific antigen (PSA) testing is controversial and has been widely debated.[1] First approved by the Food and Drug Administration in 1986 as a way to monitor prostate cancer progression, its use as a screening test increased dramatically in 1988.[2] The result has been concerns about overdiagnosis and overtreatment of men with benign prostate hyperplasia.[3] Until 2012, the Centers for Disease Control and Prevention (CDC) recommended annual testing for all men over 50 years and for men with a family history over 40. In 2012 the CDC reversed this policy to oppose PSA-based screening.[4] In 2017 the CDC modified its stance again, and it currently recommends that PSA-based screening be discussed with all men ages 55–69 using a shared decision-making (SDM) approach.

Prostate cancer is one of the most heritable cancers: an estimated 42% of the risk is attributable to genetic factors.[5] This reality leads many men with family histories of prostate cancer to be tested. But PSA screening is complex. Blood PSA levels tend to rise with age, and larger prostates make more PSA. Other factors that can elevate PSA levels include prostatitis, other urinary tract infections, benign prostatic hyperplasia, prostate biopsies, and injury.[6] Because palpation of the prostate can also influence results, PSA screening should be undertaken before any rectal exam is conducted.[7]

SDM is defined as "an approach where clinicians and patients share the best available evidence when faced with the task of making decisions, and where patients are supported to consider options, to achieve informed preferences."[8] There are four key ingredients: (1) that at least two parties—patient and physician—be involved; (2) that both parties share information; (3) that both parties take steps to build a consensus about the preferred treatment; and (4) that an agreement is reached on the treatment to implement.[9] Localized prostate cancer and benign prostate hyperplasia are two of six preference-sensitive conditions in which clinical evidence does not clearly support one treatment option, so SDM is considered particularly appropriate.[10]

Despite an extensive literature review, we could find only one study comparing PSA across sexual orientations. In a California Health Interview Survey, gay and bisexual men (GBM) had lower odds of having an up-to-date PSA test than did heterosexual men ($OR = 0.61$; CI = 0.42, 0.89; $N = 19,410$)[11] No research has documented the SDM approach recommended for PSA testing. Recent advances in technology have also changed the ways patients and physicians communicate through the electronic medical record, potentially altering how SDM is experienced. The following first-person case study, narrated by the senior author (Rosser), is provided to address these gaps in research.

CASE STUDY

Here's my relevant family history. My father died of prostate cancer on November 5, 1992. He was about 62 years old at diagnosis, and 68 at death. In his understanding, the disease progressed primarily because of hospital error. His file was lost, so he did not receive follow-up care until the cancer had disseminated. His demographics are consistent with an early-onset, aggressive prostate cancer. Following the old CDC recommendations, each year my brother and I have faithfully had a PSA test and a prostate digital exam on the anniversary of his death. We do this both to honor our father and to look after each other. So, for 18 years and half a world apart, we have undertaken this ritual and shared our results with each other. This means I have watched my PSA slowly but steadily increase, always remaining within the normal range (less than 4.0). The other relevant demographics are that I am a healthy, 59-year-old, HIV-negative, gay-identified man with a history of prostatitis. I am married to a prostate cancer survivor.

Monday, November 28, 2016. I scheduled my annual prostate exam (and general checkup with my physician), but most of the clinical visit is taken up discussing my symptoms of a severe cold and saying good-bye because he is retiring. Rather than interrupting the consultation to take blood, he suggests we just do the rectal exam first and then do the blood workup after the consult is over. Although we both know this could invalidate the results, we do it. After all, for 18 years, it's always been within the normal range.

Tuesday, November 29. I receive my results online. After three years of receiving a result of 3.19, I see that my PSA score has jumped to 5.09. Damn. I look at the finding, and then click on the graph (figure 20.1). The number tells me I'm no longer in the normal range, and the graph confirms this increase as sudden and not normal. Given that PSA testing instructions say not to palpate the prostate within 48 hours of a PSA test, it could be the first stage of diagnosis or a false positive. Part of me immediately wishes that we had not cut corners in palpating the

FIGURE 20.1 Graph of author's prostate-specific antigen screening results (in ug/L)

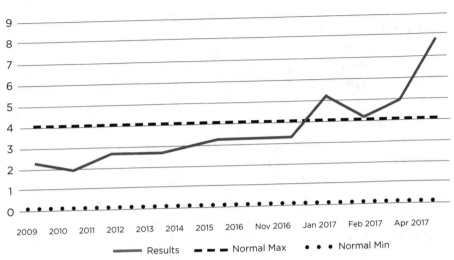

prostate first; part of me feels so bad for my physician. I read the e-mail from him in MyChart: "I usually tell people to wait a month, but a week or two might be fine too if it was just elevated due to my exam. Just schedule a 'lab only' apt anywhere for 2–4 weeks from now. Hope it goes well!" For another patient, this e-mail might sound vague; and in another era, the decision not to inform the patient in person, cold. But my doctor knows me well. It's the right call to leave it to my preference. Still, I feel that I've entered a new phase of e-medicine that is so patient-centric that even the doctor is gone. I'm aware I will receive the result alone. I decide not to be retested this year. I will wait until the new year and make a new start.

Sunday, January 1, 2017. My husband, Bill, and I are in Berlin celebrating New Year's. At midnight, all hell breaks loose, everyone's partying, and now they're firing off fireworks in all directions. It's complete joyous mayhem with ear-splitting explosions everywhere. I find myself on the sidewalk screaming my lungs out, "F**k prostate cancer! You ain't gonna get me." I feel a blessed, cathartic release from holding in all the uncertainty. It's a declaration to myself and the universe that it's a new year and time to face the reality behind the result. Whatever it is, I'm going to be okay.

Monday, January 16. We arrived back in the States on January 10. I'm at home, waiting for my confirmatory PSA test to arrive in my in-box. It will probably appear in MyChart tomorrow. On Friday, I had my second test. I'm philosophical. I figured that some time either my older brother or I would draw the short straw, and it appears that it may be me. On reflection, I am annoyed that the doctor did the rectal exam first, despite knowing that doing so could invalidate the results of the PSA test. But I realize I also bear some responsibility. I knew better and could have resisted, but I hadn't.

I expected to go through some version of stages of grief and adjustment,[12] but they have not occurred. Specifically, I neither minimized the result nor engaged in any bargaining with God—two of Kübler-Ross's classic five stages. I suspect these stages say more about her clients' religious beliefs than anything about a universal psychological process. Given that gay men are less likely to be engaged in traditional religion,[13, 14] these stages may be particularly unsuited for us. We who come to prostate cancer with a family history, and who have been tested for many years, do not necessarily feel so much shock as resignation. There was no need for denial, and, given my familiarity with prostate cancer from my husband's experience, no learning curve. Instead, what I notice is that I immediately accept the elevated results, intellectually. But it's taken me a couple of weeks, and that New Year's outburst, to emotionally accept that my PSA is elevated. On January 9, I have my first dream involving me as a prostate cancer survivor.

I want to repeat the PSA test without any preceding stimulation or palpation of the prostate. Theoretically, any rectal stimulation of the prostate, including that through receptive sex or anal stimulation in masturbation, could invalidate results. This cause-and-effect relationship has not been proven, but it is one proposed explanation for why gay and bisexual men appear to be diagnosed with prostate cancer earlier than heterosexual men. I decide first just to repeat the test. If it comes back elevated, I will wait another couple of weeks with no rectal stimulation whatsoever and have a final test.

Part of my process in adjusting to a potential diagnosis of prostate cancer is to think about potential causes and effects. To the best of current knowledge, I don't have prostate cancer because of anything I have done. Two things I love come to mind: sex and cycling. Though it's possible that repeated vigorous receptive anal sex could damage the prostate, and cycling for miles might cause persistent pressure on and ultimately

A Shared Decision-Making Approach

damage the prostate, neither is confirmed as a risk factor. (Unfortunately, this is more a statement of the lack of rigorous studies on cyclists and on gay men than a confident statement on lack of risk.) But even if either does turn out to be predictive, both activities have brought me such pleasure that I would not change my past to prevent a diagnosis.

Tomorrow I receive my confirmatory test results. While I would prefer my initial results to be a testing error and the results now to be back within the normal range, I pray only for acceptance. I've been wondering why I have not been more freaked out. Perhaps it's my personal history and context as a gay man. Health professionals need to recognize that my cohort of GBM who are being diagnosed with prostate cancer are chiseled veteran survivors. We grew up when homosexuality was deeply stigmatized. Many of us came out when homosexual activity was still illegal, and we risked jobs, family, religious damnation, and careers to claim a life worth living, forged a community, and lived through the worst decades of the AIDS epidemic. Finally, some of us were lucky enough to find happiness and contentment. I'm living a life that was unimaginable to me when I was young. So I am not afraid of prostate cancer, even if it does mean dying early. Indeed, I find myself saying, "It's only prostate cancer," which, fortunately, is a cancer with excellent survival rates.[15]

Given my research, I do not have a lot of irrational fear. What I am most afraid of is being robbed of my sexual functioning (or of cycling). Sex has brought me such joy, and I use it for so much—connecting with my husband, making love, emotional regulation, self-affirmation, and connection to my tribe. But I cannot allow myself to think that far yet. I'm learning that part of going through this process well is "One day at a time." Today is about accepting the possibility that tomorrow I will receive confirmation that I have an elevated PSA.

Tuesday, January 17. My results arrived last night, but I have not gone online to review them. (I had a tiff with Bill and need to wait until we resolve it before learning my fate.) Now that we have sorted it out, I go online and am delighted to receive a new result of 4.13. Immediately, I'm struck by how important context is. If I had not received a result of 5.09, I would be worried at its being elevated. But having received a 5.09, it's hard not to interpret this as being almost back within the normal range. My doctor's note confirms my interpretation: "It's a tough call what to do next. Almost back to normal but not quite. You could discuss this with a urologist. We could watch it and check again in a few months. We could call it close enough and check next year. What do you think?" I e-mail back with my proposal to recheck in four weeks, during which time I plan to focus on increasing fitness (the idea being to be tested under ideal conditions) and ensure a period of no direct prostate stimulation (e.g., receptive sex) before the next test. What I don't know (and suspect no one does) is just how long before a PSA test prostate stimulation can actually affect results. Given that the test says 48 hours, but adding in a highly conservative period to eliminate any doubt, I figure that seven days before retesting is a reasonable period to wait. I'm erring on the extremely conservative side. Before I start down the road of biopsies, which can be painful and have risks, I want to be absolutely sure the results warrant it.

I e-mail my doctor. I propose that if my PSA is back within the normal range within four weeks, I will go back to annual testing and attribute this whole blip to some combination of invalid testing, illness, or infection. If it shoots back up, then a biopsy would seem prudent. But if, as is most likely, it remains just slightly elevated, I'll monitor my PSA with tests every four to eight weeks. Emotionally, I'm oddly okay with active surveillance as a strategy. Before I was actually in this situation, I would have predicted that I could never choose active PSA surveillance. Personality-wise, I'm an impatient "just get it done" type of guy. But knowing the sexual challenges Bill and other GBM prostate cancer survivors live with, I'm now far more comfortable choosing active surveillance. I'm acutely aware I'm not an MD or expert in the medical aspects of prostate cancer, so I need my doctor's input as well.

Friday, January 27. It's been ten days since I got the results. Two realizations. First, going to the gym turns out to be a really helpful, useful practical assignment for guys in an active surveillance phase. I've gone seven of the ten days since the result. The hardest thing for me about waiting weeks for the next result is the waiting; it oozes powerlessness. Even if it is just a placebo, going to the gym gives me something I can physically do to fight against the PSA result. And that's powerful—physically, psychologically, and emotionally. Even if it doesn't move the PSA result, I figure the worst thing it will do is improve my general fitness.

Second, I started telling people but stopped because of the mixed reactions I received. The most important person I told was my brother. I decided not to tell my mother at this time: She's 90, powerless to help, lives in another country; she has already dealt with this with my Dad's diagnosis. I also told a colleague and my trainer, a fellow cyclist. Telling people about an elevated PSA is stressful. I'm learning that while I think of this as *only* prostate cancer, others hear it as *fatal* or *sick, old,* or just *cancer.* In the middle of this, our governor, Mark Dayton, released a statement stating he was just diagnosed with prostate cancer, so it's all over the news. I like the governor and feel less isolated. I wish him well as he sorts out treatment.

Sunday, February 12. Had a good workout today, my cold is finally gone, my sexual behavior has involved no anal stimulation, and I think it's time to have another blood test. The nice thing about active surveillance is that you get to take the tests at your own pace. I'm hopeful of a good result (within normal), but I will just have to wait and see.

Monday, February 13. Had my blood drawn at 9:00 A.M. today, and the results are back by 3:00 P.M. The result is 4.84. The note from my physicians says, "Well, it's not going back to normal. I think you should talk to urology next. The [phone] number is . . ." Damn. I agree with the recommendation.

Tuesday, February 14. I'm dealing with two principal reactions. I have an acute sense of being on my own. Even though Bill went through this eight years ago, it feels isolating. It's my body, my result, and in that sense, it's a unique door that I must go through by myself. The second immediate issue is telling others. So far, only five people know I am going through this. But each time I have told someone, I ended up needing to educate him or her about prostate cancer and PSAs. I don't need people looking at me differently or seeing me as sick. What I want most right now is someone I can talk to about what I am feeling and to help me process *my* reactions. Practically speaking, later today I will make the appointment with the specialist.

Wednesday, March 22. Attended my first urology consult today. It was in the brand-new university outpatient clinic building—all show and no heart. Checking in mirrored being at the airport, only there were no staff to answer questions or reassure the nervous. The resident who saw me seemed to be trained well and made only one unfortunate comment. (He opined that New Yorkers value their erections more than

Minnesotans, based on his experience of men requesting penile implants. No!) He never used my name, asked me about my sexual orientation, or inquired who the man (Bill) sitting beside me was. I saw three nurses, two of whom talked about how busy they were, emphasizing "too busy to follow up with patients." Finally, I see my urologist, Dr. K., who, by contrast, was kind, clear, and compassionate; he was also the first person to even acknowledge Bill's being in the room. Unfortunately, he changed his message from an earlier e-mail's reassurance that my PSA was only mildly elevated, and he explained that now that he'd reviewed my family history of prostate cancer, we would need to be more proactive. He offered me three choices: a biopsy, an advanced blood workup, or an MRI. Given that an MRI could inform a biopsy, I chose options 2 and 3.

I don't know why something called "patient-centered care" has to be so impersonal and uncentered. Why does a 20-minute consult take two hours, most of which the patient spends alone in a room, waiting anxiously? Thank goodness, Bill was there to keep me company and remember key details. Dr. K. explained that family history is everything in prostate cancer, and mine requires action. I left feeling alone, small, and scared—reactions I am sure must be common. Each nurse interaction was strictly confined to asking me health or insurance questions, taking my blood pressure, or printing something out for me. Nurses have become technologists. Two questions I had for Dr. K. were answered. He confirmed my impression that there is no link between cycling and prostate cancer. When I asked him about nutrition, he provided a complex answer. I came away with the message that red vegetables may be particularly good (or possibly bad). I will look it up. MRI on Sunday, blood work on Monday.

Sunday, March 26. Went to the MRI. The technician informs me that an MRI of the prostate is one of the longer ones—in my case, a 45-minute confinement in the machine. While I can see how the machine makes some people feel claustrophobic, I found it okay. In a weird way, lying still in the machine was an opportunity to meditate about my own mortality and accept a prostate cancer diagnosis.

Monday, March 27. Got the results of the MRI in MyChart. The good news is that they've located the suspicious areas, so if we go to biopsy they can focus on these, and even better news, there is no evidence of spread outside the prostate. There's a remark also about prostatitis, but it's unclear to me whether that refers to my history or whether I have it currently. The record tells me I'm a PIRADS 3, which it describes as "intermediate probability." The sentence I focus on is: "The presence of clinically significant cancer is equivocal." Even though I don't understand all the science, I'm glad I had the MRI done. Blood-work results haven't been released to me yet, so I have to wait until Wednesday.

Wednesday, April 5. I arrive for my follow-up. The nurse greets me but doesn't touch me or look at me. She's focused, instead, first on the weighing machine, and then on the computer screen as she asks questions and enters my responses. It feels impersonal, repetitive, as if my record is more important than I am. When I see the resident, he's more relaxed, engaging, with a nice, reassuring smile. I ask him to clarify the prostatitis result and he confirms that it's evidence of *current* infection. He reports the MRI results as equivocal and asks me what I want to do. I joke that I'm rather fond of my prostate and would prefer to keep it "if I get the option." Then I see Dr. K. He informs me that the result of the advanced blood work, called a 4KSCORE, is a 3 (also equivocal), on a scale of 1-2 (clear) and 4-5 (biopsy necessary). Putting the 4K and MRI results together, he tells me I have a 6% chance of having aggressive prostate cancer, which can be confirmed only by biopsy. I ask if the PSA and other results could have been skewed by a subclinical prostatitis and disclose that my urinary urgency has increased. I ask if it makes sense to treat the prostatitis first and repeat the PSA test to see if it is still elevated. He explains that the effects of prostatitis on PSA are unclear, although a major randomized controlled trial where the prostatitis was treated showed no improvement in results. I rationalize that one randomized trial is not a lot of evidence (especially with a nonsignificant result), and that because I want to treat the prostatitis anyway, taking a course of antibiotics and repeating the PSA is a prudent course of action. We then discuss whether I should have a biopsy. Dr. K. explains that either a surveillance period or a biopsy is reasonable. I ask what he would recommend, and he is clear he can defend either. Together we discuss the science, the quality of the evidence, and reach a plan to treat the prostatitis, repeat the PSA test, and then probably do a biopsy.

Thursday, April 27. Finished the course of antibiotics to treat the prostatitis, so I decide it's time for another PSA test. I hope it's returned to normal, but it comes back even more elevated (7.7). I call my doctor's office requesting we make the biopsy a priority. He concurs and will get me this week.

Friday, May 5. Got my biopsy at noon. Not as bad as I feared, more uncomfortable than painful, and it was all over in 45 minutes. A really helpful, reassuring medical assistant answered all my questions. Dr. K. explained everything and talked me through the procedure. He used the MRI results and sonogram to guide where to take 14 samples. Taking each core sample felt more like an itch at the time, although afterward I feel tender. I asked two questions. Dr. K. confirmed it was okay to bike even the day after, but no long bike rides (more than 50 miles) for at least a week. On gay sex, post-biopsy, we acknowledge there is no research or set of clinical guidelines, so we work together using first principles. I explain that gay men typically have three different types of rectal stimulation, each of which needs recommendations. For both fisting and receptive anal sex, Dr. K. recommended a minimum of two weeks without sex to allow time for any bleeding to heal. As for digital stimulation, he proposes it's no problem because it is unlikely to disturb the healing. For the penis, he recommends that it is fine to ejaculate "as soon as comfortable" but warns that blood is likely to be in the ejaculate for up to three months after the biopsy. We agree that at some future point, we should engage other urologists with large gay practices to seek consensus on guidance for GBM. Now I await the results.

DISCUSSION

Before discussing the implications of this case study, it is important to consider the major strengths and weaknesses of a participant-researcher, first-person, diary narrative methodology from a research perspective. Given the lack of earlier studies, case reports are a reasonable first step in documenting the types of issues that patients experience.[16] By providing firsthand accounts of what SDM is like from the patient's perspective, clinicians can better identify and anticipate the patient's experience. A researcher-authored account has the strength that it can identify and report on the most relevant information to inform clinicians (e.g., about gay-specific concerns). The principal weakness is that the experience of researchers is typically atypical. As in all first-person accounts, the reactions identified are deeply subjective, which is both a strength and a weakness.

There are three main findings from the case report. First, in the era of the electronic medical record, much of what is termed SDM is experienced by the patient as e-mail communication received when he is alone, making it harder for the specialist to gauge the patient's reactions, and for questions and answers to occur. On the positive side, major questions are shared by e-mail or text, so there is a narrative record to help the patient remember the key points. Second, SDM is ideal when all goes well, but it places at least partial burden on the patient when things go otherwise. Two instances can be observed in this narrative. First, when the initial PSA test was taken after the digital exam, both patient and provider knew better but colluded for expediency. The system is imperfect. Second, the time from initial test to biopsy was six months. A physician-only decision-making approach could possibly have saved some time. The primary benefit for the patient appears retention of a sense of control over the disease's diagnostic process and a role as his own advocate. We note, at several points, that it was the patient who initiated contact to engage the next stage of diagnosis. The roles of the practitioner are also clear: to provide data, introduce and answer questions, and help interpreting signs.

From the physician's perspective, learning about the emotions, reactions, and concerns of GBM patients can be very helpful. Often, lack of knowledge of a patient's sexual orientation may result in a physician's not paying attention to nuances of diagnosis, such as avoiding anal intercourse before PSA testing. Studies have examined the effect of a rectal exam on PSA and found that it is minimal, even if performed just a few hours before PSA testing. However, a typical rectal exam lasts a few seconds and is different from anal intercourse. It would be helpful for providers to know the sexual orientation of patients; this information is currently not sought in a systematic manner or volunteered routinely by patients (see chapter 1 of this book). Further education regarding the specific concerns of GBM regarding prostate cancer is an essential component to SDM. Finally, the need for documentation in the electronic medical record may have superseded our attention to the patient. Medical students, nurses, and doctors are now taught, "If you did not document it, you did not do it." Hence, they may worry more about documenting than about the patient. SDM is gaining importance and, with regard to PSA testing, there are proposals by the Centers for Medicare and Medicaid Services (CMS) to institute outcome SDM metrics tied to Medicare reimbursement. Doing so will further motivate all providers to use SDM.

For GBM undergoing screening, there are five recommendations. First, it is important for GBM to discuss with their providers the strengths and limitations of the PSA test. Second, it is clearly important that PSA tests be validly conducted. Providers must emphasize that there can be no direct stimulation to the prostate for 48 hours before the blood is collected. Third, repeating a PSA test to confirm a valid, reliable finding or to track trends is a valid option. Fourth, for men used to regular PSA screening, the test should not become a mere routine. Reviewing guidelines using an SDM process is necessary. Finally, we encourage GBM to write down questions or bring a spouse or friend to urological appointments (or both), as these steps are helpful to process the amount of information shared.

For therapists and others providing clinical services for GBM as they are screened, there are three clinical insights. First, a patient's reaction to testing positive is probably determined by the patient's personal connection to this disease. Asking a patient how much he knows about prostate cancer, his history of PSA screening, and contextualizing his results within this history are all critical. Second, relying on stages of grief or other models (e.g., gay adjustment to HIV) to predict patients' reactions may not be helpful. While there are doubtless similarities between diagnoses, the family history and genetic contribution of prostate cancer provide a unique context. Third, diagnosis is not an event but rather a process that may take months or years. At each stage, keeping the patient focused on the immediate decisions is most helpful. Psychologically, promoting a "one day at a time" philosophy was beneficial in this case.

Given that this is the first paper to focus on PSA screening in a gay man, there are several areas identified for future research. First, more formative research is needed to document the experience of PSA screening in GBM. This is a critical step to developing the evidence base needed to identify whether GBM have different screening experiences and needs from other men. Second, on the issue of whether to be screened, it will be important to document the reasons why GBM choose to undertake or avoid prostate checks and PSA screening. Third, we need research on how often PSA testing is validly conducted in GBM. Here, studies should investigate whether GBM know to avoid anal stimulation before blood is collected and how often providers educate GBM patients on this requirement. Fourth, more survey studies comparing GBM and heterosexual men are needed to confirm disparities in testing.

REFERENCES

1. Hayes JH, Barry MJ. Screening for prostate cancer with the prostate-specific antigen test: A review of current evidence. *Journal of the American Medical Association (JAMA).* 2014; 311 (11): 1143–1149.

2. Legler J, Feuer E, Potosky A, et al. The role of prostate-specific antigen (PSA) testing patterns in the recent prostate cancer incidence decline in the USA. *Cancer Causes and Control.* 1998; 9: 519–557.

3. Etzioni R, Penson DF, Legler JM, et al. Overdiagnosis due to prostate-specific antigen screening: Lessons from US prostate cancer incidence trends. *Journal of the National Cancer Institute.* 2002; 94 (13): 981–990.

4. Centers for Disease Control and Prevention (CDC). Should I get screened for prostate cancer? 2017; https://www.cdc.gov/cancer/prostate/basic_info/get-screened.htm. Accessed February 12, 2017.

5. Lichtenstein P, Holm NV, Verkasalo PK, et al. Environmental and heritable factors in the causation of cancer—analyses of cohorts of twins from Sweden, Denmark, and Finland. *New England Journal of Medicine.* 2000; 343 (2): 78–85.

6. American Urological Association. What men should know about prostate screening. 2017; www.auanet.org/media-toolkit-for-early-detection-of-prostate-cancer. Accessed December 12, 2017.

7. Crawford ED, Schutz MJ, Clejan S, et al. The effect of digital rectal examination on prostate-specific antigen levels. *Journal of the American Medical Association (JAMA).* 1992; 267 (16): 2227–2228.

8. Elwyn G, Coulter A, Laitner S, et al. Implementing shared decision making in the NHS. *British Medical Journal.* 2010; 341: c5146.

9. Charles C, Gafni A, Whelan T. Shared decision-making in the medical encounter: What does it mean? (Or it takes at least two to tango). *Social Science & Medicine.* 1997; 44 (5): 681–692.

10. Centers for Medicare and Medicaid Services. Beneficiary engagement and incentives: Shared Decision Making (SDM) Model. 2017; https://innovation.cms.gov/initiatives/Beneficiary-Engagement-SDM/. Accessed April 25, 2017.

11. Heslin KC, Gore JL, King WD, Fox SA. Sexual orientation and testing for prostate and colorectal cancers among men in California. *Medical Care.* 2008; 46 (12): 1240.

12. Kübler-Ross E, Kessler D, Shriver M. *On grief and grieving: Finding the meaning of grief through the five stages of loss.* New York: Simon and Schuster; 2014.

13. Halkitis PN, Mattis JS, Sahadath JK, et al. The meanings and manifestations of religion and spirituality among lesbian, gay, bisexual, and transgender adults. *Journal of Adult Development.* 2009; 16 (4): 250–262.

14. Rosser BRS. Christian and Catholic background and adherence in New Zealand homosexually active males: A psychological investigation. *Journal of Psychology & Human Sexuality*. 1990; 3 (1): 89–115.

15. American Cancer Society. Survival rates for prostate cancer. 2016; www.cancer.org/cancer/prostatecancer/detailedguide/prostate-cancer-survival-rates. Accessed February 24, 2016.

16. Radley A, Chamberlain K. The study of the case: Conceptualising case study research. *Journal of Community & Applied Social Psychology*. 2012; 22 (5): 390–399.

GLOSSARY

This glossary includes not only terms used in prostate cancer treatment, research, and sexology but also colloquial terms that have specific meanings or nuances within the LGBT community. We gratefully acknowledge the online NCI Dictionary of Cancer terms, the Oxford Living Concise Dictionaries, and Wikipedia for standard definitions. Definitions, colloquialisms, and contextual terms have been tailored to the focus of this text.

Active surveillance: A treatment plan that involves closely watching a patient's condition but not giving any treatment unless there are changes in test results that show the condition is getting worse. During active surveillance, exams and tests are done on a regular schedule.

AIDS-defining cancers: Three cancers—Kaposi('s) sarcoma, non-Hodgkin's lymphoma, and cervical cancer—are termed AIDS-defining cancers because a diagnosis of any one of them in a person diagnosed with HIV then determines a diagnosis of AIDS.

Androgen deprivation therapy (ADT): Treatment to suppress or block the production or action of male hormones. This treatment requires having the testicles removed, taking female sex hormones, or taking drugs called antiandrogens. Also called *androgen ablation* and *androgen suppression*.

Anodyspareunia: Recurrent or persistent pain experienced by the receptive partner during anal stimulation or intercourse. To meet clinical criteria, it must be (a) recurrent or persistent, (b) sufficient to cause marked distress or interpersonal difficulty, and (c) not caused by other medical or mental conditions or exclusively by other behavioral determinants (such as lack of lubrication or relaxation technique).

Antiretroviral (ARV) treatment: Denoting or relating to a class of drugs that inhibit the activity of retroviruses such as HIV. Also called *antiretroviral treatment (ART), highly active antiretroviral treatment (HAART)*, and referred to colloquially as *HIV drug cocktail* or *HIV medications*.

Aporia: In the context of prostate cancer treatment in gay and bisexual men, the introduction of doubt and distrust in the patient generated by the specialist's response (or lack of response), such as denial of the patient's experience.

Asynchronous: *Adjective*. A term used in online research to specify that the study does not require participants to complete activities at the same time. An online focus group is a typical example of a synchronous activity, whereas posting to a message board or commenting on other's posts is typically asynchronous.

Benign prostatic hyperplasia (BPH): An enlarged prostate due to normal aging. As the prostate enlarges, it can put pressure on the urethra, causing voiding problems. It does not lead to prostate cancer.

Bicalutamide: Sold under the brand name Casodex, bicalutamide is an antiandrogen medication that is primarily used to treat prostate cancer.

Biopsy: A prostate gland biopsy is a test to remove small samples of prostate tissue to be looked at under a microscope. A thin hollow needle is inserted up the rectum and through the wall of the rectum into the prostate. Most urologists will take about 12 core samples from different parts of the prostate.

Bisexual: *Adjective:* Pertaining to sexual activity with both genders. *Noun:* Someone who is romantically attracted to or sexually oriented toward both genders. *Identity label:* Someone who identifies as sexually oriented toward both genders.

Bother: One of two scales commonly used in prostate cancer research to estimate the effect of treatment on quality of life. Whereas *function* refers to the frequency of difficulties in sexual, urinary, bowel, or hormone-related behavior, *bother* refers to how big a problem it is in a person's day-to-day life. See also **Function** and **Health-related quality of life**.

Bottom: *Verb:* To engage in oral, anal, or vaginal sex as the receptive partner. *Identity label:* Someone who identifies as being or preferring to be the receptive partner (typically in anal sex).

Bowel incontinence: Inability to hold feces in the bowel. Lack of voluntary control over defecation.

Brachytherapy: The treatment of cancer, especially prostate cancer, by the insertion of radioactive implants directly into the tissue.

Butt plug: A phallic- or spindle-shaped object flanged or handled at the bottom designed to completely fill the anus.

Case-control study: A research study that compares persons with a condition or outcome of interest (cases) with persons who do not have the condition or outcome (controls), and retrospectively compares how frequently the exposure to a risk factor is present in each group.

Caverject injection: A prostaglandin injection into the penis. It works by relaxing certain muscles in the penis and widening blood vessels, which increases blood flow to the penis and helps cause an erection.

Chosen family: A term used in the gay community and sex research to denote a network of friends who function as an intimate support network (and often as a substitution for or in contrast to biological family in situations where the biological family is estranged).

Chronic disease: A condition that persists over a long period and generally cannot be prevented by vaccines or cured by medication, and one that does not just disappear.

Cisgender: A person whose sense of personal identity and gender corresponds with his or her birth sex.

Climacturia: Urination during orgasm. It is a relatively common side effect of radical prostatectomy, occurring in 22% to 43% of men after prostatectomy.

Cock ring: A penile vasoconstrictive device, often made of rubber and worn at the base of the penis, to increase rigidity and duration of penile erection.

Cohort study: A study design in which one or more groups of people (called *cohorts*) are followed prospectively and evaluated at subsequent times for a disease or outcome. The study is conducted to identify which risk factors are associated with a disease.

Coitus: Penis-vagina sexual intercourse.

Comorbidity: The simultaneous presence of two or more chronic diseases or conditions (e.g., HIV and prostate cancer) in a patient.

Controlled study: A study in which one group of people (e.g., GBM prostate cancer survivors) is compared with another group (e.g., heterosexual prostate cancer survivors) to identify differences in variables of interest (e.g., urinary function) between the groups.

Couplehood: A term used in research to describe two persons or a dyad who identify as a couple or as being in some form of a long-term relationship.

Couple's disease: A description of prostate cancer that emphasizes how the sexual and other effects of treatment have an influence on both partners in a relationship.

Cowper's glands: A pair of small pea-shaped glands located beneath the prostate that open into the urethra at the base of the penis. They secrete pre-ejaculate and add to ejaculate.

Da Vinci robot: A robotic surgical system, approved by the U.S. Food and Drug Administration in 2000, designed to facilitate complex surgery, including radical prostatectomy, using a minimally invasive approach.

Decisional (or treatment) regret: Distress or remorse about an earlier healthcare decision.

Depend: A popular brand of disposable diapers or underwear containing absorbent material that is used by persons with incontinence.

Diagnosis: The process of identifying a disease, condition, or injury from its signs and symptoms.

Digital rectal exam (DRE): An examination in which a health provider inserts a lubricated, gloved finger into the rectum to feel for abnormalities.

Discrimination: Unjust or prejudicial acts against a person or group on the grounds of an actual or perceived characteristic. In social science research, it is one of two types of stigma. See also **Stigma**.

Ejaculation: The release of semen through the penis during orgasm.

Epidemiology: The study of the prevalence, distribution, and possible control of disease and other factors relating to health at the community or population level.

Erectile dysfunction (ED): An inability to achieve and sustain erection of the penis sufficient for completion of sexual activity. In prostate cancer research, ED has been operationalized, historically, as an erection of the penis adequate for coital sexual intercourse. Also called **Impotence**.

Eunuch: A man who does not have functioning gonads. In prostate cancer treatment, there are two common treatments that result in this condition: surgical castration, in which the testicles are removed, and chemical castration, in which the production of androgen is suppressed. See also **Androgen deprivation therapy**.

Finasteride: Sold under the brand names Proscar and Propecia, among others, finasteride is a medication used for the treatment of benign prostatic hyperplasia (enlarged prostate).

Function: One of two scales commonly used in prostate cancer research to estimate the effect of the frequency of sexual, urinary, bowel, and hormonal difficulties on quality of life. See also **Bother** and **Health-related quality of life**.

Gay: *Adjective:* Referring to sexual interest in or activity with the same gender, most commonly used to describe interest or activity between two men. *Noun:* Someone who is romantically attracted to or sexually oriented toward the same gender. *Identity label:* Someone who identifies as sexually oriented toward the same gender.

Gay and bisexual men (GBM): An umbrella term to cover the population of cisgender and transgender men who are attracted to or sexually active (or both) with other men, including those who identify as gay or bisexual and those who have these attractions or behavior but do not identify as such.

Gay community: See **Lesbian, gay, bisexual, transgender, questioning, and intersex (LGBTQI)**.

Gay couple: An ongoing sexual or romantic relationship involving two men, implying a commitment to each other. Also termed a *male couple* or a *same-sex male couple*.

Gay pride: 1. A sense of dignity and satisfaction in connection with the public acknowledgment of one's own homosexuality. 2. An annual celebration by the LGBT community, usually held in June (in the Northern Hemisphere), to commemorate Stonewall, a series of violent demonstrations against a police raid from June 28 to July 1, 1969, at the Stonewall Inn, a gay bar in New York City. The demonstrations mark the birth of the modern LGBT community.

Gender and sexual minorities (GSM): A social science, legal, and policy umbrella term that identifies LGBT persons as a minority population with challenges and concerns similar to those of other racial, ethnic, and indigenous populations. See also **Gender minority** and **Sexual-minority men**.

Gender minority: An umbrella term for anyone who transcends traditional concepts of gender as binary (male-female) and does not identify with the gender assigned at birth. Sometimes it is used as analogous to *transgender* and sometimes more broadly to include anyone who may transcend or transgress gender roles.

Gender-reassignment surgery: The surgical procedure(s) by which transgender persons' physical appearance and the function of their existing sexual characteristics are altered to resemble their identified gender. It is part of the treatment for gender dysphoria (and also for intersex conditions). Also known as *gender-reassignment surgery, genital-reconstruction surgery, gender-confirmation surgery,* or *sex-realignment surgery.* For transgender women, it may involve feminizing genitoplasty, penectomy, orchidectomy, and vaginoplasty (none of which typically includes the removal of the prostate).

Gleason score: A grading of prostate cancer tissue on the basis of how it looks under a microscope. Gleason scores range from 2 to 10 and indicate how likely it is that a tumor will spread. A low Gleason score means the cancer tissue is similar to normal prostate tissue and the tumor is less likely to spread; a high Gleason score means the cancer tissue is very different from normal tissue and the tumor is more likely to spread.

Grounded theory: A method used in qualitative research involving the construction of theory through systematic analysis of data.

Gynecomastia: The swelling of the breast tissues in boys or men, caused by an imbalance of the hormones estrogen and testosterone, sometimes a side effect in hormonal treatment for prostate cancer.

Health disparities: A public health term to describe demographic differences in health outcomes. Often used to denote differences by race or ethnicity, the term also denotes differences by sex, sexual identity, age, disability, socioeconomic status, and geography. In 2016 the U.S. National Institutes of Health formally included **Gender and sexual minorities** as part of health disparities research.

Health Insurance Portability and Accountability Act (HIPAA): HIPAA is a law in the United States governing privacy standards to protect patients' medical records and other health information.

Health-related quality of life (HRQOL): The overall enjoyment of life. Many research studies assess the effects of prostate cancer and its treatment on the quality of life. The measures used in prostate cancer research typically assess the ability to carry out activities (termed **Function**) and the difficulty, pain, or challenge in doing so (termed **Bother**).

Hegemonic: *Adjective:* A social science term to denote social, cultural, ideological, or economic influence (or a combination) exerted by a dominant group. In this context, it describes how heterosexual society influences gender and sexuality norms.

Heterocentrism: A heterosexual bias or focus that may result in the discrimination, exclusion, marginalization, or neglect of LGBT persons.

Heteronormativity: The belief that people fall into distinct and complementary genders (male and female) with natural roles in life, and that this is both normal and desirable.

Heterosexism: A system of attitudes, biases, and discrimination that favors opposite-sex sexuality and relationships. It includes the presumption that other people are (or should be) heterosexual.

Heterosexual: *Adjective:* Descriptor of opposite-sex-oriented sexual attraction and behavior in humans or other species used in clinical, research, legal, and other professional communication. *Identity label:* Someone who identifies as romantically or sexually oriented toward the other gender. Also known colloquially as *straight.*

HIV/AIDS: Human immunodeficiency virus (HIV) infection and acquired immune deficiency syndrome (AIDS) comprise a spectrum of conditions caused by infection with HIV. HIV/AIDS is endemic in GBM communities and in recent decades has been the leading cause of death of GBM.

HIV-positive: Having had a positive result in a blood test for the virus HIV.

Homosexual: *Adjective:* Descriptor of same-sex sexual behavior or attractions in humans or other species used in clinical, research, legal, and other professional communication. *Identity label:* Used historically as an identity label but now dated. Currently used to identify same-sex sexually oriented individuals to pathologize, criminalize, politicize, or denigrate them.

Hormone therapy: Treatment that adds, blocks, or removes hormones. To slow or stop the growth of prostate cancer, synthetic hormones or other drugs may be given to block the body's natural hormones. Also called *endocrine therapy* and *hormonal therapy.*

Illness Intrusiveness Theoretical Framework (IITF): The study of how chronic life-threatening health conditions disrupt or compromise quality of life.

Immunodeficiency: A weakening of a body's ability to fight infections and diseases. It is either congenital (i.e., present at birth) or acquired (e.g., through infection with HIV).

Impotence: A synonym for **Erectile dysfunction.**

Incidence: A measure in epidemiology of the number of new cases during some time period, often expressed as a percentage rate within a population.

Inclusion/exclusion criteria: Criteria used in research studies to identify who is eligible (inclusion) or not eligible (exclusion) to participate in a study.

Insertive partner: In the context of gay male sex, the man or transgender woman who places the penis into another person's anus, mouth, or vagina.

Interdependence theory: A social exchange theory that examines how the rewards and costs of interpersonal relationships influence human interactions.

Internalized homonegativity: Negative attitudes (e.g., shame, guilt) that gay men have toward their own and others' gay sexual orientation. In colloquial language, it is sometimes still called *internalized homophobia* (but this term is now considered inaccurate because it does not resemble a clinical phobia or pathology).

Intracavernosal injection: An injection into the base of the penis often used to treat erectile dysfunction in men. See also **Caverject injection.**

Kegels: Exercises performed to strengthen the pelvic floor muscles, developed originally for women recovering from childbirth, but used also to combat urinary incontinence. See also **Pelvic floor rehabilitation.**

Lesbian, gay, bisexual, transgender, questioning, and intersex (LGBTQI): The LGBT community, also referred to as the gay community, is loosely defined groups of lesbian (L), gay (G), bisexual (B), and transgender (T) persons—to which queer-identified or questioning (Q) and intersex (I) are added. LGBT-supportive people or allies (A) are sometimes also added: organizations, businesses, and subcultures united by a common culture and social movements.

Libido: The sexual urge, desire, instinct, or drive.

Liminality: A transitional or initial stage of a process.

Magnetic resonance imaging (MRI): A procedure in which radio waves and a powerful magnet linked to a computer are used to create detailed pictures of areas inside the body, including the prostate. In preparation for prostate cancer biopsies, it can be used to better detect likely areas of cancer.

Marginalization: Treatment of a person, group, or concept as insignificant or peripheral.

Minority stress theory: The theory that racial, sexual, gender, and other minorities experience chronic high levels of stress through the experience of discrimination, microaggression, marginalization, and other stigma. Minority stress has been put forward as an explanation for higher rates of psychological distress in LGBTQI populations.

MyChart: An electronic medical record software that stores medical data electronically and allows both health professionals and patients to access the record remotely. It includes such features as appointment reminders, graphs of medical data, and the ability for providers and patients to e-mail each other within a secure system that complies with the Health Insurance Portability and Accountability Act (HIPAA).

Observational study: A type of study in which individuals are observed or certain outcomes are measured (e.g., a survey or interviews). Unlike clinical trials, which may test a treatment, no attempt is made to affect the outcome.

Oncology: A branch of medicine that specializes in the diagnosis and treatment of cancer. It includes medical oncology (the use of chemotherapy, hormone therapy, and other drugs to treat cancer), radiation oncology (the use of radiation therapy to treat cancer), surgical oncology (the use of surgery and other procedures to treat cancer), and psycho-oncology (focusing on psychosocial aspects of living with cancer or cancer survivorship).

Oral sex: Sexual activity using the mouth. In the context of gay male sex, oral sex typically involves mouth-on-penis (fellatio), but it can also include mouth-on-testicles (tea-bagging) and mouth-on-anus (anilingus).

Orchidectomy: Surgery to remove one or both testicles. Also called *orchiectomy*.

Orgasm: The climax of sexual excitement, characterized by intensely pleasurable feelings usually centered in the genitals. Orgasm is a central nervous system activity resulting in feelings usually of pleasure that are distinct from ejaculation (the physiologic production of seminal or other fluid). See also **Sexual response cycle**.

Outness: The quality or state of being out, originally focused on sexual orientation, but which can also be applied to how public or private a person is about having a disease, such as HIV or prostate cancer.

Ovariectomy: Surgery to remove the ovaries.

Pelvic floor rehabilitation: A series of exercises to strengthen the muscular base of the abdomen, used in prostate cancer treatment primarily to treat urinary incontinence.

Penile implant: A firm rod or inflatable device that is placed in the penis during a surgical procedure. The implant makes it possible to have and keep an erection. Penile implants are used to treat erectile dysfunction, or impotence.

Phosphodiesterase type 5 inhibitor (PDE5i) drugs: A class of erectile-enhancing medications used to treat erectile dysfunction. They work by increasing blood flow to the penis, causing an erection. Common PDE5 inhibitors recommended for the treatment of erectile dysfunction include sildenafil (Viagra), tadalafil (Cialis), and vardenafil (Levitra).

Potency: The ability to achieve an erection or to reach orgasm.

Prevalence: A count, used in epidemiology, of the total number of individuals with a condition. Common prevalence measures include lifetime prevalence (e.g., the number of men who will be diagnosed with prostate cancer over their lifetime), period prevalence (e.g., the number of men sexually active with men during the last five years), and point prevalence (e.g., the number with a condition at a specific time).

Prostate: A gland in the male reproductive system. The prostate surrounds the part of the urethra (the tube that empties the bladder) just below the bladder and in front of the rectum, and produces a fluid that forms part of the semen.

Prostate cancer: Cancer that forms in tissues of the prostate. Prostate cancer usually occurs in older men.

Prostate-specific antigen (PSA) test: A laboratory test that measures the amount of prostate-specific antigen (PSA) in the blood. PSA is a protein made by the prostate gland. The amount of PSA is typically higher in men who have prostate cancer, benign prostatic hyperplasia (BPH), or infection or inflammation of the prostate.

Prosthesis: A device, such as an artificial leg, that replaces a part of the body. In prostate cancer, an alternative term for **Penile implant.**

Quality of life (QoL): See **Health-related quality of life (HRQOL).**

Queer: Sexual or gender identity that does not correspond to established ideas of sexuality and gender, especially heterosexual norms.

Queer theory: An approach to social and cultural studies that seeks to challenge or deconstruct traditional ideas of sexuality and gender that appear based in **heteronormativity.**

Radiation therapy: The treatment of cancer or other diseases using X-rays or other forms of radiation.

Radical prostatectomy: Surgery to remove the entire prostate and some of the tissue around it. Nearby lymph nodes may also be removed.

Receptive partner: In the context of gay male sex, the man or transgender woman who has a penis or other object inserted into the anus, mouth, or vagina.

Rehabilitation: A medical term to describe the process of restoring to health through training and therapy. In prostate cancer, it denotes training and therapy to address the common sexual, urinary, bowel, and hormonal effects of treatment.

Relationality: The state of being in relationship or considered in relation to another.

Role-in-sex: In same-sex relationships, the pattern or preference to be the insertive partner (see **Top**), receptive partner (see **Bottom**), or to be in both roles (see **Versatile**). It is distinct from sex roles, which are defined as roles or behavioral patterns learned by a person as appropriate to his or her gender and typically determined by prevailing cultural norms.

Saturation: A term used in qualitative research to describe the point at which collecting more data will not yield more information on the research question(s). It is frequently used to describe the number of persons who need to be interviewed to sufficiently investigate a research question.

Seeds: Radioactive seed implants are a form of radiation therapy for prostate cancer. Also known as **brachytherapy** or *internal radiation therapy*. A doctor implants 40 to 100 seeds into the prostate gland, using ultrasound for guidance.

Semen: The fluid that is released through the penis during orgasm. Semen is made up of sperm from the testicles and fluid from the prostate and other sex glands. Colloquially known as *cum*.

Semen exchange or "gifting": Playing with ejaculate in some deliberate way, for example, licking it off a body, transferring it through kissing, or otherwise giving it from one person to another.

Serum: The clear liquid part of the blood that remains after blood cells and clotting proteins have been removed.

Sex roles: The roles persons learn as appropriate to their gender, as determined by prevailing cultural norms.

Sexual disqualification: The experience of no longer being considered, or not considering oneself, a sexual person.

Sexual dysfunction: An umbrella term covering any difficulty in performing sex across the sexual response cycle. It includes difficulties in sexual interest (libido), arousal (e.g., difficulties getting or sustaining erections, or pain in receptive sex), and orgasm (e.g., anorgasmia or pain during orgasm).

Sexual health: A state of physical, mental, and social well-being in relation to sexuality. It requires a positive and respectful approach to sexuality and sexual relationships, as well as the possibility of having pleasurable and safe sexual experiences that are free of coercion, discrimination, and violence (World Health Organization definition). See also **Sexual well-being.**

Sexually transmitted infection (STI): An infection passed from one person to another or others through sexual contact, such as oral, vaginal, or anal sex (e.g., syphilis, gonorrhea). Older terms for STI include *sexual transmitted disease (STD)* and *venereal disease (VD)*.

Sexual-minority men: Men whose sexual identity, orientation, or practices are different from those of the majority (i.e., exclusively heterosexual men). The term is used primarily to refer to the LGBT population but also includes persons who engage in sex with men, but may not identify as lesbian, gay, bisexual, or transgender. In demography research, *gender and sexual minority* is becoming the preferred term; it denotes the population of persons whose gender identity or sexual identity, orientation, or practice is different from the majority's. The term *gender and sexually diverse persons* is also sometimes used.

Sexual mode: An Australian term for **Role-in-sex.**

Sexual orientation: An enduring pattern of romantic or sexual attraction to persons of the opposite gender (heterosexual), the same gender (homosexual, gay, or lesbian), or both or more than one gender (bisexual).

Sexual response cycle: A physiological model describing human sexual behavior across distinct phases of sexual expression, from desire to arousal and excitement, to plateau, then to orgasm and resolution.

Sexual subcultures: Subgroups of people, often with distinct sexual beliefs or interests. As used in this text, gay sexual subcultures might include such groups as leather men, the bear community (hairy men), the polygamous community (multiple sex partners), S&M (giving and receiving pain during sex), and party and play (sex with party drugs).

Sexual well-being: The state of being comfortable, healthy, or happy with one's sexuality and sexual life. The term *well-being* is sometimes used to reflect a broader meaning not narrowly defined by physical health or functioning; it is often used by clinicians working with patients diagnosed with chronic disease.

Shared decision-making (SDM) model: A structured approach to patient-centered care whereby clinicians and patients work together to make decisions that balance risks and expected outcomes with patient preferences and values. In the United States, prostate cancer treatment is one of six conditions for which SDM is recommended.

Spatiality: Any property relating to or occupying space.

Stigma: Something with a significant negative association attached to it. Social science distinguishes at least two types of stigma: enacted stigma (e.g., experience of **Discrimination**) and felt stigma (e.g., **Internalized homonegativity**).

Surveillance: A public health term for the ongoing systematic collection, recording, analysis, interpretation, and dissemination of data that reflect the current health status of a community or population.

Survivorship: In cancer research, survivorship focuses on the health and life of a person with cancer after treatment and extending until the end of life. It covers the physical, psychosocial, and economic issues of cancer beyond the diagnosis and treatment phases. Survivorship includes issues related to the ability to get healthcare and follow-up treatment, late effects of treatment, second cancers, and quality of life. Family members, friends, and caregivers are also considered part of the survivorship experience.

Temporality: The state of existing within, or having some relationship with, time.

Tenesmus: Cramping rectal pain. Tenesmus makes a person feel that he needs to have a bowel movement, even if he just had one.

Top: *Verb:* To engage in oral, vaginal, or anal sex as the insertive partner. *Identity label:* Someone who identifies as the insertive partner (typically in anal sex).

Transgender: A person whose personal identity and gender do not correspond with the sex assigned at birth. It is also an umbrella term for anyone whose gender identity is not exclusively male or female. Colloquially the term *trans* is commonly used.

Transgender woman (TGW): A person who was assigned male at birth because of being born with male genitals (and with a prostate) who now identifies as a woman and who may have had gender-reassignment surgery.

Transsexual: A term historically used to describe transgender individuals.

Tumor-nodes-metastasis (TNM): A grading system used in prostate cancer treatment. It describes a tumor on the basis of how abnormal the cancer cells and tissue look under a microscope and how quickly the cancer cells are likely to grow and spread. Also called *tumor grade* and *histologic grade.*

Urinary incontinence: Inability to hold urine in the bladder, a lack of voluntary control over urination.

Urinary leakage during sex: A common symptom following prostate cancer treatment whereby a man who cannot sufficiently tighten the muscles that close off the urethra releases urine at some time during sex or at orgasm. See also **Climacturia.**

Urology: The surgical specialty that deals with the treatment of conditions involving the male and female urinary tract and the male reproductive organs (including prostate cancer).

Vacuum pump (vacuum erection device): A pump consisting of a plastic tube, which fits over the penis and creates a vacuum to help the penis become erect, and a tight band (or constriction ring) to maintain the erection.

Versatile: *Adjective:* Engaging in oral, anal, or vaginal sex as both the insertive and receptive partner. *Identity label:* Someone who identifies as preferring to be both the insertive and receptive partner or having no preference (typically when referring to anal sex between two men).

Viagra: See **Phosphodiesterase type 5 inhibitor (PDE5i) drugs.**

Watchful waiting: Closely watching a patient's medical condition but not giving treatment unless symptoms appear or change. Watchful waiting is sometimes used in conditions that progress slowly. It is also used in advanced cancer patients when the risks of treatment are greater than the possible benefits. See also **Active surveillance.**

ABOUT THE EDITORS AND CONTRIBUTORS

Donald Allensworth-Davies, PhD, is an assistant professor with the School of Health Sciences at Cleveland State University, where he is also the coordinator for the Consortium of Eastern Ohio Master of Public Health Program. He served as co-investigator for one of the first national surveys in the United States of gay prostate cancer survivors funded by the National Cancer Institute, and he continues to focus his research efforts on GBT prostate cancer survivorship as well as health disparities among LGBT elders.

Jonathan Bergman, MD, MPH, is assistant professor of urology and family medicine at UCLA, and at Olive View–UCLA Medical Center and the Veterans Administration Greater Los Angeles. His research and clinical focus includes health services research, population health, and end-of-life care.

Thomas O. Blank, PhD, is professor emeritus in the Department of Human Development and Family Studies at the University of Connecticut. His article in the *Journal of Clinical Oncology* in 2005 was the first to identify the specific needs and issues of gay men with prostate cancer. He and his colleagues Marysol Asencio and Lara Descartes have contributed a number of chapters and articles to the literature on gay men and prostate cancer and, more generally, LGBTQ communities and cancer.

Perry Brass's nineteen published books include the best-selling self-help books *How to Survive Your Own Gay Life* (1999) and *The Manly Art of Seduction* (2010), the futurist novel *Carnal Sacraments* (2007), and the coming-of-age novel *King of Angels* (2014), a finalist for a Ferro-Grumley Award from New York's Publishing Triangle, set in Kennedy-era Savannah, Georgia. In 1969 he coedited *Come Out!*, the world's first gay liberation newspaper, published by the Gay Liberation Front. In 1972 he cofounded with two friends the Gay Men's Health Project Clinic, the first clinic specifically for gay men on the East Coast, still operating as the Callen-Lorde Community Health Center. Brass's work deals with issues of sexual freedom, personal authenticity, and liberation politics that have emerged from his continuing involvement—ever since the Stonewall Rebellion—with the movement for what is now called LGBT rights..

Benjamin D. Capistrant, ScD, is an assistant professor and social epidemiologist in the Division of Epidemiology and Community Health at the University of Minnesota School of Public Health, Minneapolis. He specializes in aging research, including examining the social support and caregiving needs of GBM prostate cancer survivors, their spouses, and support networks.

Lynae Darbes, PhD, is a psychologist and behavioral scientist whose primary focus is the influence that partners and relationship dynamics have on health behavior. Her career has also focused on investigating the relationship context of sexual minorities, especially same-sex male couples. She has been principal investigator on several NIMH-funded grants to develop and test interventions focused on couples, including same-sex male couples.

Brian de Vries, PhD, is a professor of gerontology at San Francisco State University; he received his doctorate in life-span developmental psychology from the University of British Columbia in 1988. Dr. de Vries is a fellow of the Gerontological Society of America and past board member of the American Society on Aging. He has edited five books, authored or coauthored over 100 journal articles and book chapters, and given more than 150 presentations to local, national, and international professional audiences on the social and psychological well-being of midlife and older LGBT persons, among other topics.

Gary W. Dowsett, PhD, is a professor, deputy director, and chair at the Australian Research Centre in Sex, Health, and Society at La Trobe University, Melbourne. A sociologist, he has specialized in HIV/AIDS research, both internationally and in Australia's gay communities. He has also worked in sexuality and masculinity studies and men's health. He is a fellow of the Academy of the Social Sciences in Australia.

Murray Drummond, PhD, is a professor in sport, health, and physical activity and the director of the SHAPE Research Centre at Flinders University, Adelaide, Australia. His research interests are in qualitative health research, with a particular focus on men and masculinities within the context of sport, health, and body image.

Duane Duncan, PhD, is a lecturer at the University of New England, New South Wales, Australia, and an adjunct research fellow at the Australian Research Centre in Sex, Health, and Society at La Trobe University, Melbourne. His work as a sociologist explores broad shifts in the performance of masculine identities in relation to consumer culture, neoliberal governmentality, and wider transformations in gender relations characterizing late modernity.

Daniel R. du Plooy, MPhil, is a PhD candidate and research officer at the Australian Research Centre in Sex, Health, and Society at La Trobe University, Melbourne. His current research is on migrant well-being in Australia.

Shaun Filiault, PhD, holds an LLM in U.S. law and is currently pursuing a doctorate in law at the University of New Hampshire, having previously been awarded a PhD in health sciences. He is a professor of psychology at River Valley Community College in New Hampshire and a judicial law clerk in the U.S. District Court for the District of Massachusetts. He previously held a position as a lecturer in health promotion at Flinders University, Adelaide, Australia.

Clement K. Gwede, PhD, MPH, RN, FAAN, is a senior member and professor of health outcomes and behavior and population sciences at Moffitt Cancer Center and the University of South Florida's Department of Oncologic Sciences in the Morsani College of Medicine, Tampa. His research addresses health disparities and informed and shared decision making across the continuum of cancer control, including the role of patient preferences, toxicities, and quality of life in treatment decisions among patients with newly diagnosed localized prostate cancer.

Crystal Hare, BSc, is completing a master's degree in clinical psychology at Ryerson University, Toronto, Canada. Her primary research focus is psychosocial oncology, including changes in sleep patterns and fatigue levels associated with cancer diagnosis and treatment.

Tae L. Hart, PhD, CPsych, is professor of psychology at Ryerson University, Toronto, Canada. Tae's research centers on psychological factors associated with adjustment to illness in chronically ill individuals, primarily quality of life, psychological distress, and symptom burden in patients who have been diagnosed with cancer, multiple sclerosis, or gastrointestinal disorders.

Ross Henderson, Grad Dip Couns, is currently completing his master's in Gestalt psychotherapy. He is a counselor and psychotherapist in private practice in Sydney, Australia. He has over 20 years' experience in adult education and has delivered training as both lecturer and tutor to undergraduate and postgraduate students in counseling psychology. He has worked for a variety of corporate and nongovernmental organizations in both managerial and counseling capacities over the last 30 years.

Michael A. Hoyt, PhD, is an associate professor in health psychology and clinical science at Hunter College of the City University of New York. His work focuses on biobehavioral processes related to psychological adjustment and coping with chronic illness, emotion regulation, cancer survivorship, gender, and evidence-based intervention.

Shanda L. Hunt, MPH, is an assistant librarian and data-curation specialist at the School of Public Health at the University of Minnesota, Minneapolis. She conducted the structured literature search cited in chapter 1.

Charles Kamen, PhD, MPH, is a clinical psychologist with a strong background and training in behavioral medicine, health disparities, and dyadic interventions. His program of research focuses on (1) cancer-related health disparities affecting sexual- and gender-minority cancer survivors, and (2) behavioral interventions to address these disparities. He is currently principal investigator on an NCI-funded grant focused on sexual- and gender-minority cancer survivors and their caregivers.

Andrew Kellett, BPsych, is a researcher and doctoral candidate in the Translational Health Research Institute, School of Medicine, Western Sydney University. His focus is on mixed-methods research into health inequalities and marginalized groups.

Nidhi Kohli, PhD, is an associate professor in the Department of Educational Psychology, College of Education and Human Development, at the University of Minnesota, Minneapolis. Her research focuses on the development and improvement of statistical methods for analyzing longitudinal data, and she is the research methodologist and statistician on the Restore study.

Badrinath R. Konety, MD, MBA, is a professor and chair of the Department of Urology and director of the Institute for Prostate and Urologic Cancers at the University of Minnesota Medical School, Minneapolis. A board-certified urologist, fellow of the American Cancer Society and the American Urological Association, and research expert in biomedical aspects of prostate cancer treatment, he has been listed as a Best Doctor in America since 2009.

David M. Latini, PhD, MSW, is an associate professor of urology and psychiatry at Baylor College of Medicine, Houston, where he teaches medical students human sexuality and LGBT health, and a private-practice psychologist. His research work focuses on genitourinary cancer survivorship, symptom management, and health literacy. With Tae Hart, he led the first study of the effect of prostate cancer on gay men in the United States and Canada.

Mark S. Litwin, MD, MPH, is professor of urology, public health, and nursing at UCLA, where he practices urologic oncology, teaches, and conducts research in translational population science, including outcomes, quality of life, costs, and quality of care. He directs a large state-funded program that provides free care to low-income, uninsured men with prostate cancer in California.

Emilia Lombardi, PhD, is an assistant professor in Baldwin Wallace University's Department of Public Health, Berea, Ohio. She has a PhD in sociology from the University of Akron and has been examining health disparities among lesbian, gay, bisexual, and transgender populations since the mid-1990s.

Brett M. Millar, PhD, is a postdoctoral researcher in Health Psychology and Clinical Science Program at the City University of New York and Hunter College's Center for HIV Educational Studies & Training. His work focuses on the health of gay and bisexual men, including understanding self-regulation in health behavior and decision making.

Darryl Mitteldorf, LCSW, is an oncology social worker. He is the founder of two U.S.-based national cancer survivor support and advocacy nonprofit organizations, Malecare and the National LGBT Cancer Project.

Gerald Perlman, PhD, is a clinical psychologist, certified psychoanalyst, and certified bioenergetic therapist in private practice in New York City. He is a former supervisor and director of psychology internship training at Manhattan Psychiatric Center. Currently he is on the faculty and organizing committee of the New York Society of Bioenergetic Analysis.

Janette Perz, PhD, is a professor of psychology and director of the Translational Health Research Institute at Western Sydney University, Australia. Her research is in the area of gendered sexual and reproductive health. She has been co-investigator with Jane Ussher in a significant research program in psycho-oncology, including cancer carers, sexual experiences and interventions for couples facing cancer, and changes to fertility across a range of cancer types.

Garrett P. Prestage, PhD, is an associate professor at the Kirby Institute, University of New South Wales, Sydney, where he has worked since 1992. He has been active in gay community life in Australia since the mid-1970s. He pioneered HIV behavioral surveillance work and major cohort studies among Australian gay and bisexual men.

Gwendolyn P. Quinn, PhD, the Livia Wan Endowed Chair, vice chair of research, and professor in the Departments of Obstetrics and Gynecology and Population Health and at the Center for Biomedical Ethics at the New York University School of Medicine. Her research focuses on patient-physician communication, health disparities, and reproductive health and cancer.

Duncan Rose, GradDipPsych, MClinPsych, is a registered and practicing clinical psychologist. He was previously a research officer in the Translational Health Research Institute at Western Sydney University, Australia, where he was involved in research examining gay and bisexual men's experience of prostate cancer.

Michael W. Ross, PhD, MD, MPH, MHPEd, MSt, is a professor and the Jocelyn Elders Chair in Sexual Health Education in the Department of Family Medicine and Community Health at the University of Minnesota Medical School, Minneapolis. Dr. Ross is a prodigious researcher, having published over 500 peer-reviewed publications, mainly on LGBT health.

B. R. Simon Rosser, PhD, MPH, is a professor and clinical-research sexologist specializing in gay men's health in the Division of Epidemiology and Community Health at the University of Minnesota School of Public Health, Minneapolis. He pioneered the study of sexual function and dysfunction in gay and bisexual men (GBM); most recently, he led Restore, one of the first NIH-funded studies of prostate cancer in GBM.

Matthew B. Schabath, PhD, is an associate member in the Department of Cancer Epidemiology at Moffitt Cancer Center and associate professor in the Department of Oncologic Sciences in the Morsani College of Medicine, Tampa. He specializes in cancer epidemiology research, including health disparities among sexual and gender minorities and knowledge and attitudes of healthcare providers toward LGBTQ populations.

James Smith, PhD, is an associate professor and Equity Fellow with the Office of Pro Vice Chancellor—Indigenous Leadership at Charles Darwin University, Australia; he is also co-lead of the Indigenous Leadership Research and Evaluation Network. He has worked in men's health policy, practice, and research contexts in Australia for more than 15 years, with notable contributions in areas relating to men's health promotion, men's health policy development, and men's help-seeking practices and healthcare use.

Kristine M. Talley, PhD, RN, is an associate professor and codirector of the Center for Aging Science and Care Innovation at the University of Minnesota School of Nursing, Minneapolis. She is a certified gerontological nurse practitioner. A strong focus of her research is on rehabilitation for urinary incontinence, including that experienced after prostate cancer treatment.

M. Beatriz Torres, PhD, MPH CHP, is an associate professor of communication studies at Gustavus Adolphus College, in St. Peter, Minnesota. She specializes in health communication and health disparities. She was involved as a qualitative researcher in the data analysis of the Restore study (Aim 1).

Jane M. Ussher, PhD, CPsychol, is a professor of psychology in the Translational Health Research Institute at Western Sydney University, Australia. Her research focuses on examining subjectivity in relation to the reproductive body and sexuality, and the gendered experience of cancer and cancer care. As a trained clinical psychologist, she has also made a contribution to the integration of research and clinical practice in gendered health, and she has developed psycho-educational interventions in the field of cancer care, addressing sexual changes after cancer, fertility concerns, and the needs of cancer carers.

Andrea Waling, PhD, is a research officer at the Australian Research Centre in Sex, Health, and Society at La Trobe University, Melbourne. She specializes in the study of masculinity, bodies, men's health, and sexuality.

Richard Wassersug, PhD, is a prostate cancer patient and a research scientist, based in Vancouver, British Columbia, who spent most of his career as a professor of anatomy and neurobiology at Dalhousie University, Halifax, Nova Scotia. He is the lead author of the 2014 book *Androgen Deprivation Therapy: An Essential Guide for Prostate Cancer Patients and Their Loved Ones.*

William "Bill" West, PhD, is an instructor in the Department of Writing Studies, University of Minnesota College of Liberal Arts, Minneapolis. He specializes in health communication, including technical and professional communication, online pedagogy, the rhetoric of medicine, and communication in the patient-physician dyad.

Erik Wibowo, PhD, completed his doctoral studies at Dalhousie University and a post-doctoral fellowship at the Vancouver Prostate Centre. He is now working at the British Columbia Cancer Agency on a project, led by Dr. Tsz Kin (Bernard) Lee, to develop a questionnaire that can be used for assessing sexual function of men who have sex with men with prostate cancer.

Daniela Wittmann, PhD, LMSW, is an assistant professor of urology and a certified sex therapist at the University of Michigan Medical School. Her clinical work and research focus on couples' sexual recovery after prostate cancer treatment. With funding from the Movember Foundation, she is leading in the United States a multisite trial of a web-based intervention for men and couples recovering sexual intimacy after prostate cancer treatment.

ejaculate loss: emotional reactions, 57; gay sex/sexuality and, 24, 48, 55; multiorgasmic capabilities enhanced by, 166; personal experiences, 265–266, 268, 298–299; as prostate cancer treatment side effect, 24, 39, 47–48, 55, 56, 102, 275; radiotherapy vs. radical prostatectomy, 218, 221, 227–228; relationships and, 55, 57. *See also* non-ejaculatory orgasms

ejaculation, 322; retrograde, 299

ejaculatory bother, 87–88

Elator (penile support device), 172

e-mail, 304

EMBASE, 13

emotional reactions, 56

employment, 200, 204

epidemiology, 322, 325

epigenetic markings, 93

equipoise, 229

erectile dysfunction: anal sex and, 25, 59–60, 61, 105; bother from, 174–175; condom use and, 109; defined, 322–323; gay identities and, 38, 41–42; gay sex/sexuality and, 55, 56, 57; illness intrusiveness and, 203; masculine identity and, 111, 296; partnerships and, 174–175; personal experiences, 264, 292–293, 295–296, 298; as prostate cancer treatment side effect, 3, 25, 39, 55, 56, 57, 102, 153, 164–165, 261; quality of life considerations and, 155; radiotherapy and, 289; radiotherapy vs. radical prostatectomy, 218, 219, 221–223, 227, 228; relationships and, 39, 44–46, 55, 57; sexual aids/toys assisting with, 167–173, 186; sexual disqualification because of, 44–46;

support group discussions about, 220, 301

erotic electrostimulation, 183–187

eroticization, 174

estrogen therapy, 165–166, 167, 235, 237

ethnicity, 152

eunuch, 323

Europe, northwestern, 151

Evans, Andrew, 288

familial support, 24, 25, 74–75, 90–91

family, "chosen," 91–92, 321

Family and Medical Leave Act (FMLA; U.S.), 125

family history, 316

fatty diet, 15

feces, blood in, 286

fellatio (blow job), 165

Fergus, K. D., 16 *t. 1.2*

finasteride (Propecia), 15, 285, 323

Flomax, 297, 298

Florida, 151

Food and Drug Administration (FDA), 305

foreplay, 60, 169

"forgetting," 104

function, 321, 323

funfactory.com, 171

gay/bisexual men (GBM): defined, 323; health promotion strategies for, 119; HIV/AIDS deaths among, 3; pharmaceutical industry and, 253; prostate cancer diagnoses among, 12; prostate cancer risk among, 2, 15–23;

Healthy People 2020, 13

hegemony, 324

Henderson, Ross, 272–282

heterocentrism/heteronormativity:
defined, 324–325; GBM sexual
rehabilitation/recovery and, 181–182;
HCPs and, 132, 133–134, 137–138,
143–144, 175, 248; pharmaceutical
industry marketing and, 253; in
prostate cancer literature, 105, 106,
123, 132, 137, 277; in prostate cancer
research, 100

heterosexism, 55, 261–262, 292,
294–295, 325. See also discrimination; homophobia; stigmatization

heterosexual coping, 69–70, 73, 78, 91

heterosexuality, 3, 325; assumptions of
(see heterocentrism/heteronormativi-
ty)

heterosexual marriage, 69

heterosexual men: anal sex and, 61, 105;
emotional reactions of, 300, 301;
interdependence theory and, 73;
long-term vs. short-term outcomes of
prostate cancer treatments for, 219;
masculine identity and, 63; openness
to discussing sexual practices, 59;
with postmenopausal partners, 57;
pro-inflammatory biomarkers
among, 93; PSA testing among, 15,
305; research focused on, 3, 81, 93;
sex toy use of, 166–167; as sexually
promiscuous, 45, 119; single, 203;
social support of, 73, 74, 91, 201, 301;
survivorship roles of, 150. See also
sexual rehabilitation/recovery—GBM
vs. heterosexual men

HIV/AIDS: activism, 248; ARV treatments for, 79; cancers resulting
from, 19, 320; deaths from, 3;

defined, 325; diagnosis of, and
prostate cancer risk, 15–23, 152, 233;
epidemic, 309; gay sex/sexuality and,
109–110; as GBM healthcare
challenge, 92; health messages
regarding, 119; interdependence
theory and, 70; pharmaceutical
industry and, 253; safe sex and, 259;
transmission risk, 25

homonegativity, 326

homophobia, 70, 73, 110, 119, 123, 133,
175, 238. See also discrimination;
heterosexism; stigmatization

homosexuality, 309, 325

hormone therapy, 3, 14, 156, 235, 288,
294, 325

Horn, Mark, 286, 289

hot flashes, 156, 288

hotoctopuss.com, 171

Hoyt, Michael A., 79

Hu, Jim, 239, 289

Huntley, A. L., 201

Iceland, 250

illness intrusiveness, 200, 202

illness intrusiveness and social support:
future research in, 211–212; IITF and,
200, 202–203; moderation analyses,
206–208, 207 fig. 12.1, 208 fig. 12.2,
209 t. 12.3; relationship status and,
200, 203–204, 206 t. 12.2, 208–212;
research literature on, 201–202; as
underresearched, 200

Illness Intrusiveness Ratings Scale
(IIRS), 203–204

Illness Intrusiveness Theoretical
Framework (IITF), 200, 202–203,
210, 325

oral sex, 42, 60, 105–106, 165, 169, 237, 327

orchidectomy, 3, 14, 327

orgasms, 172; absence of, 164; changes in, following prostate cancer treatments, 166–167, 265–266; defined, 327; radiotherapy vs. radical prostatectomy, 227. *See also* non-ejaculatory orgasms

outness, 327

Out with Cancer groups, 252

ovariectomy, 327

Ovid, 13

panic symptoms, 238

partnerships: cancer survivorship and, 69; illness intrusiveness and, 200–201; sexual recovery role of, 165, 174–175

patient buy-in, 304

patient-centered healthcare, 312

PDE5 inhibitor drugs, 105, 169, 181, 190, 192, 193, 327. *See also* Cialis; Levitra; Viagra

pelvic floor rehabilitation, 62, 327

pelvic lymphadenectomy, 236

penile implants, 105, 169, 180, 181, 187, 191–192, 327

penile injections, 180, 181, 190–191, 192, 193

penile prosthesis, external (dildo), 170

penile sleeves, 171–172

penile support device, external, 172

penis-casting products, 170

penis size reduction, 38, 39, 42–44, 156, 219, 220–221, 227, 228–229

Perlman, Gerald, 100–101, 292–302

personal development, 200, 203

Perz, Janette, 19 *t. 1.2*, 23 *t. 1.3*, 75, 145–146

Pfizer, 295

pharmaceutical companies, Malecare work with, 252–253

phosphodiesterase type 5 inhibitor drugs. *See* PDE5 inhibitor drugs

polyamorous relationships, 69

potency, 327

prejudice, 68, 72, 75, 78, 79, 90, 91, 152

prevalence, 327

Propecia, 15

prostate: defined, 327–328; enlarged, 274, 285 (*see also* benign prostatic hyperplasia (BPH)); as erogenous zone, 39, 46, 122; loss of, 24; physical trauma to, and PSA testing, 24

prostate cancer: as "couple's disease," 322; deaths from, 287; defined, 328; fear of recurrence, 267, 268; localized/early stage, treatment options for, 152–153, 236; physiological/psychological demands of, 86; predicting progression of, 287; rates of, 2–3, 13–14, 151, 259; risk factors for, 15, 151–152, 287, 305, 308–309; survival rates, 267–268, 309; testing age, 273. *See also* gay men with prostate cancer; GBM with prostate cancer

prostate cancer diagnosis/diagnoses: comprehensive care model for, 233–235; emotional reactions, 219–220, 284, 294, 299, 300, 308; faulty, 288; perceptions of, 72, 74; personal experiences, 258–260, 272–274, 278, 284–289, 292–294, 306–314; rates of, 2, 3, 13–14; shared decision-making (SDM) model used following, 304 (*see also* shared decision-making (SDM) model)

Prostate Cancer Foundation of Australia (PCFA), 50, 145, 250, 282

prostate cancer screenings: comprehensive care model for, 233–235; rates of, 15; research literature on, 15. *See also* prostate-specific antigen (PSA) testing

prostate cancer treatments: access to, 90–91; challenges of, 24–25; comprehensive care model for, 236–238; culturally competent, 92, 125–126, 158–160, 159 *t. 9.1*; decision-making regarding, 294–297, 302, 304 (*see also* shared decision-making (SDM) model); five-year survival rates after, 3; gay sex/sexuality following, 103–106, 121–123; GBM dissatisfaction with, 133, 193–194; illness intrusiveness and, 202–203; negative effects of, 3, 38–39, 78, 101–103, 152–156, 237–238, 275–276 (*see also* sexuality, post-prostatectomy); perceptions of, 68, 72, 74; phases of, 232; psychological effects of, 24, 86; sexual function changes following, 165–167; sexual recovery following, 164 (*see also* sexual rehabilitation/recovery); treatment options, 152–153, 236, 274–275. *See also* brachytherapy; prostatectomy; radiotherapy

prostatectomy: anal sensitivity following, 61; average age for, 266; celebrities opting for, 294; decision-making regarding, 260–262, 278–279, 288–289, 297; defined, 328; erectile dysfunction following, 164, 261; orgasmic changes following,

166–167; personal experiences, 259, 262–263, 280; prognosis for recovery/survival following, 261; regrets following, 153, 239, 304, 322; as treatment option, 275; urinary incontinence following, 261. *See also* GBM with prostate cancer—radiotherapy vs. radical prostatectomy effects; sexuality, post-prostatectomy

prostate massage, 287

prostate-specific antigen (PSA), 153–154

prostate-specific antigen (PSA) testing, 15, 24, 328; active surveillance approach and, 296; average age for, 293; as controversial, 288, 305, 306; in GBM, research needs for, 316–317; GBM vs. heterosexual male rates of, 305, 317; HIV infection and, 109; personal experiences, 259–260, 268, 273, 274, 282, 284–286, 292, 293, 306–307, 307 *fig. 20.1*, 308, 309–310, 313–314; research studies involving, 109; SDM model and, 304, 305–306

prostatitis, 285, 305, 313

prosthesis, 328. *See also* penile implants

protectiveness, 58–59, 63–64, 69

proton beam therapy, 294

psychiatric morbidity, 233

psychological adjustment: contributors to, 89 *fig. 8.1*, 90–92; epidemiological surveys of, 87–88; models of, 86, 87; research directions for, 92–94; understanding factors behind, 88–90

psychological interventions, 93

psychotherapy, 289

PsycINFO, 13

PubMed, 13

Pulse (vibrator), 171

quality of life, 3, 87, 88, 93, 133, 153, 154, 174, 201, 233. *See also* health-related quality of life (HRQOL)

Queensland Cancer Council, 262

queer, 328

queer theory, 328

racial background, 151, 152, 156, 204–205, 233, 287–288

racial minority identities, 92

radiation proctitis, 223

radiotherapy: burn damage from, 289; decision making regarding, 152–157, 288–289; defined, 236, 328; late radiation effects, 292, 298–299; personal experiences, 292, 297–299; side effects of, 164, 166; as treatment option, 274–275. *See also* GBM with prostate cancer—radiotherapy vs. radical prostatectomy effects

Rastinehad, Art, 284, 285, 286–287, 288, 289

receptive partner (bottom), 328

recreation, 200, 204

rectal anatomy changes, 221, 223

rectal irritation/pain, 24–25, 153

rectal toxicity, 153

Regan, T. W., 70

rehabilitation, 328

relationality, 328

relationships: adjustments in, 153; configurations, 69, 106; ejaculate loss and, 55, 57; erectile dysfunction and, 39, 44–46; illness intrusiveness and, 200, 203–204, 206 *t. 12.2*, 208–212

religious activities, 203

Reproductive Health Matters (journal), 258

research literature: gaps/inconsistencies in, 39–40, 55, 69–70, 175; on GBM/HCP communication, 134–136, 135 *t. 8.1*; on GBM with prostate cancer, 12, 14 *t. 1.1*, 55–56; heteronormativity and, 100; heterosexism and, 55; inclusion/exclusion criteria in, 325; on partnerships and cancer survivorship, 69; on psychological adjustment, 87–88; qualitative studies, 16–19 *t. 1.2*, 39, 324, 328; quantitative studies, 20–23 *t. 1.3*, 39; on sexual/gender minorities, 13; on TGW, 12; on treatment outcomes, 154

Restore Aim 1, 22 *t. 1.3*

Restore Aim 3, 22 *t. 1.3*

retrograde ejaculation, 299

rimming, 165

role-in-sex, 218, 223–224, 328

role-play, 237

Rose, Duncan, 75, 91, 145–146

Rosser, B. R. Simon, 18 *t. 1.2*, 22 *t. 1.3*, 56–57, 63, 151, 201–202, 237, 306–314, 307 *fig. 20.1*

RxSleeve, 171

safe sex, 259

same-sex marriage, 77, 106, 124–125, 175

Sandoe, David, 250

Satisfaction with Support, 204

saturation, 328

Schindler, Paul, 284

Schover, L. R., 195

seeds, 288, 294, 328. *See also* brachytherapy

self-esteem loss, 24, 173, 220, 227

NOTES

NOTES

NOTES

NOTES

NOTES